The Scientific Practice of Professional Psychology

APPLIED CLINICAL PSYCHOLOGY

Series Editors:
Alan S. Bellack
University of Maryland at Baltimore, Baltimore, Maryland
Michel Hersen
Pacific University, Forest Grove, Oregon

The Scientific Practice of Professional Psychology

Steven J. Trierweiler

University of Michigan
Ann Arbor, Michigan

George Stricker

Adelphi University
Garden City, New York

Plenum Press • **New York and London**

Library of Congress Cataloging-in-Publication Data

Trierweiler, Steven J.
    The scientific practice of professional psychology / Steven J.
  Trierweiler, George Stricker.
        p.   cm. -- (Applied clinical psychology)
    Includes bibliographical references and index.
    ISBN 0-306-45654-0
    1. Clinical psychology--Research. 2. Clinical psychology-
  -Methodology.   I. Stricker, George. II. Title. III. Series.
    [DNLM: 1. Psychology, Clinical. 2. Research Design.
  3. Empiricism. 4. Logic.   WM 20 T826s 1997]
  RC467.8.T74 1997
  616.89--dc21
  DNLM/DLC
  for Library of Congress   97-34813
                                                            CIP

ISBN 0-306-45654-0

© 1998 Plenum Press, New York
A Division of Plenum Publishing Corporation
233 Spring Street, New York, N.Y. 10013

http://www.plenum.com

10 9 8 7 6 5 4 3 2 1

Printed in the United States of America

Preface

A workable vision of scientific practice has proven to be an elusive, if laudable, goal for professional psychology. The field cannot be faulted for failing to seek scientific wisdom, but it has been slow to integrate that wisdom fully with the wisdom of practice. This has proven to be a major oversight for, despite psychology's long-standing commitment to science, practitioners are unlikely to think scientifically if the methods and products of science are described in ways that make it impossible to do so. Unfortunately, the rhetoric of science too often has done just that: So focused has it been on the problem of distinguishing good science from bad that it has inadvertently defeated any hope of a practical science developing in our field.

We offer one remedy for this situation: This book is about scientific thinking for the professional psychologist. Specifically, it is a primer on the application of scientific logic to professional practice. We argue that the professional needs a more straightforward and realistic scientific identity than heretofore has been available. The professional consciously must become a local clinical scientist, bringing all the power of scientific thought to the specifics of the clinical situation. Contrary to forces in psychology that promote uncritical acceptance of science as given by academic researchers or, alternatively, that encourage criticism and ultimate disregard of the scientific endeavor, we call for a redoubling of efforts to incorporate scientific thought into practical professional inquiry. The oft-mentioned pillars of science for the practitioner, outcome evaluation and direct application of scientific findings to clinical problems, are important but incomplete benefits of science. In addition, specific extension of scientific forms of thought into the realities of practice is required. In elucidating this idea in the book, we focus on the implications of scientific methodology for inquiry in actual practice situations.

One goal of our work is to offer a hopeful perspective for those who wish seriously to have it all—both the intellectual and empirical integrity of science and the received knowledge and skill originating in professional traditions. We value freedom of inquiry and openness to possibility above theoretical predilection, intellectual pretense, and expert expressions of certainty. We envision a professional who is comfortable managing the boundary between art and science and who holds allegiance to evidence and truth above dogma, be it professional or scientific in origin. Becoming such an individual requires a lifetime of effort and the most rigorous and conscientious attention to the logical foundations of modern science. Methodology, both traditional and innovative, when considered in light of the realistic complexities of professional practice, becomes something more than a recipe for credible science:

It becomes a guidebook for thought, critical questioning, and reflection in specific situations.

Insofar as our focus is on fundamental issues, this book should be beneficial to all professionals seeking to bring scientific thought into their everyday work. We draw heavily on examples from individual and family psychotherapy. However, the ideas could apply to a wide variety of professional activities. We do not consider this work to be the last word on scientific practice; we hope it contributes to renewed scrutiny of the role that science must play in clinical practice.

The book is divided into three parts. Part I begins with a brief history of the science–practice debate in professional psychology. This is followed by a summary of the local clinical scientist model. Part II explores the logic of traditional scientific approaches as they pertain to local practice. Included here are issues in the philosophy of science, the logic of research design, and statistical approaches to inquiry. Part III examines nontraditional approaches, which in many ways harken back to the most basic questions about the meaning of science for practice. Here we discuss topics such as qualitative methods, critical thinking and logic, and framework development and offer concluding thoughts.

Our presentation is intended to be thorough; we attempt to be as complete and straightforward as possible without compromising the actual complexities of the issues presented. In the course of writing the book, it proved necessary to outline many background details of methodological topics as we explored their fundamental logic. A good deal of this material is abstract, consistent with its historical origins. We believe that great errors have been made, in the name of clarity of presentation, in trying to present methods as simple, taken-for-granted rules of conduct: In the process, whole traditions of thought and doubt have been lost to us. We do not repeat these errors here. As a result, some will find aspects of the presentation difficult, and more than one reading may be required. Others who have more background may be able to skim some of the details—although we hope these readers will find the material presented in a different light than is customary. We have not presented everything, nor have we shied away from difficult topics, especially in the chapters on philosophy of science (Chapter 3), statistics (Chapter 5), and logic (Chapter 8). The reader is encouraged to study this material carefully and to read other works on the topics. Above all, we hope readers recognize that the logic of science is exciting, has enormous implications even for the most mundane observations in practice, and resides among the deepest roots of our professional culture.

Many individuals have contributed both spiritually and substantively to this project over its many years. Special thanks goes to Roger L. Peterson and Russell Bent, who set the context for the development of the local clinical scientist model. Roger L. Peterson's contribution of incisive intellect and limitless support was particularly important early in the conception of the project. Many colleagues and friends provided useful commentary on various ideas represented herein. Included here are Peter Carino, Morris Eagle, Lorraine Mangione, David Singer, Colborn Smith, Mitchall Thomeshaw, and Joel Weinberger. In addition to intellectual assistance, Donna K. Nagata, Christopher Peterson, and Tamara Lyn read chapters and provided invaluable feedback that greatly improved the presentation. Numerous students, some of whom are now full-fledged professionals, were similarly helpful, including Ronald Berg, Cleary Donovan, Ann Drake, Jerry Gold, David Goldfinger, Sharon Gordon, Jennifer Hillman, Jeremy Leeds, Tamara Lyn, Vagdevi Meurier, Curie Park, Katherine Rosenblum, Marianne Ruggeri, Aaron Sardell, Jennifer Stevens, and Melanie Tallie. Finally, in addition to the many outstanding scholars whose works are cited throughout the book, there is more than one generation of excellent teachers represented herein. Their influences are legion, albeit now difficult to identify as they have become intertwined with our intellectual and professional lives. For Steven Trierweiler these include Bruce L. Baker, Stephen L. Golding, Fredrick Kanfer, James T. Lamiell, Gordon Paul, Julian Rappaport, the late Donald T. Shannon, and Harry Triandis. For George Stricker these include Emory L. Cowen, Gordon F. Derner, and Melvin Zax. It is impossible to thank these important figures adequately, but we hope that we have carried on something that was meaningful to them without distorting it too seriously. Finally, we would like to thank our families for tolerating our extended, book-related distraction. We hope that we have set a foundation to make future excursions less consuming and obsessive.

Steven Trierweiler
George Stricker

Contents

The History of Scientific Research Training and the Local Clinical Scientist

The Problem of Integrating Science and Practice

Something and nothing produce each other;
The difficult and the easy complement each other;
The long and the short off-set each other;
The high and the low incline toward each other;
Note and sound harmonize with each other;
Before and after follow each other.
Therefore the sage keeps to the deed that consists
in taking no action and practices the teaching
that uses no words.
—LAO TZU (1963, p. 58)

The years following World War II were heady times for U.S. psychology. An ambitious program for developing psychology's professional side, adopted at the Boulder Conference, recommended that psychologists be trained as scientist-practitioners (Raimy, 1950). They would embody the intelligence, values, skills, and burgeoning promise of both psychological science and psychological intervention as each embarked on a period of striking growth. New ideas, of substantial intellectual, social, and practical consequence, abounded in both arenas. Psychological science—careful, conservative, and increasingly assertive about its logical-empiricist foundations—promised to bring both mind and body under the secure fold of twentieth-century science. Similarly, psychologists were discovering that their knowledge and interests could contribute to the development of nonmedical interventions for mental dysfunction, and to improving the overall mental health of U.S. society. The notion of integrating these two aspects of psychology, science and practice, and of enhancing psychology's social credibility at the same time was a spontaneous and obvious acknowledgment of the state of the discipline.

THE PROBLEM

Unfortunately, having a good idea is one thing; implementing it is quite another. Even today the promise of a unified psychological profession, born in the spirit of the postwar era, has yet to be realized. Rather, two distinct lines of training exist: One consists of traditional academic programs, mostly housed in research universities, that openly allege their adherence to the scientist-practitioner model (Belar & Perry, 1992); the other, the professional school movement, emphasizes a practitioner training model that is innovative, and these programs usually are housed in university and freestanding institutions that may not have a longstanding tradition of doctoral education (e.g., R. L. Peterson, 1992). There is overlap among these types of programs, but it is extremely limited; in large part, both physically and culturally, they represent differing organizations and political interests within organized psychology. As recently as 1990, each group had its own conference in which the problems of curriculum development and of research training in professional psychology were addressed (Belar & Perry, 1992; R. L. Peterson et al., 1992).

The history of the scientist-practitioner model, as enacted by psychology training programs, has not corresponded well with the integrative ideal elaborated at the 1949 conference. What could have gone wrong? It seems so obvious that knowledge production should be connected with implementation. In a field like professional psychology, where much of practice is inherently ambiguous, based as it is on human interaction, what could be more reasonable than to temper it with the care and rigor of the scientist? In turn, would not a science informed by the problems of practice proceed in a more directed, practice-relevant fashion?

Complex political, economic, and intradisciplinary issues surround this matter. Broadly speaking, however, the record is clear: The promise and rhetoric surrounding the Boulder Model notwithstanding, a large number of practitioners argued that the traditional training system was not paying sufficient heed to their needs and interests (D. R. Peterson, 1985). Science, and particularly research training, they asserted, was overemphasized at the expense of responsible attention to practical experience. When traditional programs were unwilling or unable to respond to these concerns, practitioners developed an explicitly professionalized version of training wherein the training culture, in comparison with Boulder Model programs, was relatively more practice oriented and relatively less research oriented. Today these practitioner programs train a substantial proportion of new professional psychologists, and their impact on accrediting bodies and on the ways training is conceived in this country is undeniable. The debate goes on as some continue to assert the priority of traditional interpretations of the Boulder Model, as though they were never in doubt (e.g., Belar & Perry, 1992; O'Sullivan & Quevillon, 1992), even as others point to the failure to implement the model adequately (Stricker, 1992). At the same time, the newer practitioner-oriented training programs, many of which view themselves as closer to the scientist-practitioner ideal than traditional programs, are showing signs of maturity (Bourg, Bent, McHolland, & Stricker, 1989; R. L. Peterson et al., 1992).

The problem with debates of this sort is that they tend to feed on stark contrast: Contrary to the spirit of the Boulder Conference, science is pitted against practice and practice against science. People, their interests and identities as psychologists, their institutions, and their accomplishments, become cardboard figures on an artificial stage, where serious examination of the identity problems attendant on the integration of science and practice becomes impossible. Fortunately, there are recent attempts to solve these problems. Authors from a variety of persuasions, encompassing both academic and professional backgrounds, are attempting to breathe renewed vigor into the science–practice relationship, and to delineate more exactingly how scientific training might contribute to a practitioner's everyday activities (e.g., Hoshmand & Polkinghorne, 1992; Kanfer, 1990). Notably, these include authors from explicitly practitioner-oriented programs, where the concern has never been to exclude science, but rather to place it into proper perspective relative to the realities of training in professional practice (e.g., D. R. Peterson, 1985, 1991; Stricker & Trierweiler, 1995; Trierweiler, 1987; Trierweiler & Stricker, 1992). For the most part, these are integrative attempts to expose the fallacies in viewing scientific products as irrelevant to practice or clinical formulations as lacking in rigor. These proposals have involved the adaptation of scientific method and thinking to clinical contexts (e.g., Kanfer, 1990; D. R. Peterson, 1991; Shakow, 1976) or, more sweepingly, the critique of logical-empiricist science in favor of a more constructivist-hermeneutical variety (e.g., Hoshmand & Polkinghorne, 1992; R. L. Peterson, 1992).

THE LOCAL CLINICAL SCIENTIST

These are positive developments, but culture and identity problems remain that are endemic to training in science and practice (see Stricker & Keisner, 1985a). On the whole, psychology is not a field with unambiguous ties between basic science and practical technology, and it is unlikely to become such a field in the foreseeable future. Students long have needed more direct assistance in managing the complexities of our knowledge base and praxis. In this book, we will address these neglected aspects of professional psychology training by discussing how research methodologies can be viewed as frames for critical thinking in realistic clinical contexts.

This discussion will be based on preliminary work by Trierweiler and Stricker (1992; Stricker & Trierweiler, 1995) that offered a pedagogical solution to the science–practice problem in a discussion of how science and research methodology training should be presented to professionals. We focus on the natural linkages that exist between scientific and professional forms of practice and thought, rather than on how practice should be modified to be more scientific or on how science should be modified to be more practical (see Stricker, 1992). In addition, we emphasize the local realities of clinical practice, and the problems professional psychology students face in blending the various aspects of the discipline into their professional identities, even as we discuss basic methodological concepts.

Our approach might be termed *critical-pedagogical*. Rather than concentrating on socializing the students to a particular form of problem solving, as is often the case in research curricula, we begin with the question of what professional psychologists should know about scientific inquiry and how they should use it. Attention to this question places our own theoretical predilections and beliefs about the epistemological adequacy of various forms of scientific and clinical inquiry in the background, secondary to didactic goals. Having identified what we want to teach, we then explicitly select and focus the discussion of this material on an image of professional identity that is compatible with the realities of professional practice. We have termed this image the *local clinical scientist*: Practitioners are viewed as critical investigators of local (as opposed to universal) realities who are knowledgeable of research, scholarship, personal experience, and scientific methodology. They also are able to develop plausible, communicable formulations for understanding essentially local phenomena using theory, general world knowledge including scientific research, and, most importantly, their own abilities as skeptical scientific observers.

This definition will be elaborated in Chapter 2. Briefly, in this view, scientific research training in professional psychology is as much an exercise in critical thinking and attitude development as it is preparation to conduct scientific research. As we will show, this is a belief that has an extended history in doctoral-level clinical psychology training, and was implicit in the Boulder Model (Raimy, 1950). However, it has received little direct implementation in training in science and methodology. Neglect of this training perspective may be one reason why the split between science and practice remains.

Our central thesis is that the difference between "hard-nosed" scientific and everyday clinical inquiry is a matter of emphasis. Traditional science, by its nature, seeks consensus: It attempts to be completely public in the ways questions are framed and in the ways they are answered. The so-called "scientific method" is an approach to problems that promises answers that are altogether public, general, and unambiguous. In contrast, the clinical method is fundamentally private (personal) and localized (i.e., the relevant information is often completely unique to the situation; see Chapter 2). Although, in principle, many aspects of a clinical inquiry could be described publicly, doing so requires great effort and rarely is accomplished in practice. Individual clinical efforts usually require more attention to unique circumstances than to universal scientific laws. As a result, our public representations of the complexities of clinical work (e.g., psychotherapy outcome research and clinical judgment research) remain only rough approximations, seldom offering unambiguous guidance for specific circumstances.

Clinicians need skills in the application of the scientific metaphor to the local context; a thorough understanding of science and scientific values, and the ability to generate internally consistent formulations that are logically consistent with detailed local data. A critical-pedagogical approach requires that all methods be considered tools that have strengths and weaknesses for particular inquiry requirements. Thus, we will deal directly with both traditional and nontraditional approaches to psychological inquiry. As we develop throughout the book, the clinician needs to be a natural scientist of the clinical situation, like a Sherlock Holmes of clinical problems.

RESEARCH TRAINING IN CLINICAL PSYCHOLOGY: SOME HISTORICAL BACKGROUND

To better understand how the science–practice dilemma came to be, a closer look at the context and details of the Boulder Model will be helpful. This discussion draws heavily on the historical presentations of Stricker (1992) and Stricker and Cummings (1992).

The more one examines Raimy's (1950) work on the Boulder Conference, and its farsighted, even brilliant, precursor, the Shakow Report (American Psychological Association, Committee on Training in Clinical Psychology, 1947), the more amazing it becomes that these have not been retained as required reading for all professional psychologists. Taken together, they are among the most radical and inspired documents in the history of the professions, and they provided the spadework needed to establish the profession of psychology as legitimate in the eyes of the general public. They are contemporary documents in that they reveal the rationale for many of the structures and attitudes underlying current professional psychology training practices. They do not cover all of the ground one needs to cover in professional training, and their authors certainly could not anticipate the changing economic and political landscape of psychology and mental health care. Nonetheless, the powerful image of the scientist-practitioner has long been the standard for training psychologists to fulfill the multiple roles inherent in our diverse field.

Two Streams of Development of Professional Training

The Boulder Model's influence on training can be thought of in terms of two developmental/historical streams, the political and the pedagogical.

The Political Stream

The political stream has to do with actions associated with consensus building and policy development in the context of intellectual diversity. Psychology has long been an extremely diverse discipline, and so it was during the postwar years. Psychology training was occurring in major universities throughout the country, embodying the complete range of distinctions one can make among institutions in terms of region, academic status and influence, economic resources, public versus private, and so on. The difficulty in bringing academic departments together to work collectively on something they were already doing in their own various ways should not be underestimated. Raimy (1950) pointed out that attitudes among Boulder conferees ranged from the view that there was no scientific basis for the professional practice of psychology to those wishing to establish completely professionalized training. The unification of the scientist and practitioner identities was a brilliant political symbol for rallying consensus amid the open divergence of opinion existing in the field. At the same time, it was not a compromise and it was more than a symbol: The scientist-practitioner model was an affirmative direction for training in clinical psychology.

The Pedagogical Stream

The pedagogical stream involves the Boulder Model as an educational ideal, and as a guide to professional training program development. Although the conference clearly contributed to this idealized image, a curriculum was designed, and broad educational guidelines were established, one must go to the Shakow Report to understand the theoretical vision implicit in the model. Integrative models like this one have a certain eloquent common sense that inspires, lends legitimacy, and leads one to conclude that the best of both worlds will be retained and expressed in something new. The possibility that such an image may be more aspirational than actually accomplished is easily lost in the enthusiasm of political consensus.

The Social Context for the Boulder Conference: The Forcing Event

The scientist-practitioner model did not arise simply out of the good will and social consciousness of academic psychology. The federal government played a significant role, as it has in scientific and social welfare efforts throughout this century (see also Rappaport, 1992; Weiss, 1992). Following World War II, the Veterans Administration (VA) and the U.S. Public Health Service sought to expand the ranks of professionals available to treat the psychological distress of World War II veterans. Experience with World War I suggested that this distress would peak in the early 1970s. Until the late 1940s training in clinical psychology had been loose and haphazard, almost an avocation for the academically trained psychologist. Professional training experiences were, for the most part, constructed by the student in sites similar to current internships and through the pursuit of individualized supervision. The VA wanted something more precise than this state of affairs. Professionalizing psychology was the answer, an idea already existing in some psychology departments before World War II (e.g., Columbia University; see Shakow, 1948), in an association devoted to applied psychology, and in the existing practice of psychology. The VA requested that the American Psychological Association (APA) identify the boundaries of competent clinical psychology training and establish mechanisms for accreditation. This request led to the formation of the Committee on Training in Clinical Psychology, under the leadership of David Shakow. Thus, the Boulder Conference resulted from government funds, the work of this committee, and the force and sensibility of the resulting Shakow Report (American Psychological Association, Committee on Training in Clinical Psychology, 1947).

Research Training in the Political Stream: The Boulder Conference

Three perspectives toward the relationship between research and practice were represented in Boulder, as discernible in Raimy's (1950) documentation of the conference: (1) the evaluation and development of existing clinical technologies, (2) the search for new conceptualizations and technologies growing out of professional efforts, and (3) the adoption and implementation of the scientific attitude in professional work. Unfortunately, these perspectives, and the important training emphases they imply, were not uniformly represented by the different departments attending the conference. Rather, they described the diversity of interests represented at the conference.

Most importantly, the view implicit in the first two perspectives, that too little was known to justify psychological practice, was carried most clearly in the tone and discussions of how science and practice relate. Academic psychology was, as it continues to be, confident about its research traditions, but less secure about the rigor of practice. Insufficient attention was given to the third perspective, and the problems implicit in Raimy's recognition that

> much of the time, thinking in a practical, clinical setting requires suspension of highly critical, analytical concern over constructs, especially where immediate problems of human welfare are involved. The clinical psychologist ordinarily functions in a social setting in which abstract ideas cannot be debated at all times, but where practical decisions must be reached by a number of persons with differing backgrounds and skills. Realization of the need for adaptability should, in the long run, free the clinical psychologist from feelings of guilt over the "unscientific" demands of clinical reality, if at the same time he has had the opportunity to learn how to analyze personality concepts in terms of their systematic implications. There cannot be overindoctrination in the scientific attitude. There can be an illusory oversimplification of the problems faced by the clinical psychologist who is also a scientist. (Raimy, 1950, p. 86)

Of course, science is supposed to be conservative, so some degree of debate was to be expected. This was an age when case studies were prominent in a field dominated by psychoanalytic thinking (Stricker, 1992). As the rules and logic of creating more formally rigorous research designs became more widely available (e.g., Campbell, 1957; Underwood, 1949, 1957), it was reasonable for statistically minded scientists to wonder about the intense individually focused activities of clinicians. Even more suspect, from a scientific perspective, was the tendency for clinicians, like medieval scholastics, to find status and legitimacy through their links, via personal psychoanalysis, with great minds of the past. Unlike science, where, in principle, research techniques and findings are presumed to be completely open to the public, clinicianhood seemed a private club where only a few cognoscenti could grasp what was really going on. Or perhaps, as many scientists feared, even clinicians did not know: As one Boulder conferee quipped, "Psychotherapy is an undefined technique applied to unspecified problems with unpredictable outcome. For this technique we recommend rigorous training" (quoted by Raimy, 1950, p. 93).

Thus, a major rationale for the scientist-practitioner model at the Boulder Conference was to encourage the use of scientific methods to evaluate and improve clinical approaches. Without the promise of government funds, it is doubtful that even this cautious nod would have been given (Rappaport, 1992; Weiss, 1992). In any case, far from the solid foundation for professional training usually imputed to the model, the impression one gets from the discussion of research training for clinicians is more tentative and hopeful than visionary; there clearly was much work to be done. Consider the tentative quality of the reasons given for combining training in research and practice.

1. Graduate students, it was agreed, should receive training in both research and practice in order to develop interest and background in both areas. Following completion of training, some persons might well continue to be active in both areas; others might concentrate on one.
2. The manifest lack of dependable knowledge in clinical psychology and personality demands that research be considered a vital part of the field of clinical psychology. Participants at the Conference displayed considerable humility with respect to confidence in present techniques.
3. There is little evidence to show that interest and competence in both areas are unlikely to occur in the same person. There is considerable evidence that certain individuals are capable of both. With the number of applicants far in excess of our training facilities, selection can be aimed at students capable of being trained in the double role.
4. Effectively performed service functions to provide an avenue for bringing psychologists into intimate contact with the significant problems of research.
5. Effectively performed service functions have provided in the past, and probably will provide in the future, a means whereby research in clinical psychology and psychiatry will obtain much needed support for the initiation and continuation of research projects. Competence in service does not insure competence in research, but recognized competence in service is likely to provide support for research as a means of obtaining better answers to current problems. (Raimy, 1950, pp. 80–81)

Interestingly, the charm and power of the idealization ring out even in so tentative a presentation. Of course the hidden question—hidden even to this day—concerns exactly what this person is supposed to be like. One can only speculate what course training might have taken had Boulder conferees actually developed professional case studies of individuals consensually identified to embody the model. However, it is doubtful that such a consensus would have been possible given the politics of the time. There was recognition of the didactic problems the model presented.

Students lack confidence in their abilities to do research, and their clinical interests make research appear as a noncontributory, time-serving requirement. The educational task faced by psychology departments seems to be one of stimulating interest in research without stifling or frustrating the student's spontaneous interest in problems of personality diagnosis and therapy. The Conference felt that the task is one that requires a frank facing of the motivational problems rather than a forcing of students into compliance. (Raimy, 1950, pp. 81–82)

How familiar this sounds to those of us engaged in contemporary professional training. As such, how it underscores our point that the tasks implicit in the model have never been satisfactorily accomplished. The solution at the time, which was politically sound, was to keep things as they were: Like other graduate students, professional students would be trained in research and statistics courses and work under the sponsorship of active researchers, completing a master's thesis and a doctoral dissertation. The only hint of anything different is that they would be trained to make "relevant analyses" of clinical phenomena (Raimy, 1950, p. 85), to bring new ideas into research; and to make "careful definition of concepts as a check upon the 'intuitive' judgment often required in such practical situations as staff meetings and clinical reports" (Raimy, 1950, p. 86).

Research Training in the Pedagogical Stream: The Shakow Report

If Raimy's (1950) report of the Boulder Conference carries the politics of the times, the Report of the Committee on Training in Clinical Psychology of the American Psychological Association (1947) carries their educational spirit and aspirations. This document is often referred to as the Shakow Report, which Raimy wisely included as an appendix to the Boulder Conference volume (from which citations are drawn below). Here, science is an attitude to be instilled in good people, to be used sensitively for the good of the public. Early on it was clear that the envisioned integration of science and practice would require considerable effort.

We are cognizant of the great difficulties which a shift from an academic to a professional program involves in a university setting. We recognize that this change must take much effort and time and that even were it possible to set up a fairly fixed schedule of training, such a step would at present be both premature and ill-advised because of the great need for experimentation in ways of implementing a sound program. We are therefore emphasizing the goals and principles of what we consider a desirable program rather than attempting to lay out a detailed blueprint. (Raimy, 1950, p. 210)

It would be work of a pedagogical nature carried out by individuals dedicated to training high-quality clinical psychologists.

In that wise volume, 'Medical Education,' (Flexner, 1925, p. 176), Abraham Flexner says '. . . the medical school cannot expect to produce fully trained doctors; it can at most hope to equip students with a limited amount of knowledge, to train them in the method and spirit of scientific medicine and to launch them with a momentum that will make them active learners—observers, readers, thinkers, and experimenters—for years to come. . . . The general arrangement of the curriculum, if sound, can make this task a bit easier, or if unsound, a bit harder; but in general much more—very much more—depends on teacher and student than on curriculum mechanics or teaching devices.'

If we substitute clinical psychology for medicine, this statement expresses the essential point we wish to make in this report. Our task is to find good teachers to give good students good training that will start them off in the first stages of their careers as clinical psychologists. (Raimy, 1950, p. 211)

And it was fully expected that this emphasis on teaching would impinge on standard ways of operating in academic settings. For example, in discussing some general principles for training, the committee notes:

Departments of psychology have perhaps been too much concerned with providing their instructors with freedom to organize their courses as they saw fit under an assigned title. This has frequently resulted in considerable duplication in courses and in the omission of important areas. In either case the student suffered. Without in any way infringing on the instructor's fundamental freedom, it would seem possible . . . for instructors to lay out courses which are complementary and supplementary to the others given, rather than overlapping because they are ignorant of the general content of colleague's courses. . . . The student should come in contact with a number of instructors representing a variety of points of view and types of experience. (Raimy, 1950, pp. 217–218)

The program should be oriented toward enhancing both the personal and professional growth of the student as a psychologist.

The general atmosphere of the course of training should be such as to encourage the increase in maturity. . . . The environment should be 'exciting' to the degree that the assumed 'insatiable' interest in psychological problems is kept alive, the cooperative attitude strengthened, and the passivity usually associated with so much traditional teaching kept at a minimum. The faculty must recognize its obligation to implant in students the attitude that graduate work is only the beginning of professional education. (Raimy, 1950, p. 219)

And a scientific attitude plays a prominent role in this formulation.

Throughout the course of training there should be an emphasis on the research implications of the phenomena with which he is faced, so much so that the student if finally left with the set constantly to ask 'how' and 'why' and 'what is the evidence' about the problems with which he is faced. There is probably no more important single task placed on the teaching staff than this direction towards research. (Raimy, 1950, pp. 219–220)

Taken together, the Boulder Model and the Shakow Report offer a sound, but preliminary, guidebook for training—more an aspirational direction than a precise training model. The scientist-practitioner model was and is a great idealization. However, as we have suggested, problems abide in the distinction between the model as an educational aspiration, and the model as a description of actual training practices in real, political, and diverse educational institutions. Boulder participants were only beginning to evaluate the notion of combining psychological science with practice: They could not know how practice would develop over the years, nor the directions in which science would lead them (Stricker, 1992). History suggests that the doubts, concerns, and political controversies underlying the model are still operating. The scientist-practitioner model, as an idealization rather than as a reality, is invoked too often as a tacit solution to problems that have not been considered carefully. Meanwhile, as a pedagogical theory for training that was in need of serious articulation and development, it has, for the most part, lain dormant, captive to the same politics and academic conservatism that contributed to its widespread rhetorical adoption (Stricker & Cummings, 1992).

From Boulder to the Present

As years passed, a growing number of graduates of Boulder Model programs became practitioners who operated outside and independently of academic institutions. Their professional skills and services were well received, and their confidence grew (Stricker, 1992). New approaches to therapy were developed that were linked directly to experimental psychology (e.g., Paul, 1967; D. R. Peterson, 1968), suggesting that one day practice would indeed involve implementation of the truths discovered in the laboratory. By the late 1960s, many psychologists, both within and outside training institutions, felt that the legitimacy of practice was established and they began to ask why the technical and professional aspects of practice were not more fully the focus of clinical psychology training.

Stricker (1992) suggested that scientific research has indeed influenced practice, but not always in the direct ways one might expect. Rather, since the Boulder Conference, scientific methodologies have created a cultural context within which practice activities, like psychotherapy, are interpreted and modified. As case study methods gave way to experimental designs, the questions we asked about therapy changed from treatment demonstrations to controlled outcome studies. The questions raised by these studies, in turn, lent legitimacy to the explosion of creative approaches to psychotherapy we witnessed in the 1960s. Later, in the 1970s and 1980s, more flexible, comprehensive, and time-sensitive methodologies came into widespread use, including multivariate analysis, meta-analysis, time-series analysis, and latent variable models, shaping the possibilities for the scientific analysis of psychotherapy process currently found in the literature, and raising prospects for integration across approaches heretofore deemed impossible (e.g., Stricker & Gold, 1993). From this perspective, methodological science plays a central role in the process of social legitimation of professional activities.

Yet, at the same time as these scientific questions were being raised, occasionally answered, and often forgotten, practice went on, changing to some extent, but mostly expanding into new arenas for enacting psychological intervention. The most blistering attacks by science could never completely disable a mode of practice that people liked, and what appeared to be the strongest endorsement by science could not raise a particular approach into preemptive ascendance over its counterparts. Quite independently of the attacks, endorsements, and diffidence of scientific psychology, we still find a broad range of approaches to psychological intervention thriving. Ranging from psychoanalysis to behaviorism to humanism to family systems to community psychology, these approaches exist as subcommunities within the larger discipline, belying the unity and scientific certainty sought at Boulder. Science and practice have remained largely separate endeavors.

Consistent with this picture, the story of training across this period of our history resides mostly in the political stream. Problems with research training in the existing scientist-practitioner programs played a central role in the push for explicitly professional education. Even in the mid 1960s, an APA-convened committee composed of prominent researchers, scientist-practitioners, and practitioners concluded that research training overemphasized research production at the expense of training in research consumption for clinicians (American Psychological Association, Committee on the Scientific and Professional Aims of Psychology, 1965). Rodnick (1966) observed that much of the research training activity for clinicians was irrelevant to their professional training, and the report coming from the Chicago Conference criticized an overemphasis on laboratory experimentation and scholarly production at the expense of creative applications of research methodology to clinical problems (Hoch, Ross, & Winder, 1966). The movement for professional training grew and became organized, leading to the current well-established professional programs that graduate at least a third of the students obtaining degrees in clinical psychology (D. R. Peterson, 1985; Stricker & Cummings, 1992).

Exploration of a pedagogy for implementing the Boulder vision did not occur during this heavily politicized period, at least in the public forum. Much was written about how clinicians were not great research producers, and not even great consumers (e.g., Barlow, Hayes, & Nelson, 1984; Cohen, Sargent & Sechrest, 1986; Goldfried, 1984; Strupp, 1981). Yet commitment to science has remained strong: Contrary to stereotypes, professional schools uniformly implemented research training programs, and research training has played a prominent role in curriculum development throughout the rise of the professional training movement.

SCIENCE AND METHODOLOGY IN CONTEXT

The purpose of this history is to give the reader a clear context for understanding why and how research training in professional psychology is what it has become. It is now time throughout this field to pursue the goal, not only of making professional work scientific, but also of making scientific work *professionalistic*. Method does not function independent of time and context, nor is it necessarily limited to that context. Indeed, there is a sense in which method carries the true creative spirit of science at its best, better than does the substance of scientific knowledge. In the remainder of this book we strive to convince the professional reader that methodology is an art form of great beauty and elegance, and that it has unlimited potential for guiding clinical thinking in the hands of the creative professional. It is an art form created in the history of the profession, in the context of heated debate, and in the passionate love of practice. As the reader will see, our pedagogy will strive constantly to maintain contact with this history so as to understand and justify the intellectual work required to grasp difficult methodological theory.

The Local Clinical Scientist

> The object of reasoning is to find out, from the consideration of what we
> already know, something else which we do not know. Consequently,
> reasoning is good if it be such as to give a true conclusion from true
> premisses, and not otherwise.
> —C. S. PEIRCE (1877/1955, p. 7)

> A poet's hope: to be,
> like some valley cheese,
> local, but prized elsewhere.
> —W. H. AUDEN (1991, p. 853)

The problem of integrating science and practice in professional psychology involves
two overarching issues: professional identity and methodology. Consider some definitions of these terms: *Professional identity* refers to a manifold context for understanding the problems of inquiry and method in professional practice, for relating to
the body of scientific methodologies currently existing in psychology, for relating to
scientific knowledge and the various other information sources affecting the professional's work, and for guiding professional action. It is a view of the self as a
professional (Singer, Peterson, & Magidson, 1992) as an instrument of inquiry that
must be pursued actively in one's training, and it is an ideal for the conduct of
professional practice that is achieved uniquely in each successive clinical intervention. *Method*, in this context, suggests a means for accomplishing the goal of enacting
a professional identity. It is interesting to note that the definition and etymology of the
concept of *method* encompasses both means and ends. Skeat (1989) identified the
concept as referring to an "arrangement, system, orderly procedure, [or] way." It
comes from the Greek *meta* (μετα), meaning "after," and *hodos* (οδοσ), meaning "a
way." Literally translated, it is "a way after," or "a following after" (p. 373).

What about a method for a scientific clinical practice? "A way after" what?
Clinical research scientists have identities framed in the culture of their workplace,
typically the research university. This culture values certain goals and there exists a
body of methods by which these goals can presumably be realized. Values, goals, and
appropriate methods also exist within the culture of the clinician, but they diverge
from those of the research scientist. As we saw in the last chapter, both of these
cultures predated the Boulder Conference, and have changed and developed in
striking ways since then. Within the constraints of everyday practice, neither the goals
nor the means by which they are to be pursued need modification for either researcher

or clinician and, sadly, there is a sense in which scientists and professionals can and do function quite independently of one another. To be a scientist, one must feel like a scientist; the cultural separation between science and practice has made this difficult for serious clinicians.

In this chapter we discuss this problem as we pursue the central aim of this book: the development of methodology for the local clinical scientist. We begin with a discussion of some contemporary thinking about the problem of science and practice that both informs and complements the model we will propose. We then discuss in greater detail the local clinical scientist model as an identity for the pursuit of scientific values in local clinical contexts. This background will set the stage for the discussion of methodology in the remainder of the book.

THE RECENT LITERATURE

There are two explicit approaches in the recent literature to the problem of the scientist–practitioner split, reflecting the historical response to the Boulder Model: (1) attempts to integrate traditional science with professional practice and (2) attempts to envision a new science that would be aligned more closely with practice. In this section, we discuss these two approaches, which roughly reflect the science-to-practice and practice-to-science ideals associated with the original Boulder Model. In addition, we discuss a third, more quiet tradition that we believe is more directly the legacy of the Shakow Committee's original vision: the notion of the clinician as a thinking natural scientist. Despite its limited representation in the literature, this third approach is the immediate progenitor of the local clinical scientist model.

Integrating Traditional Science

The notion that science should be integrated with practice dates back to the Boulder Conference itself. The implicit identity guiding this thinking has long been the university research scientist. In this view, traditional scientific approaches to knowledge production are considered inherently superior to other forms of investigation (cf. Hoshmand & Polkinghorne, 1992), with knowledge emanating from the laboratory through scientifically based technologies to final applications with particular clients (D. R. Peterson, 1991). Scientifically controlled studies determine what is possible and what is not. Applied psychologists are expected to bring their actions in line with these findings. By implication, the identity of the professional, working in a world of chaos and uncertainty relative to his or her scientific counterparts, is necessarily a compromise of the preferred—from a scientific perspective—identity of the university scientist. The secondary scientific status of the clinician is particularly notable relative to the preeminent scientific identity: that of the experimental scientist engaged in laboratory research, where the highest levels of scientific control of extraneous influences can be approximated. In its most extreme forms, which were quite prominent in many training programs in the decades immediately following the Boulder Conference, this thinking carried the belief that if a professional idea or technique could not be scrutinized in the laboratory, it was "soft-headed" and not worthy of support by the profession.

Today these views may be moderating, but the underlying issues remain. As professional schools began to draw high-quality students, scientific clinical psychologists became increasingly interested in bridging the gap between academic science and clinical practice. Stricker (1992) noted that some felt that science and practice already were intimately related, mutually informing one another in every decision and action made by the professional (e.g., Singer, 1980). Others, such as Matarazzo (quoted in Barlow, 1981, p. 148), expressed exactly the opposite point of view; research and practice did not touch one another save in the most minimal and trivial ways. As scientific findings increasingly came to support the efficacy of psychotherapy (e.g., Smith, Glass, & Miller, 1980; Strupp, 1986), the need for academic psychology to make some move to accommodate rising professionalism became increasingly apparent.

Paul's (1967) implementation of an experimentally controlled psychotherapy outcome study was a major methodological development in this context, the importance of which cannot be overstated. Science and practice were given a way to relate directly to one another in this work. In addition to Paul, researchers such as Kanfer (1970), D. R. Peterson (1968), Ullmann and Krasner (1975), and numerous others demonstrated that the methodological behaviorism that informed much of the psychological research of the 1960s and 1970s was fertile turf for the development of psychological interventions. The costs were the adoption of a more limited range of acceptable approaches to professional intervention and a sense of the professional as a technician implementing scientifically legitimized technologies rather than the broad-ranging, intellectual healer envisioned by Freud and others (e.g., Freud, 1959; Gay, 1989).

Barlow and colleagues' (1984) book on the science–practice link illustrates how implicit professional identity assumptions have informed integrative attempts over the years in its emphasis on evaluation. The key scientific concern for the scientist-practitioner was the evaluation of the efficacy of interventions, using acceptable scientific methodologies adapted to clinical evaluation problems, and the acceptance of accountability for the quality of service delivered. Case studies, single-subject research designs, and several other creative methodological frameworks were suggested as means to these ends. The focus was on the generation of evaluations of professional services that are observable and, therefore, independently verifiable. Presaging the present discussion, and following Cronbach (1975a), these authors pointed to the need for intensive local observation to assess the effects of interventions. Still, there was no suggestion that clinical work might itself offer substantive contribution to scientific psychology, nor that it even involves scientific thinking apart from scientific evaluation procedures.

More recently, some discussions have recognized more explicitly the extensive cultural and identity differences that exist between academic scientists and professionals. There is a growing awareness that simple, direct translation of the scientist identity into clinical contexts is not viable. Kanfer (1990) discussed the science–practice split in terms of a bridge needing constant attention. He suggested that there must be groups of individuals in the field who explicitly devote their attention to linking scientific and clinical findings to one another. Similarly, D. R. Peterson (1991) pointed to the complementarity between scientist and practitioner identities, but recognized their fundamental difference with respect to the goal of inquiry. Both Kanfer and D. R. Peterson recognized that the primary concern of the clinician is the welfare of the client, and that this concern modifies the notion of science in the applied context. Each offered a flow chart model for the process whereby clinicians, starting with the condition of the client, use scientific and experientially acquired understanding to assess, plan, implement, and evaluate interventions. The recognition of the role of experientially acquired understanding is a major addition to the evidentiary base of the traditional scientist—experiments, in effect, are not the only pathway to knowledge.

These efforts to expand traditional science to accommodate clinical realities remind us that science is a very powerful public institution despite the many critiques leveled against it over the years, as we discuss below and in Chapter 3. At a commonsense level this is rightly so; a well-designed experiment can greatly affect our view of the world. Moreover, these discussions show that science, which is often seen as overly conservative, is adaptable, holding out the promise that it can inform a broader range of contexts and questions than many realize. This adaptability is critical to any solution to the scientist–practitioner split.

Developing New Science

Although some have emphasized the relationship between traditional science and practice, other psychologists have expressed concern that traditional science is, at best, incomplete as a knowledge base for professional psychology. At worst, it can be downright misleading. This critical position is rooted in a long history of public critique of scientific psychology and particularly in the role the philosophical position of logical positivism has played in science (Chapter 3). It is part of a much larger tradition of criticism operating throughout the social sciences even as they were coming into prominence in the 1950s, 1960s, and 1970s. Much of the critique has been directed toward the behaviorism that dominated scientific psychology up through the 1960s, when it gradually gave way to cognitivism (e.g., Allport, 1967; Gergen, 1985; Koch, 1959; Lamiell, 1987; Rychlak, 1981).

Although largely compatible with approaches to the science–practice problem already discussed, the implicit identity that accompanies this point of view is that of a philosopher of science who is critical of past perspectives, particularly those that are in some sense politically entrenched. Usually these critiques seek to expand the range of phenomena acceptable in scientific analysis, the range of methods available for investigating those phenomena, the criteria by which conclusions are drawn and evaluated, and the range of participants in the investigatory process. More recently, these critiques have focused on the limitations of the implication that only a certain elite group has access to the primary means of knowledge production (Hoshmand & Polkinghorne, 1992).

The major thrust of these positions is that traditional science, focused as it has been on observable phenomena and the investigation of populations, is not sufficient for the serious examination of individuals (e.g., Polkinghorne, 1983). Other useful "ways of knowing," such as those attained through clinical, historical, biographical, or interpretive analysis, have been overruled inappropriately in the name of scientific certainty, whether science actually addresses the phenomenon under investigation or not. Doubts are raised about the claims of science to have endorsed humanistic values and a commitment to human welfare. Following as it has the assumptions of logical positivist philosophy in asserting the primacy of sensory data, logic, and mathematics in scientific formulations (see Chapter 3), the science of the twentieth century is thought to have become too detached, conservative, critical, and conceptual. Many have argued that this positivist thinking, which was the philosophical foundation for many of the currently existing research methods, needs to be replaced by a position more sensitive to human realities (e.g., Bateson, 1972). Prior to the 1980s, this line of dissent focused on the restrictive qualities of behaviorism (e.g., Rychlak, 1981). During the 1970s and 1980s, as cognitivism became widespread in science, concerns shifted to the social adequacy of scientific approaches, to the limitations of so-called nomothetic science, which was singularly rooted in the assumptions of applied statistics (e.g., Lamiell, 1987; Lamiell & Trierweiler, 1986), and to a social constructionist theory of knowledge creation in psychology (e.g., Cushman, 1990; Gergen, 1985; R. L. Peterson, 1992) that suggested a broader array of methods might indeed be appropriate. Throughout this book, we will discuss this historical trend in the philosophy of science and its impact on professional psychology.

Critical perspectives are important in reminding us that just because science has not yet addressed a clinical issue, or has addressed it in a particular way that is not well coordinated with action in the clinical realm, it does not follow that a phenomenon, or a view of a phenomenon, should be dismissed as having no legitimacy for the profession. Rather, there are numerous ways of viewing professionally relevant phenomena, some of which capture qualities of human experience and action that defy simple scientific scrutiny, yet that may be central to a professional inquiry. Additionally, science operates in a sociopolitical context that affects both inquiry and the sense of what is important for scientific investigation in a particular time and place. Critical philosophy has played a central role in making scientists aware of these issues in the past 25 years.

A modicum of caution is beneficial in pursuing a critical line of thinking: There can be a tendency to criticize a position simply because it is espoused by some established authority. There is little in the social sciences that found acceptance without an extended history of doing battle with some previous authority. Analogous to the artistic innovations of late nineteenth-century Europe, the academy, more or less explicitly defined, has set the standards for acceptability of achievements in the psychological and social sciences. This was as true for positivism supplanting metaphysics as it was for psychoanalysis supplanting ignorance, behaviorism supplanting psychoanalysis, and cognitivism supplanting behaviorism. It continues to be true as postmodern thinking attempts to gain a foothold. In fact, no useful approach to human psychology has been completely replaced, but rather, each has its day only to lose its temporary position in the mainstream to some promising—usually perceived as new—competitor.

Our position with respect to this struggle is that it is inherent to the profession, and it is the ferment that will keep clinicians forever engaged with intellectual life— for their own good and the good of their clients, we might add. Indeed, we can use this disciplinary diversity to learn something: A critical pedagogical position suggests that neither science nor philosophy, in itself, provides a definitive basis for affirming or rejecting a method or its potential applications. Our task is to understand the assumptions and functional properties of methods, and to determine what they can and cannot accomplish within their own specific domain of applicability.

THE CLINICIAN AS A THINKING SCIENTIST

In contrast to the traditions outlined above, the third position, based in the Shakow Report (Chapter 1), endorses the legitimacy of practice within its own frame, rather than from within an academic discipline such as science or philosophy. It focuses on the educational stream and the identity of the professional as a scientific thinker operating within the natural world for the benefit of clients. Although an important conceptual foundation for the Boulder Conference, this perspective is the least developed approach. Even cursory examination suggests that it reflects the notion of integration better than the other two positions. We suspect that this third position has received less attention because it focuses on the integrity of training, rather than on science or practice itself. In so doing, it tends to ignore the political stream of power and influence that has been so determinative a force in our profession.

Shakow (1976) represented one version of this identity, which in his mind was what the scientist-practitioner identity was all about. His article is remarkable in that the professionalization of clinical training was already well under way at its publication, yet Shakow hoped to defend the scientist-professional model by showing that it adequately encompassed the needs of clinicians. Shakow saw the scientist-professional as a knowledgeable generalist,

> a person who, on the basis of systematic knowledge about persons obtained primarily in real-life situations, has integrated this knowledge with psychological theory, and has then consistently regarded it with the questioning attitude of the scientist. In this image, clinical psychologists see themselves combining the

idiographic and nomothetic approaches, both of which appear to them significant. (1976, p. 554)

The thinking clinician is a rigorous observer who emphasizes theory rather than technique, and who operates very much in everyday reality. Scientific training for such individuals would emphasize observation, and Shakow distinguishes four types:

- *Objective observation*, taking the perspective of the naturalist observing events from outside the subject and the situation
- *Participant observation*, requiring the clinician to be aware of how he or she affects the situation, and how the situation affects the observation itself
- *Subjective observation*, wherein the observer attempts to gain empathic understanding of the patient's feelings about self and others
- *Self-observation*, essentially self-awareness gained through careful self-examination under guidance

The message for the thinking clinician is clear: She or he must be ready to adopt and to integrate multiple perspectives, to be aware of and sensitive to the experiences of self and others, and to be ever questioning and skeptical about her or his own perceptions and beliefs.

As Shakow was well aware, observation is only part of the story, for the clinician operates within intellectual and professional traditions as well as the face-to-face situation. As a result, the clinician entering the field not only needs observational skills, but also the ability to select from and integrate a bewildering, and often disparate, array of information sources. These include:

- Clinical and psychological theoretical writings, which are ever changing and constantly being embellished by highly persuasive rhetoricians
- Research reports, which often have the character of relevance and importance but which typically are not translated into the experiential language of the practitioner
- Clinical case studies
- Colleagues and supervisors
- The clinician's own experience
- Institutional clinical and business practices
- Cultural and societal conceptions and misconceptions
- Clients themselves, who have the ability to influence the course of events quite apart from the clinician's abilities as a scientific observer

The apparent impossibility of this task is a well-kept secret in the profession. Most clinicians find a solution to this problem by selecting one or two ways of looking at the world that fit their style and personality, and these approaches encompass clinical psychology for those individuals.

We believe the implicit priority placed on personal preference in training, as opposed to the larger corpus of psychological knowledge and theory, is a mistake and a major problem for training in clinical psychology. An explicit pedagogy of critical thinking in professional psychology is needed, one that shows students how to make sense of the diverse and internally inconsistent information culture in which they operate. A strong case can be made that, on the whole, research and practice operate synergistically in advancing our field, and, therefore, scientist-practitioner status is a possible, albeit rarely exhibited, achievement. A lasting solution to the science–practice gap depends on our open recognition of this potential in our training, professional, and political activities (Stricker, 1992; Stricker & Keisner, 1985b; Stricker & Trierweiler, 1995; Trierweiler & Stricker, 1992).

THE LOCAL CLINICAL SCIENTIST

Definition of the Model

The local clinical scientist model is halfway between old and new science; as a pedagogical position, there is no requirement to reject one position in favor of another except on practical grounds for a particular goal. These grounds must be defined within the particular context of the inquiry. The local clinical scientist identity is a means for focusing on clinical phenomena, both in their specific local form and in their relationship to more general formulations of science.

The local clinical scientist model was developed so that the research and evaluation training might encourage critical, scientific thinking in professional pursuits, as well as research itself (Trierweiler & Stricker, 1992). Different theories and traditions within professional psychology suggest different methods of inquiry for local practice, and encourage attention to particular sources of knowledge within psychology. The local clinical scientist model is one such view coming from scientific methodology rather than from a substantive tradition.

The model begins with a conception of science that provides a context within which a professional must develop competency (Trierweiler & Stricker, 1992). Psychological science can be viewed as "a systematic mode of inquiry involving problem identification and the acquisition, organization, and interpretation of information pertaining to psychological phenomena. It strives to make that information consensually verifiable, replicable, and universally communicable" (McHolland, 1992, cited in Trierweiler & Stricker, 1992, p. 103). This formulation emphasizes that science has sought to generate knowledge that pertains to the general case, where *general* means "involving or applicable to the whole" (*Webster's*). In contrast, the local clinical scientist is an individual who strives toward these goals in an individual, local context, even though such contexts present practical realities that may prevent traditional scientific goals from being strongly realized (e.g., privacy).

The local clinical scientist is a critical investigator who uses scientific research and methods, general scholarship, and personal and professional experience to develop plausible and communicable formulations of local phenomena. This investigator draws on scientific theory and research, general world knowledge, acute observational skills, and an open, skeptical stance toward the problem to conduct this inquiry.

In emphasizing the process of scientific clinical inquiry within the realistic constraints of clinical practice (see also Hoshmand & Polkinghorne, 1992), this model is a sensible identity frame both for the professional psychologist and for the researcher who is engaging in the professional practice of psychology. The model involves a variety of professional functions, and much work will need to be done to develop its potential. To date, we have concentrated on three areas directly pertaining to the professional student's grasp of science and scientific methodology in professional psychology. These include: attitudinal skills, critical thinking skills, and methodological skills (Trierweiler & Stricker, 1992). In the final section of this chapter we elaborate some of this thinking as a context for the discussion of methodology that follows. Before doing so, however, we must look briefly at some definitions that will be important for the exposition that follows.

Some Definitions Relating to the Local Clinical Scientist Model

The Local Clinical Scientist as an Identity Model

The focal point of the model is the image of the professional standing alone amid an ambiguous reality that must be explored, understood, and influenced positively by professional action. When standard concepts and tools of inquiry are inadequate, the professional's own critical judgment becomes increasingly important. We believe that scientific training should be designed to improve this sort of on-the-spot judgment. Thus, one primary function of the local clinical scientist identity is to guide the development of scientific forms of thinking in clinical contexts. Other goals emanating from the scientist-practitioner model, such as applying scientific knowledge to clinical practice, and using clinical practice and observation to inform the scientific knowledge base, are viewed as important but secondary to the development of critical scientific thinking in local contexts. In this way the local clinical scientist identity is a pedagogical and pragmatic frame for incorporating the entire corpus of psychological knowledge, theory, and method as it applies to the identifiable realities of particular circumstances.

The Clinical Situation

The clinical situation is the naturally occurring laboratory for the local clinical scientist; it is any situation wherein a prospective client seeks assistance from a trained psychologist. This definition is intended to be completely general with respect to types of problem and treatment (e.g., individuals, couples, families, groups, and organizations). The help-seeking action by the client makes the clinical situation different from the typical scientific laboratory: All observation, conceptualization, and intervention must be understood within this context. A particular practical outcome is expected that can set limits on the time frame and thoroughness of an inquiry.

Open versus Closed Systems.   Clinical situations, occurring as they do in the natural world, tend to be open rather than closed systems. It is rarely possible to specify completely the information universe pertaining to the identified problem. In the ideal laboratory, a scientist can exert nearly complete control over discernible influences on the phenomena of interest. The laboratory is an artificially closed system designed specifically to make such control possible: Quite literally, "walls" are put up to keep out influences that can affect scientific observation in ways extraneous to the questions being asked. In contrast, clinical situations, as open systems, allow no such walls. Therefore, the psychologist's control of the situation is inherently limited. Other influences affect the condition of the client, both positively and negatively, and the professional's access to information concerning the case can be restricted.

Observation

Although we will use the notion of observation in the traditional sense of using vision to perceive a phenomenon (e.g., Weick, 1968), we also seek to expand the definition to include any situation where the psychologist recognizes something to be true in the clinical situation, be it through vision or some other means. Thus, in our usage, observation is more similar to the notion of *apprehension*, which involves both perceiving and understanding (*Webster's*; Chapter 9), or to the traditional psychological concept of *apperception*, which involves recognition of relationships between a perception and something else, including a body of knowledge (Chaplin, 1985). What is often called "clinical intuition" is also observation, albeit observation that is more difficult to verify and communicate to others than is more physicalistic observation (Chapter 8). Most importantly, we view professional observation as directly analogous to measurement in science, which we discuss in Chapter 5. In scientific measurement, the conditions for assigning a scale value to an observation are presumed to be very precise and clearly specified, so any of a particular class of observers would make equivalent assignments. Much work is devoted to the problem of establishing the reliability of the measurement. Similarly, in professional observation, deciding that an observation means something important to one's intervention— metaphorically assigning a scale value on a given construct—is a problem of reliability of judgment. Here, however, the path to follow in establishing reliability, and indeed in determining what reliability means, is not so clear as in traditional science.

Local

At its most basic level, the concept of *local* should be contrasted with the notion of *universal* or *general*. These latter terms suggest concepts and methods that apply to each and every member of some larger whole. For example, if a scientist wishes to investigate depression, a population is identified, and each person is measured on the construct of depression. In effect, the construct of depression is deemed to be relevant to everyone, even those who are not depressed in any obvious sense. In turn, interventions are designed that might affect depression for each and every individual so identified.

In contrast, local inquiry may or may not involve such a general frame of reference. The concept of local involves four information settings that need to be assessed. These information settings reflect several related concerns that regularly confront clinicians, and, hence, they will guide our discussion in the remainder of the book.

Local as a Particular Application of General Science. In general science, the problem of identifying (measuring) an individual (be it person, event, structure, or process) on a particular attribute is pervasive, and a sophisticated logic and methodology are available to handle questions of reliability and validity that arise in making these measurements. As we will see in Chapters 4, 5, and 6, however, most of this theory and technology was designed to handle aggregated information. Aggregation is one logical way of seeking generality in one's scientific formulations. In contrast, clinicians regularly deal with individual inquiries and interventions. Even in applying general science, such local inquiry raises a question about the integrity of a specific measurement in a particular case. This is a question that cannot be answered based solely on aggregated data (Cronbach, 1975a, 1982; Lamiell, 1987). Rather, it involves the quality of a single, unique measurement act. Not only is the assignment of a trustworthy and meaningful indicator of a general category to the case important, but consideration of the local nature of the assignment also raises a question of whether this particular observation (measurement) is the best way to characterize the case (e.g., Bem & Allen, 1974). Clinicians know general scientific knowledge sometimes is very useful, but sometimes it is not.

Local Cultures. Cultures operate locally, sometimes in identifiable ways, and sometimes in tacit ways hidden in unique circumstances (Geertz, 1983; Polanyi, 1958, 1967/1992). Local scientists judge the nature of realities in relation to general science, and the integrity of a formulation of persons, objects, and events functioning within a specific context (e.g., this child's score on an aptitude test). Further complicating the inquiry of the clinician, judgment occurs in relation to a local understanding of the nature of reality as it exists in a local culture—including the ways people speak about and understand the events of their lives (e.g., a local culture's perspective on aptitude and its importance in life). Moreover, professionals actually bring the culture of science into preexisting locally manifest cultures (which also are open systems). Professionals must recognize how this affects what they observe and how observations are understood in local context, so as to work effectively with the situation. Localized views of particular situations can exist in communities, within small subgroups of people, or even within families. Failure to understand these naturally occurring interpretations can greatly impede communication with a client. For example, within the culture of a family, putting up with a father's blustery temper may be an accepted way of managing everyone's doubts and fears about their collective viability. To fail to recognize this tacit nod to the father's authority and protective function may be to miss important sources of resistance to change in the family.

Local as Unique (Not Broad or General). Standing in the midst of the clinical situation, it is a virtual certainty that some aspects of what one observes will fall outside the pale of available science. The local clinical scientist model reminds us that professionals regularly deal with information that is not general, and because of its limited availability, applicability, and interest, it never will be so. These are the idiosyncratic or idiographic aspects of life, such as the particulars of a personal biography, of a local community's history, or of events in an individual's recent past. Sometimes they involve special, relatively unique conjunctions of events that have no simple scientific explanation (e.g., the identity and life goal issues of a young woman born to a poor, and now separated, mixed-race couple). Even more disturbing, some of the unique information directly available to the professional, who is involved in an ongoing relationship with the client, is not generally communicable to others no matter how hard one tries. Nonetheless, we must recognize that, along with this unique, highly circumstantial information, there may be information reflective of as yet unrevealed generalized mechanisms, such as the outcomes of adaptive evolutionary processes (Barkow, Cosmides, & Tooby, 1992), that might guide our work once this relationship is understood. In suggesting that some information is not general, we are also suggesting that the professional be ever alert to the dialogue between the general and the specific operating in open systems. We will revisit this dialogue repeatedly in the chapters that follow.

Space-Time Local. The space-time local information setting is the most extreme formulation of local information in that it refers to the physical and temporal properties not only of the "thing" being judged but also of the specific space-time context of the act of judgment itself. Each observation occurs in a specific space-time context. Usually, conditions remain constant enough (we tend to make them that way) that time's effect is minimally disruptive. However, because human events are time extended and cannot be reviewed (save in memory, see Chapter 9), it is possible for today's observation of ostensibly the same phenomenon to differ from tomorrow's— even though expectation and bias may lead us to see them as similar. This can make it difficult to notice change or the unusual. For example, each session (and moment within a session) with a depressed patient is a unique event in space and time, even though we tend to see the same depression (and patient) from session to session. If the patient were not depressed in the observed manner between sessions, meaning the manifestation observed is specific to the treatment setting (e.g., patients often report that others do not notice the pain they exhibit in their therapy sessions), or if the depression itself differs in subtle ways from time to time, a clinician may not be prepared to notice the differences.

Unfortunately, the changing temporal landscape of the local clinical situation may be even more problematic than is the general concern about reliability of measurement on which scientists have concentrated their efforts. Science assumes that phenomena in the world are orderly, and that this order, with sufficient care, can be accessed consistently. Even if this assumption holds in general, it may not be cleanly and clearly realized on a space-time local scale. Consider, for example, that many of the signal aspects of important events in life are often emergent from unique space-time convergences between events (e.g., one's rumination about which college to attend is suddenly shaken free in the eleventh hour by an out-of-the-blue call from a long-lost friend). There are reasons to believe that temporally emergent properties of events are generally important in interpersonal perception, interpretation, and memory (Baron & Misovich, 1993; Trierweiler & Donovan, 1994). Fortuitous events and event sequences also affect the professional in the act of conducting her assessments (e.g., having recently attended an important lecture on this very topic, or yesterday's flareup of long-ignored relationship problems). Such complexities are ubiquitous. They affect all interpretive activities, including the interpretation of scientific data. For example, a borderline test score may be interpreted more negatively on some occasions than others; an ever so slight look of dismay on the face of a stressed clinician can have a major effect on the experience of the patient. Adding to the problem, these very specific events cannot be simply dismissed as error in the local clinical situation, as they can be in research studies, because they need to be recognized and corrected if possible.

Our ideas about measurement need to be revised to accommodate this complexity. Practical measurement occurs in a space-time context that can greatly affect both the reliability of judgment, from a general scientific perspective, and the adequacy of the clinician's vision of the local reality, from a local scientific perspective. Each momentary observation may be more or less influenced by (1) the fundamental order of naturally occurring phenomena, which is of interest to the clinician, and (2) temporally local chaos, which requires attention whether a clinician likes it or not. The space-time specific circumstances of the observations and interpretations made by the practitioner may be as important in understanding a case as are the results of those observations. Yet, few scientific and theoretical formulations take these local contexts into consideration. Instead of bemoaning the fact that all clinician judgment does not conform to the requirements of traditional scientific instruments, local clinical scientists need to be aware of these influences and incorporate them into their formulations.

We will discuss these four settings of local information further in later chapters.

Extrapolation

Cronbach (1982) used the term *extrapolate* to describe the process of making an external inference from a research finding (Chapter 4). Here we use the term to describe the process of extending forms of methodological thought, created in the pursuit of general science, to inquiry in the local clinical situation. In so doing, we will show how the goals and practices of science can inform local inquiry without compromising local realities. Additionally, we will see points of similarity and difference between general and local science, and raise interesting questions about the applicability of specific scientific findings to local contexts.

The Problem of Audience and Consensus

The task of the local clinical scientist is to comprehend the general and unique qualities of the local clinical situation, and their combination. We are required to relate space-time localized experiences to general science. However, the consensus-generating operations typically used to satisfy the scientific audiences often have no direct application in the face of such informational complexity (e.g., averaging, random assignment, and so on; Chapters 4, 5, and 6). At the same time, professional responsibility demands accurate interpretation and beneficial action. Therefore, we must depend on pragmatic operations that are consistent with science while also integrated with local realities in each of the senses of local described above. On occasion, a case may conform sufficiently to a general scientific formulation that it can guide the treatment; we do sometimes find cases that match diagnostic prototypes rather precisely. On the other hand, far more often there are significant divergences from such generalized formulations. Often these divergences hinge significantly on local information that may never be subject to general public scrutiny. For example, the implicit knowledge one gains about a person through extended contact and the interpersonal relationship that develops are rarely specifiable as general types, save in a superficial way, and even narrative formulations are seldom up to a serious and comprehensive portrayal. Thus, the audience for one's inquiry and formulation can range from the very local to the very general, with different case narratives pertaining across the span. Similarly, the standards for consensus about formulations can change with these differing audiences (see Chapter 9 for an expanded discussion of this point).

The local clinical scientist must develop some rather broad-ranging inquiry and communication skills to manage this complexity. In the local clinical situation, interpersonal and affective skills are as important to the scientific endeavor of understanding the situation as they are to the clinical intervention. The problem with the traditional assumptions that practice is simply applied science (see Chapter 9), and that professional inquiry must be governed solely by scientifically validated concepts and technologies, is that the need for interpersonal and affective skills is rarely given due heed.

By the same token, there never will be a professional inquiry that is completely local, because the existence of the profession implies the existence of a more general occupational frame of reference. Professional inquiry involves a modus operandi and language that is designed to make communication public, and that is central to the operation of any intervention. In effect, our professional language looms both large and local reflecting the combination of generalized and completely unique concepts that characterizes case formulations.

The Local Clinical Scientist Model as a Pedagogical Perspective

The local clinical scientist model addresses the problems just outlined by focusing on three broad skill areas relevant to handling information in open systems, namely, attitudinal, critical thinking, and methodological skills. Taken together, they provide a pedagogical model, and an identity context for relating to science and methodology.

Attitude and Judgment Skills

The local clinical scientist's attitude is critical, in that it is discerning, empirical, and open (see Chapter 8). It renders a judgment that avoids premature foreclosure on an inquiry, and constantly is alert for new, more precise evidence in support of, or against, a formulation. It is an active effort to be influenced more by evidence than by conjecture, social conformity, professional fads, or particular theoretical viewpoints. It is a position of actively seeking situations in which the possibility of change to a better position exists—as locally defined, based on evidence. Ideas about the nature of evidence abound in the scientific and professional communities, and they are implicit in all cultures and subcultures within which professionals operate. One goal of a local clinical scientist is to bring these various viewpoints together, so the professional can learn better how to analyze professional problems.

Achieving such an attitude and drawing on it to aid local understanding is no small matter. Trierweiler and Stricker (1992) suggested some possible ways in which training in methodology might contribute to this sort of attitude development. These involve seeing even the most technical matters in terms of their implications for localized understanding. In this way, methods training becomes a vehicle for the development of:

> (a) openness and receptivity to the multiple ways of looking at a problem (as opposed to dogmatism) and the various strengths and limitations of these approaches; (b) respect for the empirical support (either local support or support offered in the scientific literature) for a particular viewpoint tempered by a healthy skepticism about the certainty such support affords and the appropriateness of its application to particular circumstances; (c) a sense of professional knowledge, responsibility, and authority (professional voice) with respect to the conduct of an inquiry that facilitates timely decision making and action while explicitly eschew-

ing professional arrogance; (d) explicit recognition of one's own biases and predilections and how these might serve to limit an inquiry in deleterious ways; (e) explicit recognition of the interplay between ethics and scientific inquiry especially with respect to special issues that arise in local circumstance; and (f) explicit recognition of the need for collegial input and feedback in any inquiry however routine. (Trierweiler & Stricker, 1992, p. 106)

Critical Thinking Skills

As we will see in the methodological discussions in the following chapters, critical thinking involves consideration of the nature of evidence, the use of logic and clear communication to generate consensual formulations of phenomena, and the design of consensus-building scenarios. However, it also involves several assumptions about the nature of the inquiry process itself. The assumption that one can approximate conditions of clarity (even certainty) by seeking and achieving evidence is fundamental to critical thinking (Chapter 8). A collection of methods, and logical linkages between theories and methods, helps specify the nature of the evidence needed in a particular case, but ultimately the inquiry cannot depend solely on technically derived understanding. Rather, the attitude, judgment, and perspective of the investigative natural scientist and clinician determine the quality of the inquiry. In our view this individual must ever be in search of new ways to explore a situation, and new, more incisive ways to delve deeper into the qualities of the evidence supporting a proposition, be it conceptual in the traditional sense, or narrative (e.g., Bruner, 1990). Moreover, it is a practiced awareness of being embedded in a reality that transcends any particular formulation. It is active attention to the richly textured net of linkages that exists between objects and events extending through space and time, from past through the present and into the future. This attention to one's embeddedness in a reality greater than one's conceptualization—or even one's ability to conceptualize—is important in that it focuses the recognition that one's beliefs about the world (constructions) must be subservient to the realities one seeks. Thus, for the professional, critical thinking is intimately related to the attitude of humility and responsibility described above; it is a seeking to achieve the most defensible portrayal of local circumstances as is possible. The act of pursuing local realities, and of seeking such portrayals, is understood to be an inherently public process, however localized and unique it may seem. Local clinical scientists are not simply authorities on the nature of things, they are servants of that nature, pursuing a reasonable relationship with it in the hope of gaining some insight into pathways to healing change.

Methodological Skills

Methodological skills for the local clinical scientist involve implementation of the attitudes, critical thought process, knowledge, and observation provoked by a clinical situation. In some sense, this involves specific technical skills. Professional psychologists develop these skills throughout their scientific and clinical apprenticeship. But more broadly, we take the perspective of Kaplan (1964) that any notion of methodology is related intimately to the nature of the knowledge we seek. "I mean by *methodology* the study—the description, the explanation, and the justification—of methods, and not the methods themselves" (Kaplan, 1964, p. 18). Thus, from our perspective, knowledge of the ways things might be verified under certain hypothetical circumstances is as important to the course of a scientific inquiry as is the real course of events.

The local clinical scientist uses methodological understanding to approach a problem as effectively and as openly as possible. Naturalistic methodological skills are used to develop a vision of oneself in relation to a surrounding transcendent reality. Methodological skill may involve the implementation of specific scientific methods, such as limited surveys or participant observation, or such personal inquiry skills as the ability to suspend belief in the service of new insights, or the application and adaptation of scientific forms of analysis to local problems. It involves actively maintaining open inquiry so as to avoid the serious problem of shutting down before all of the evidence is in. And, it involves active recognition of the importance of careful entry into a relationship with information ecology presented by the clinical situation. Stepwise models, such as those of Kanfer (1990) or D. R. Peterson (1991), can guide this process, and we will offer some additional considerations later in the book.

THE REST OF THE BOOK

The remainder of this book offers an overview of methodology for the local clinical scientist. Our approach will be to examine various scientific methodological issues with an eye to their attitudinal, critical thinking, and methodological implications for a local clinical science. In so doing, we attempt to retain the identity image of the professional described above as the primary problem focus, and extrapolate the implications of problems in scientific research methodology for local scientific analysis. Our strong focus will be on how the methods are presumed to work rather than on how they are implemented.

The remainder of the book is divided into two parts reflecting: (1) extrapolations from traditional science, including philosophy of science, research design, and statistics, and (2) extrapolations from nontraditional science, including qualitative methods and innovative approaches to inquiry. The reader is invited to meld ideas of local and general in ways that are, perhaps, unfamiliar, and that require an equal valuing of both forms that is different from previous rhetoric and controversy. In this way, we hope that professional inquiry is seen clearly for what it always has been, a special and very important problem in the larger scientific goal of seeking reasonable truths.

II

Extrapolations to Local Science from Traditional Science and Scholarship

Issues in the Philosophy
of Science

Psychology has never succeeded in taking philosophy to itself nor in leaving
it alone.
—BORING (1929, p. 660)

Not knowing how near the truth is, people seek it far away,—what a pity!
—ZEN MASTER HAKUIN, in SUZUKI (1960, p. 151)

In this chapter, we discuss the place of philosophy of science in the work of the local
clinical scientist. Our goals are twofold. First, we provide the reader with basic
background in philosophy of science so as to set a foundation for later discussion of
the relationship between scientific methodologies and critical thinking in the professional psychologist. Second, we propose an extrapolation model that describes how
philosophical analysis can be used to raise questions about the information a professional seeks in the local clinical situations. We use the term *extrapolation* as elaborated in the last chapter: It involves extending a concept beyond its existing domain of
applicability into a new, or in our case, a more specific domain.

The study of philosophy of science is an important prerequisite for the development of critical clinical thinking (Miller, 1992a; D. R. Peterson & R. L. Peterson, in
press; Polkinghorne, 1983). We approach this material from an aerial perspective,
standing somewhat above the debates of philosophy of science so as to grasp how
philosophers approach the problem of inquiry. Three broad themes, or trajectories for
analysis (see below), that characterize recent philosophy of science are emphasized.
We believe these themes will continue to influence psychological science and professional practice in significant ways as we move into the next century.

The sections that follow will describe: (1) the philosophy of science and its
relationship to a local model of clinical practice; (2) the need for a critical-
pedagogical approach to philosophical material; (3) the basic themes that can be
discerned in the philosophical and psychological literature, which include the
positivistic/empirical approach, the idealist/paradigmatic approach, and the socio-
cultural/constructionist approach; and finally, (4) our extrapolation model and its
usage with some examples from professional inquiry. Overviews of each historical
trend will give the reader a basic understanding of its origins. However, it should be
understood at the outset that these are not exhaustive characterizations. Rather, they

are used here for expository purposes. Some may find the historical material rather abstract. However, such material is a necessary backdrop for linking philosophical thought to local clinical inquiry.

WHAT IS PHILOSOPHY OF SCIENCE?

Taken at face value, science presents itself in tidy packages: Problems flow endlessly, with apparent self-evidence, from theory and the literature. The methodological tools of science seem ever ready to shed light on even the most distressing complexities. Science is a remarkable approach to problem solving that is rooted in natural philosophy (e.g., Miller, 1992a). It has become the major source of professional legitimation in our field. Yet, professionals rarely understand how this has come to be. Captive to the immediacy of practice and the urgency of clinical problems, they often concentrate on the artistry of professional tradition, not feeling that their interests are well represented by science. Perhaps scientific packages are too neat; professional work certainly is not.

Philosophy of science is reflective study that probes deeply into the logic of how science works and into the adequacy of the assumptions supporting scientific thought and action. It explores scientific methods asking how, why, and if they accomplish what they claim to accomplish. It is concerned with the broader sociocultural implications of scientific formulations and scientific methods, and with limits on the applicability of science. Philosophy of science also explores the taken for granted, or ignored, and seeks ever greater precision in answers to basic questions, even to the point of questioning the questions themselves. It asks how inquiry might best proceed and how we might best think about what we do.

Philosophy of science has changed markedly over the course of this century. Two general approaches can be discerned: formulations designed to identify the best, or most definitive, way science can attain truth, and formulations attending to how science actually seems to operate. The former have been devoted to the elaboration of a set of epistemological and methodological "shoulds," the latter to the critique of these shoulds based on what seems to be the actual history of science. The twentieth century has been a very productive time; many ancient philosophical themes concerning the nature of knowledge have been revived and updated (see Miller, 1992a), and scientific knowledge has increased dramatically.

For much of this century, philosophers of science have searched for a solid empirical foundation for science, both to understand what had taken place in the dramatic scientific and technological progress of the previous century, and to establish a canon for all scientific endeavors as a way of evaluating the quality of knowledge produced by science. Their work is a chapter in the long development of naturalistic and humanistic philosophy in Western civilization, and the decline of an organized spiritual authority at the center of social life. With almost holographic consistency, we find the same themes enacted at various levels of intellectual discourse within the academy, and at differing times as we move across disciplines. These themes include:

- Objective versus subjective
- Empirical versus conceptual
- Individual versus collective
- Physical versus metaphysical
- Pragmatic versus definitive
- Restrained versus expressive
- Skeptical versus accepting

Philosophy and the Professional

Philosophy of science contributes to the scientific endeavor by raising higher-level questions about the nature of knowledge and certainty in scientific inquiry. Yet, for a variety of reasons, psychologists have not widely embraced philosophical inquiry (e.g., Meehl, 1978; Miller, 1992a; Rychlak, 1981).

There are two major positions that clinicians seem to take with respect to the concerns raised by philosophy of science: the *indifferent* position, where one ignores the problems identified by philosophical critique and goes about one's business; and the *promotional* position, where a particular perspective is embraced intensely along with an explicit critique of some rival, often well-established, and reputedly inferior perspective (cf. Miller, 1992a).

The hallmark of the indifferent position is a belief that philosophy is too abstract, difficult to grasp, and irrelevant for it to have actual implication for clinical and scientific practices. Philosophers tend not to be action oriented, so what could they possibly know about practice? This perspective cannot simply be ascribed to intellectual lassitude on the part of clinicians; philosophy, itself, has contributed in no small part. For one thing, the study of philosophy can seem a restless and dissatisfying journey through a daunting wilderness where one is always lost, and always searching for something more precise, more definitive—the ultimate and better way. Professionals like things clear, manageable, and utilitarian. Instead, in the conceptual forest of philosophy, trees are so thick and tall that it can be impossible to get one's bearings even with extended exploration. Making matters worse are academic traditions that can be alien to the clinician's nature: Some of the trees aggressively seek to grow taller and wider than all others, to absorb all of the light and push their competitors into the shadows. Professional psychologists, being inclined to approach problems from a position of understanding and acceptance rather than competition, often find philosophical discourse and debate irritating and distracting. With few exceptions (e.g., Miller, 1992b; Rychlak, 1981), the unique needs of the professional have been ignored in discussions of philosophy of science, which tend toward debate, overstatement, and occasionally hyperbole about views of science often perceived to be of little value to the professional.

On the other extreme is the promotional perspective, which embraces the rhetoric and contentiousness of philosophical scholarship. Often when psychological scholars and scientists are attracted to philosophical analysis, they are drawn into the debate for its own sake and may lose contact with the original psychological questions that motivated the exploration. As a result, critique prevails: Scientific progress becomes the replacement of the offending intellectual objects of a misguided past with something perceived to be new and better. Unfortunately, rarely are the phenomena identified by prior positions and the problems they sought to solve, better understood by the new perspective. Thus, introspectionism and psychoanalysis are critiqued as nonscientific by behaviorists, who, in turn, are critiqued by cognitivists and biological psychologists, and so it goes. Each new perspective introduces a new set of questions and quickly dismisses those of the old, based, at least in part, on claims of a superior philosophy of science. Like a serpent swallowing its own tail, the past is covered over by the advancing present without the entire project of psychological science clearly being nourished.

From our critical pedagogical standpoint, the tendency to lose perspective in our science is a serious problem. Inasmuch as philosophical discourse is designed to preempt and to dominate its rivals completely in the belief that this is the best way toward truth, it tends to close down one's thinking rather than to open it up. It is easy to fall prey to the rhetoric, and professional psychologists are fond of asserting the scientific and philosophical superiority of their favorite perspective while rarely specifying with any cogency how it informs their work. In truth, the history and philosophy of science in this century alone are such daunting bodies of literature that assertions of superiority are little more than capitulation to the complexity of it all. It is easier to accept a comfortable rhetoric, if one is to accept a position at all, than it is to explore the entire problem. More commonly, as we have suggested, practitioners simply put aside the many, longstanding appeals for psychologists to attend to matters philosophical (e.g., Grünbaum, 1983/1992; Koch, 1959; Mahoney, 1991; Manicas & Secord, 1983; Wachtel, 1984/1992) and go about their business, trusting that professional traditions are as they should be.

In considering the material that follows, the basic question for you, the reader, is not about which philosophical position is correct, but how these traditions of scholarship, observation, and interpretation of scientific research fit with your own beliefs about being a scientist, and how you can use them to enhance your scientific skills. It is a question of how a personal view might be affirmed in the context of a broader affirmation of the major concerns of philosophical and historical scholarship, and how each of these can be linked to professional identity.

HOW DO WE KNOW?

How does a professional psychologist come to know something in the clinical situation? We are especially interested in the kind of knowing that exists within a particular context, what we called *space-time local* in the previous chapter. And we are interested in how this local knowing relates to the larger knowing of the profession, to general knowledge, and to those aspects of the particular clinical situation that will become part of the record of professional discourse, such as a diagnosis or a case summary.

Later in the chapter we will consider how various forms of inquiry described in philosophical discussions might apply to an analysis of the problem of repressed memory in psychotherapy. A heated debate exists in the literature about whether or not certain dramatically recalled traumatic memories of physical or sexual abuse should be considered repressed, but authentic, or "false memories" for events that never happened (Loftus, 1993; Ofshe & Waters, 1994; Terr, 1994). The question of what is known by the clinician in evaluating a clinical phenomenon such as a memory narrative is necessarily complex and raises many of the questions about truth that have preoccupied philosophy in this century.

Before taking on so complex an issue as memory in psychotherapy, however, it will be useful to begin with a clinically relevant, but simpler example that sets the stage for the background material. Consider a scenario. You are walking to work in a clinic where you function as a therapist. On the way, you notice a young man walking toward the clinic door, but still some distance away. He looks directly at you, giving you brief pause as your eyes meet. You barely notice this, walking on to the clinic door and entering well before him. You go on about your business, not giving the moment any further thought. Later in the day, after several hours of clinical work, you find that you have a new appointment the following day in a time slot that had not been filled earlier. It is a man, age 22, who identifies himself as having a problem with relationships and as feeling very depressed. He has been referred by a colleague across town who has been working with the young man's former girlfriend. Suddenly, the image of the brief encounter, hours earlier, pops into your mind. Somehow you know it was this young man whom you saw earlier, or at least it seems like you know. You recognize that there are many other individuals who might come to the clinic and whom you have not seen before. But the paper says your referral came in person to set the appointment, and given the age and the look on the face of the man on the walkway, you have a sense this is who you will see the following day.

What are we to make of this type of "knowing"? Certainly it is not the same as knowing something scientifically. Or is it? If this is indeed the young man who comes to your appointment, then your momentary hunch seems to be confirmed. Moreover, there may be some narrative the young man could tell about seeing you as he came to make the appointment. Was he able to recognize you? Had he seen you before? How does this seeing relate to his feelings, hopes, and plans about coming to therapy? Or, maybe he did not even notice the event, or maybe you only thought he looked at you. Perhaps the look you noticed only reflected his overall apprehension about entering the clinic. Or was he actually looking at something beyond you? What if, later, you find out you remind him of someone in his family? He still may have no recall of the moment on the walkway to the clinic, but now the look may seem to indicate some more intriguing meaning that is effectively unconscious—even though he might have told you about it had you been in a position to ask at the time.

Obviously, there is much that can be made of such moments; some interpretations may prove useful, some not. Observation and speculation will be more connected to the reality if handled judiciously. If, for example, the new client is not the young man on the walkway, then too much early speculation is really off the mark. One might go so far as regularly to put such speculations out of one's mind, thereby avoiding any possibility of errors. At a minimum, responsible practice seems to suggest that we not put too much stock in such speculative information. But, then, what if our observational instincts turn out to be correct; might this not be simply good, connected scientific observation and reasoned inference? This example illustrates the simplicity and complexity of local clinical science. A major concern for local clinical science has to do with the extent to which it is best executed from positions of caution and doubt, versus positions of speculation and active theory development.

How is this example different from determining that an individual is depressed after a diagnostic interview, from determining that a child's behavior problems call for a combination of individual and family therapy, or from assessing whether or not a memory has been repressed or simply forgotten? Clearly, these latter actions are ostensibly more well defined in terms of existing modes of practice, some of which have come into being on the basis of scientific thinking. For example, with the establishment of the DSM-III in the early 1980s, the diagnostic interview for depression has increasingly become focused on relatively more accessible and specific symptoms, compared with interviews in the 1950s, 1960s, and 1970s. Although it is widely recognized that such interviews and the diagnostic criteria themselves are not simply based in science (e.g., Schacht, 1985), they are relatively more so than the glance at the young man on the walkway. Yet glances, diagnoses, memory narratives, and much more are all part of the observational realities of professional practice. Whether we forget that such events occur, relate them to a formal theory (such as a theory of momentary eye contact), or simply accept them as part of the unaccounted-for uniqueness of a particular case, they constitute the domain of local clinical inquiry.

THE MAJOR THEMES IN PHILOSOPHY OF SCIENCE
AS TRAJECTORIES FOR INQUIRY

We divide philosophical thinking, as it has influenced psychology, into three basic themes that can be thought of as trajectories guiding local inquiry. The term *trajectory* is used to suggest a direction, or a tendency for an inquiry to pursue a particular form, style, or emphasis. It differs from method in being less precise and necessarily more abstract a strategy—capturing nicely the distant but focused stance that accompanies our aerial perspective metaphor. Imprecision has the positive feature of allowing that the trajectory may be expressed differently in different situations.

The three trajectories in our model include (1) an empirical/positivistic trajectory, (2) an idealist/paradigmatic trajectory, and (3) a sociocultural/constructionistic trajectory. Below we give an overview of each of these trajectories, followed by discussion of the philosophical tradition in which the trajectory is rooted. Because of the inherent abstractness of some of the material to follow, we beg the reader's forbearance if all does not seem clear initially, on our word that it will be (more) so by the end of the chapter.

The Positivistic/Empirical Trajectory

The positivistic/empirical trajectory emphasizes observable phenomena—phenomena directly given in some basic, usually perceptual, way—and the extent to which an inquiry can be framed in observational terms. It involves the information that we believe would be most directly available to observers similar to ourselves, operating under similar assumptions and circumstances (see Manicas & Secord, 1983). In most clinical situations, this information boils down to empirical events in the real world, such as what a person says or does that we can see and describe. Note here that the notion of trajectory does not necessarily imply that we define *observable* in any particular way, even though some psychologists have chosen to emphasize physically specified behavior as a means to this end (e.g., Skinner, 1987). Rather, it reflects a direction in which to push an analysis. Behavior may be part of such a push, but it may not be the whole story and will not even be available to the inquiry in some situations.

Consider, for example, a situation where a description of an action is designed to illuminate the actor's motive more than to render a precise description of behavior. For example, a teenager says, "My father didn't want to speak to me because he didn't come to the door as I was leaving." The father's behavior may be important, but so might the father's actual intent in "not coming to the door," which might, in turn, shed light on how the teen interprets situations.

The positivistic/empirical trajectory is primarily devoted to building consensus around a particular viewpoint within a community of scientists. Consensus building is a particular strength of the positivistic trajectory. An example of the positivistic trajectory in clinical diagnosis might be the direct hearing of a report that a patient has engaged in recent buying sprees that exceed his income, and considering this information as it pertains to the diagnosis of bipolar illness. Obviously information that extends beyond the report is needed to assess its veracity, but the fact of the report itself is given directly. Therefore, others can hear this or similar reports from the patient as evidence in support of the diagnosis. The extent to which the report must be pushed to even greater precision depends on who is making it (e.g., a family member or the patient him- or herself) and on what other information is available (see also Chapter 8).

The Idealist/Paradigmatic Trajectory

The idealist/paradigmatic trajectory involves a step away from the empirical. It is based on the recognition that even empirical observation involves assumptions about events, and qualities of events that are unseen and largely unseeable (Polanyi, 1958, 1967/1992). It is the recognition that our knowledge is influenced in great and small ways by theory, general world knowledge, research results, common sense, personal experience, and various implicit and explicit forms of guidance provided by experts in one's area of endeavor. It involves reflection on how the community of scientists and clinicians operates to generate statements about the nature of phenomena involved in one's work and how, in so doing, they have affected one's thinking and experience of the clinical situation. It involves methods and traditions for linking theoretical beliefs to application and action. Finally, it involves the ways an idea, or more generally speaking, meaning, is attributed to the direct experience of an object or event. This trajectory perhaps best captures the everyday world of the professional, where we learn proper comportment as apprentices to skilled practitioners.

For example, in making a clinical diagnosis, the professional community might have decided that a combination of direct empirical observation—in effect incorporating the empirical trajectory—and theoretically driven inference is required for accurate judgment. A set of questions designed to illuminate a diagnosis, such as bipolar disorder, becomes the accepted mode of pursuing the diagnostic problem.

The idealist/paradigmatic trajectory involves the analysis of such traditions, how they influence the outcome and process of a particular inquiry, and how they might be applied optimally in particular circumstances. In contrast to the positivist/empirical trajectory, which views knowledge as grounded and justified in empirical observation, the idealist/paradigmatic views it as intimately tied to the culture of the scientist.

The Sociocultural/Constructionist Trajectory

The sociocultural/constructionist trajectory for analysis encourages us to move one very large step further beyond the culture of the scientist and professional into the realm of knowledge as a product of a larger social process. This trajectory involves consideration of how the larger cultural, political, and economic trends in society, including social critiques and personal self-interests, affect the inquiry. It encourages attention to how particular viewpoints have come to evolve in a particular sociocultural milieu and to how one has come to use them as tools for producing knowledge about the world. It encourages reflection on how one is embedded in a social matrix extending beyond disciplinary matters. This trajectory leads one to seek enlightened (or enlightening) self-awareness and modifications of formulations and their implicational structure based on this awareness (e.g., greater understanding of those culturally different from oneself may accompany a serious examination of one's own values). It involves a search for the social limits on the generality and meaning of a particular formulation so that one can deal with these limits in an enlightened manner. In so doing, it necessarily takes one into the realm of moral and ethical questions, both as they pertain to the manifest outcomes of one's science and to those things absent in that science. In the past 25 years or so, for example, much concern has been generated about diagnostic categories as they are applied to particular social groups, such as women and minorities, and how these categories may have been generated under the shadow of sociocultural assumptions that are unfavorable to these groups. A recent example is the controversy generated by the diagnosis of *self-defeating personality* because it could be used to pathologize women in abusive relationships.

In the next sections we discuss the history of the trajectories we have identified. Relatively more time will be devoted to logical positivism because of its importance as a philosophical justification for modern science, and because it points to problems essential to any scientific formulation of professional inquiry.

HISTORICAL BACKGROUND
OF THE POSITIVIST/EMPIRICAL TRAJECTORY

Logical Positivism

To read the current social scientific literature, traditional scientific thinking, once a great symbol for hope, emancipation, and mastery, has become a domineering, hegemonic discourse that oppresses as much as it emancipates, occludes as much as it illuminates. Positivism is widely held to be discredited as a means for the creation of knowledge. Yet there is irony in such conclusions: Auguste Comte (1880), who was the founder of positivist philosophy and who coined the term *positivism*, was a social reformer interested in seeing individuals and societies live in harmony. He placed special emphasis on the important moral role of women in society and the need for their status and educational prospects to be raised. Rather than depending on theology or metaphysics to govern the course of intellectual development, both of which were the province of elites, Comte envisioned a world in which knowledge arose out of an increasingly "positive" intimacy with directly given scientific phenomena and societal needs. This intimacy arose across the hierarchy of disciplines, which Comte identified and which remains a subject of great debate today, starting with mathematics, astronomy, physics, chemistry, biology, and on to sociology (another term coined by Comte). The point of positivist philosophy was simple: Knowledge of both the social and the physical world should arise out of the natural realm, from what can be seen directly and which is therefore available to all, and it should be applied to fulfill the needs of society.

Logical positivism arose in Germany and Austria early in the century as a group of scientists and philosophers attempted to specify how science worked. Consistent with the trend away from metaphysical philosophy that had been operating since the nineteenth century; and following the tradition of Bacon, who believed that knowledge should be practical and verifiable, and Locke, Hume, and others who held that verification was an empirical process; the positivists sought to blend the formal and analytical aspects of thought and language with the empirical and synthetic aspects of successful science. As Stevens (1939/1976) put it, "The name Logical Positivism quite properly suggests the union of the formal and the empirical—a union which, in a well-ordered scientific household, is possible and legitimate" (p. 16). The specification of how scientific language is structured, and of how empirical statements are meaningful, was a central goal of logical positivist efforts.

The positivists distinguished three types of terms that might exist in a scientific theory: (a) logical and mathematical terms, (2) theoretical terms, and (3) observation terms. Later versions of this thinking, which has been called the *received view* (Suppe, 1974), essentially describe contemporary scientific work in psychology and are prominent in the seminal work of MacCorquodale and Meehl (1948) on the admissibility of hypothetical constructs in psychological theory, and Cronbach and Meehl (1955) on the construct validity of psychological tests—which is the best articulation of received view science existing in the psychological literature (see Chapter 6).

Initially, positivist thinking was dogmatic and restrictive, emphasizing the notion that the meaning of any concept is exhaustively specified in the operations associated with its measurement. This *operationism* (Stevens, 1939/1976) still is widely taught in the introductory chapters of methodology textbooks. As the first third of the century passed, however, the strict positivist position gave way to an increasing loosening of the standards by which linguistic propositions were seen to be grounded in the particulars of experience. It was recognized that, in fact, science depended regularly on historical descriptions and on imputed linkages between observation, operation, and theoretical terms that did not fit a rigid positivist canon very well. Thus, in the final version of the received view, the standards for verification were loosened to allow a broader interpretation of the role of observation in supporting or refuting a theory.

In psychology received view science has involved a variety of positions coexisting from the 1920s through to the present, ranging from a relatively rigid and exclusive radical behaviorism (e.g., Skinner, 1971, 1974) to broad theoretical systems demonstrating minimal concern about the problem of verifiability, in the positivist sense, as in certain schools of psychoanalytic thought (Grünbaum, 1983/1992; Meehl, 1976). Today, we find proponents in this strong scientific tradition settling into what has been termed *critical realism* or *fallibilist realism*. Critical realism recognizes that, although strict verificationist thinking is flawed as an absolute standard for science, the attempt to link theoretical concepts logically to observational concepts remains a useful, if nondefinitive, endeavor (e.g., Cook & Campbell, 1979). Scientific approaches continue to use behavior, or its artifacts, as a means to the end of operationalization.

Positivist Thinking in an Ambiguous World

Positivist positions attempted to move the source of knowledge out of the metaphysical realm of mind and spirit into that of the concrete and the physical. Local clinical scientists need to understand how positivism in the current received view form came to be, its power in the generation of consensual views of phenomena, and its fundamental weakness, which is often discussed in the contemporary literature. To do so, let us look more closely at how common sense and dogmatic certainty become strangely juxtaposed in the strong form of the positivist perspective, actually underscoring its failure to establish a definitive foundation for science.

Consider a specific example that illustrates the problem with empirical observation as a singular foundation for science. Look at the number of this page. This would seem a reasonable request on our part, as authors, to make of you the reader, because we can be reasonably certain that there is a number on this page. Yet it immediately illustrates the problems associated with the extreme positivist position. First, is there any sense that your looking at the page number has the same empirical status as our request that you do so? Well no, because we have no idea, as we write this, which number this page will have. You can see the number, we cannot. Therefore, our prediction that there will be a page number must depend on our general knowledge of books and a reasonable extrapolation to this book. But, you might say, we are effectively seeing the same thing because our inference is merely a low-level generalization from other books we have had before us, on which page numbers were indeed an empirical fact, just as it is for you, and there is a sense in which we share this fact. Additionally, there are other points of overlap, such as a basic understanding of what the number means, how it identifies a page, and a page's location, and so on. And furthermore, the number has a certain structure we might be able to communicate even if one of us could not read the mark as a numerical symbol on the page. However, if that were the case, and the nonreader were you (it could also be one or both of us if this passage were being dictated), then the whole proposition of looking at the number on the page—which is an observation-level proposition—would be in doubt. All of this is by way of saying that, in the end, we must make certain assumptions about your basic observational capacities, some of which are conceptual, even to bring the discussion to the observational level. The problem for positivism was in applying its own verificationist principle to these assumptions, which of course it could not, and the loosening described above began.

But there still is the ink on the page. If you were to deliver your book to us, we could share a gaze at the number. Actually, we could only say we shared it for, short of seeing through one another's eyes, we could never share precisely the same gaze even in the most mundane sense of photons of light falling on a retina. Moreover, this says nothing of the symbolic and interpersonal impact of having an unknown reader actually go to the bother of bringing the page number to our attention (at some future time as this is written), which would necessarily be a different experience for us, from our perspective, than it would be for you as a reader. But, you could insist, there still are molecules of ink clinging to fibers of paper (or computer screen pixels illuminated in a particular configuration) that compose this page number, that have some reasonable permanence through time and a reasonable level of shared meaning to observers. As you did so, we would nod, and probably make some remark about how that is precisely how positivism contributes to a local clinical science, in making us aware that although there are no uninterpreted givens, there are levels of discussion where the differences that can be generated about what is being interpreted become trivial. At the same time, however, our approach to certainty itself becomes increasingly stretched and trivial, as is amply illustrated by this example. Even more, we could argue that, in a space-time local sense, your first glance at the page number—perhaps after reading our suggestions in the text, perhaps before—was different from each and every glance that followed as your perspective, knowledge, and purpose changed with the movement of time. All is in flux. There is no simplicity in the idea of sharing observation outside of an agreed-upon way of communicating about the things we see. This complication has wreaked havoc on the positivist aspirations to be the ultimate standard for knowledge.

A Positive View of Positivism?

Positivism's influence on scientific thinking and methodology in twentieth-century psychology has been profound: The image of scientific psychology provided by the received view, particularly as articulated by Cronbach and Meehl (1955), is one in which scientific meaning is established through the logical connection between scientific formulations and observations. If we expand our definition of appropriate scientific empiricism, then one implication of a positivist trajectory is that there exist observational moments in a local clinical event that can be coordinated with particular theories. We might think of these metaphorically as hooks or anchors in the time stream of an event. An obvious example is a symptom in a psychiatric disorder. To the extent the diagnostic system is working as planned, there should exist identifiable moments in the time stream of a clinical situation during which particular behaviors, observations, or self-reports occur that are identifiable as indicators of symptoms associated with particular syndromes. The implications of the received view extend beyond this, however, into both formal and informal identifications of a variety of clinical phenomena.

For example, when is a transferential moment, or trend in a relationship, manifested and identifiable? What evidence suggests that a memory is repressed? How does a school psychologist infer that motivation is a problem in evaluating the validity of a child's intelligence test score? The positivistic/empiricist trajectory involves a continuous search for observational-level evidence, to the extent it is possible. It strives to keep unspecified leaps of inference to a minimum as a formulation is used. Additionally, it implies an effort to make the information publicly available, in the sense of being communicable to colleagues and other relevant parties. Positivist thinkers have invented an impressive array of methodologies to ensure that scientific statements are grounded in directly experienceable and replicable realities. We will discuss these at length in later chapters.

HISTORICAL BACKGROUND OF THE IDEALIST/ PARADIGMATIC TRAJECTORY

Depending on one's background and predilections, the skepticism required to accept or reject the positivist position may be difficult to grasp. As the page number example shows, for us to assume that such an observation were in any way useful to communication, the fundamental observation itself must be based on existing knowledge. It is physical and sensory only in a limited sense. The physicalistic experience involved in so simple an operation cannot meaningfully be said to stand, in and of itself, as a foundation for higher-level statements one might make with reference to the observation. Moreover, there is no sense in which such an observation will lead necessarily to any particular theory via logic (deductive or inductive) and, therefore, in the extreme skeptical position, no inferences about the nature of what is observed are, in any sense, justified (see Ayer, 1952). Put differently, both our request and your response to it depended heavily on who we are and who you are, and they are tied to a real world only in a limited sense. This loading of the responsibility for the nature of an observation on the observer—or more precisely, on a class of observers—is an essential feature of a different perspective on science, where attention is directed more toward the actual history of science than toward the establishment of an ideal model for science. This perspective is perhaps best represented in the writing of Thomas Kuhn.

Kuhn's Scientific Idealism

Few single works in the history and philosophy of science in this century have had the widespread impact of Kuhn's (1970) *Structure of Scientific Revolutions*. Kuhn intended to write a history of scientific change and progress that dealt realistically with the existing historical record (Hoyningen-Huene, 1993). He observed that notions of simple, linear progress in science did not fit the record very well. Rather, change in science seemed to involve transitions between periods of relative stability and periods of dramatic change. For example, the move from viewing the earth as the center of the universe, as in the centuries-old Ptolemaic system of cosmology, to the Copernican system, in which the earth revolves around the sun, was seen to be revolutionary in Kuhn's history. Strikingly, and in contrast to positivistic characterizations of science, Kuhn recognized that the observational basis for scientific change often had existed long before a new system of thought was accepted. The possibility that existing thought and observation may be at odds just prior to scientific change led him to interpret scientific thought as a kind of culture or world view, which he termed a *paradigm*. In this culture, individuals share a vision of the world and a system of problems to be solved. The paradigm supplies a set of scientific puzzles, theories and methods for working on the puzzles, and standards for evaluating proposed solutions. Usually, the major scientific puzzles are clearly articulated in mathematical or some other shared scientific language, such as the problem of developing a single unified theory of different forms of attractive force (such as gravity, electromagnetism, and strong and weak subatomic forces) in physics or of seeking a way of interpreting genetic code in biochemistry. Part of the everyday work of science within the paradigm, which Kuhn termed *normal science*, is to identify such puzzles and to implement the accepted approaches to their solution.

Kuhn identified times when puzzle solving within a paradigm ceases to be successful or yields results that are inconsistent with major theoretical ideas comprising the paradigm. The seeds of historical change are sewn when the work of normal science reveals a set of *anomalies*, which are situations—usually observations or experimental results—that cannot be accounted for within an existing paradigm. Initially these anomalies may be ignored or deferred, often for extended periods of time, as science awaits their explanation. Rarely do they just disappear, and their return to the spotlight may be dramatic. If someone develops a theory that can account both for the anomalies and for everything understood in the previous paradigm, the possibility for a *scientific revolution* is in place.

A scientific revolution is a historical transition with far-reaching ramifications; a change not only in theoretical understanding, but actually in the way the world, the substance of science, and the nature of scientific practice are viewed. A dramatic example in this century is the change brought about by Einstein's elaboration of relativity theory in physics. Kuhn suggested that such changes are not simply the adoption of a new, more encompassing theory from which the old can be derived. Rather, the basic meaning of fundamental concepts is changed.

For example, in contrast to Newtonian mechanics, matter became convertible to energy in the Einsteinian universe. Scientific revolutions involve a kind of "you can't go back again" shift in perception (Kuhn drew heavily on the metaphor of seeing the world differently) that can take generations for broad acceptance. In this sense, science changes, and even progresses, but not in the fashion of the simple linear theoretical and technological progress common in the rhetoric of science. Scientific change is, instead, a matter of fits and starts, puzzles and social transformations that cannot be reduced to the machinations of mathematics, logic, observation, or any simplistic notion of a scientific method—however useful such a tool might have been to problem solving on a smaller historical scale.

Over the last 25 years, Kuhn's work has frequently been used to question traditional scientific work, particularly in the social sciences, and to support the assertion that revolutions are needed or are actually in progress. Note, however, that Kuhn's actual published material does not encourage such interpretations; it is not so much a critique of scientific conduct as it is a description of how the social institution of science seems to operate (Hoyningen-Huene, 1993). Instead, his strong interest has been in the problems of changing perception and the incompatibility between theories (which he termed *incommensurability*).

From a Kuhnian perspective, professional psychology remains preparadigmatic in the sense that the puzzles and methods for their solution existing in our profession are multitudinous and highly variable with differing theoretical perspectives. Some have argued that the shift from behaviorism to cognitivism in the past 25 years constitutes a paradigm shift (e.g., Baars, 1986), but, even so, there is little evidence to suggest a major unifying shift in thinking across the diverse elements of our discipline. The major implication of Kuhn's work for critical thinking in local clinical science is the need for reflective consideration of how the many paradigms of psychological science and clinical practice permeate our work as professionals. In this sense, the local clinical scientist model can be seen as a paradigm for applying scientific and philosophical thinking to clinical inquiry.

The Structure of Scientific Communities

Kuhn's (1974) elaboration of the notion of *disciplinary matrix*—a constellation of group commitments—is particularly interesting for our purposes. This constellation has four components. First, it involves symbolic generalizations, which are basic propositions accepted by the group without question or disagreement. In the physical sciences, these often will be mathematical formalizations of basic constructs and relationships. The more developed the science, the greater is the number of such propositions. Although professional psychology has few such propositions that are universally accepted, within regions and training networks we find clear traditions that, if articulated, would be comparable to Kuhn's concept of symbolic generalizations (e.g., psychodynamically oriented clinicians tend to agree that the unconscious has important implication for clinical progress whereas behavioral clinicians do not). A major task for the local clinical scientist is to articulate these assumptions and to discern how they affect particular inquiries.

Second, Kuhn suggested that scientific groups share basic models of the phenomena in which they are interested. Strength of commitment to these models may vary within the community from belief that the model simply serves heuristic value to strong ontological beliefs that they describe the true nature of things. In professional psychology, such models range from instincts acting like pressures, to behaviors acting like discrete elements in an omnipresent economy of actions and rewards, to relationships acting like fences constraining the freedom of participants' actions. Identifying the models, how they operate in particular practice circumstances, and how one's commitment to a model waxes and wanes in practice are central to a local clinical science.

Third, scientific communities were seen to consist of shared values. These are high-level preferences and evaluations that are shared broadly within a community of scientists. They unite the groups even though they may be applied differently by different members and subgroups. Thus, for example, a value of precision may be considered more or less adequately manifest in a particular measurement circumstance, although all scientists will share the value. In professional psychology, emotional connection with clients, the ability for self-analysis, or the ability to bound and define a professional task are values of major concern depending on the particular interests and expertise of a professional group.

Fourth, Kuhn noted that scientific communities use a set of particularly cogent exemplars to define their interests, to guide future operations, and to socialize new members. Professionals tend to use both broadly shared exemplars, such as famous case studies, and exemplars of more limited distribution, such as examples provided by supervisors and colleagues or from one's own experience, to guide future work.

HISTORICAL BACKGROUND OF THE SOCIOCULTURAL/ CONSTRUCTIONIST TRAJECTORY

The third trajectory for our consideration has created a great deal of excitement in the psychological community in the past decade or so, even though it has been around for some time.

Social Constructionism

The third trajectory can be called *social constructionism*, following an important paper by Gergen (1985). Its basic tenet is that knowledge is not a function of an ever-refined narrowing of the gap between theory and the contours of reality but rather that knowledge is a product of social-historical process. The social construction of reality is intrinsic to communication and human interaction in a historically situated social domain. Extreme versions of this position have recently been called *postmodernism* (Gergen, 1991, 1992). Knowledge is thought to be constructed relative to any grasp of external reality or, indeed, relative to no external reality at all. Different societies, and the same societies at different times in history, reside in different realities, all fundamentally legitimate and none superior in any respect, because all human realities spring from the same fundamental social processes. As such, the social constructionist position represents a serious challenge to the notion that science is a singularly perfected path to enlightenment. Science is simply one among a potentially endless variety of constructive mechanisms human societies have developed to legitimize and, quite literally, create what we take for granted as reality. This position moves beyond Kuhn in pointing to a general sociocultural process that transcends the small society of scientists that was the focus of Kuhn's inquiry. Indeed, the very existence of such a scientific society in a culture illustrates how social construction operates to create a means of designing and propagating knowledge.

Like many exciting new ideas, or new versions of old ideas, social construction-ist thinking has played different roles at different stages in its development. In earlier parts of this century, this thinking was not about philosophy of science at all—just as Kuhn's work was more a historiography than a philosophy of science—but rather it was about using sociological analysis to understand how meaning was created. Mannheim's famous work, *Ideology and Utopia* (1936), for example, analyzed how societies create ideological positions that inform members about their place in the world and about the goals of the society. Alfred Schutz (e.g., 1967), in an extensive body of often stunningly brilliant essays, showed how experience itself is rooted in microsocial processes that teach individuals what is appropriately taken for granted in the social world and how to understand and communicate about their experience.

More recently, the foundation of the currently existing view of social construc-tion was articulated in a landmark book by sociologist Peter Berger and theological historian Thomas Luckman (Berger & Luckman, 1966). This foundation has several important characteristics relevant to a local clinical science, and for understanding more recent thinking about the social constructionist position. Berger and Luckman offered a way of conceptualizing the interpenetration existing between formal scientific knowledge and the common sense of everyday life. They emphasized that the province of sociology of knowledge is not that of theorists defining the range of applicability of their theories, nor of intellectuals identifying the importance of formal theories in everyday life. In this sense they differed from Kuhn's focus on the disciplinary matrix of science. Rather, their sociology of knowledge, directed as it was toward the fundamental processes by which social reality is created, was concerned with the construction of everyday reality itself. This ensures that the liberation of knowledge is intrinsic to the discipline: Sociology of knowledge is not about who is right or wrong, but rather about how people come to understand the reality they experience.

Clinicians will recognize this to be basic to the clinical attitude one takes toward clients (e.g., Shakow, 1976). Thus, not surprisingly, the social constructionist position has become a major interest for clinicians. But there is more to the position than the equal valuation of the many views of reality that might exist in a social unit. Berger and Luckman emphasized a theory of social construction processes that transcends particular outcomes or viewpoints. They unequivocally stated that the social construction of reality is a theory grounded in empirical observations of how people experience their worlds, and communicate about this experience. It is about the phenomenology of social knowing and, in turn, how that phenomenology, when collectivized in society, yields social structures and processes that are of basic interest to sociologists. It is a descriptive, empirical science that, although distinguishable from formal science with its heavy emphasis on behaviorism and developments in statistically based population studies, is a science nonetheless.

Implications of Social Constructionism for Local Clinical Science

These qualities of Berger and Luckman's social constructionist theory—it is concerned with everyday knowing, it is phenomenological in orientation, it is a descriptive theory, and it is empirical science—are important for our interest in a local clinical science. Questions about the relationship between formal scientific knowing and the realities of individuals and diverse social groupings are pervasive today, and they certainly pervade the interlinking of formal clinical theory and the local clinical context. We will continue to address these matters throughout the book, drawing on the social constructionist position in a variety of ways. But a bit of reflection makes it clear that this position has major implications for philosophy of science and for the project of identifying methods that best achieve the aspirations to truth of scientific inquiry. It has been suggested that it questions the very nature of the truth to which scientific inquiry aspires (e.g., Gergen, 1985, 1992). Berger and Luckman acknowledged but sidestepped the epistemological implications of their work, particularly the implication that the science of sociology itself is a constructed phenomenon, as implied in Kuhn, that might well have no greater fundamental legitimacy than any other position one might wish to take toward the nature of social knowing [e.g., a behaviorist position as in Skinner (1974) where knowing is secondary to contingent relationships existing in an environment between behavior and its consequences].

Although this is an important concern raised by the social constructionist insight, it can be easily overstated and lead to a confusion of philosophy's wish for certainty with the positivist vision of a foundation for science in sensate experience. These aspirations are not equivalent and, as we have implied throughout, the rejection of empiricism as a foundation for science does not necessarily imply that empiricism should be rejected as a useful knowledge production strategy. Berger and Luckman's recognition that their work was empirical suggests a view of empiricism in science that is broader than many would accept, one that works for their domain of inquiry, sociology, and that seems quite consistent with the intent of naturalistic philosophers like Bacon or Locke. The notion that we cannot accept experiential data as definitively foundationist also does not necessarily put a social constructionist perspective in opposition to empiricism. To the contrary, they are quite compatible perspectives where, for example, we can endorse the theory of social construction via careful observation, as do Berger and Luckman, and socially agree to privilege good empirical observation based on its power to facilitate social consensus. At a minimum, we are safe in suggesting social constructionism is a good theory, with clear observational consequences, of how societies construe various aspects of their reality.

From a historical perspective, however, the insight that science itself is subject to the same social construction operations as any other form of knowing, has become a major theme in recent thinking about social constructionism and philosophy of science as it is translated to psychology (e.g., Belenky, Clinchy, Goldberger, & Tarule, 1986). In so doing, it has strongly challenged any notion that scientific methods, particularly those rooted in positivism such as behavioristic approaches, are sounder than other means of inquiry (e.g., Gergen, 1985). The positivist notion of an uninterpreted empirical given has been rejected, as has the idea that certain methods identify causal relationships between events that have universal applicability to like events (see Manicas & Secord, 1983). This has increasingly opened methodological doors to more qualitative, interpretive (hermeneutic), and phenomenological approaches that are quite comfortable for the clinician (Hoshmand & Polkinghorne, 1992). We will discuss related issues in Chapter 7.

IS REALITY REAL, A SOCIAL ILLUSION, OR BOTH, AND HOW CAN WE LEARN MORE ABOUT IT? SOME RECENT THINKING

The sensible professional reader will say this is pretty much a mess. But before you rush off to your next clinical hour, let us try to convince you that there is a way through this morass that is fruitful and compatible with the local science perspective. Actually, there are two useful perspectives that exist in modern philosophy. These include a revival of pragmatism as a philosophical position justifying science (Hoshmand, 1994; Rorty, 1982) and a new-look version of realism that promises to integrate these concerns (Bhaskar, 1978, 1979; Harré, 1986; Manicas & Secord, 1983). If we add the simple perspective—itself pragmatic—that psychological science, for all it lacks in ultimate validity, is not doing badly in terms of moving our thinking about psychological matters along, then there are actually three solutions. Each of these overarching perspectives is implicit in the model we will propose in this chapter, and in similar proposals concerning other methodological issues made throughout this work. Each is presented briefly below.

Pragmatism

The pragmatic perspective on science resides somewhere between the strong empiricist and the idealist positions in that it weighs observation and ideas about equally in an analysis. As originally stated by the U.S. philosopher Charles Peirce, pragmatism was a way of thinking about how concepts are defined. "Consider what effects that might *conceivably* have [the] practical bearings you *conceive* the objects of your *conception* to have. Then, your *conception* of those effects is the whole of your *conception* of the object" (Peirce, 1905/1955, p. 290). This statement implies that objects are defined by what we can do with them. Note, however, that this idea runs deeper than simply being a position of accepting that which works, although this too is an implication of the pragmatist perspective. Rather, it is concerned with the way meaning is grounded in human action. Peirce was not interested in any notion of verification, nor in any metaphysical ruminations about the ontological status of ideas or any other reality. Rather, thinking and action were intimately tied to one another. Peirce was thus paving the way for the operationism that exists in modern scientific thinking. James expanded this thinking to include emotional "objects" as well. Dewey believed that pragmatics was a general means for evaluating the clarity and logic of concepts with evaluation being the ultimate driving force in the advancement of thought (Bynum, Browne, & Porter, 1981). Hence, there is no meaningful distinction between theory and action as the two blend in an overall evaluation as a concept is recognized.

More recently, Rorty (1979, 1982), who wrote from a purely philosophical perspective, confronted what he regarded an excess in philosophy: the creation of a system wherein matters of truth are determined completely on the basis of metaphysical argument. Like earlier pragmatists, Rorty saw ideas as historically situated and defined according to their usage rather than according to some empirical or rational standard. In effect he questioned the whole extended history of the truth-seeking enterprise, ultimately suggesting that, because ideas come and go with the times anyway, why not just allow them to exist as part of the human landscape.

Professional psychology needs to explore more deeply the nature of pragmatic inquiry at the local level (e.g., Hoshmand, 1994), a notion highly compatible with the practical orientation of the local clinical scientist model. Undoubtedly a historical perspective on thought and practice, as implied by Rorty, would be of great value in local inquiry if properly adapted to the local clinical situation. Historical awareness could free us to use ideas without bearing the burden of asserting their ultimate truth value—an attitude common in evaluation of psychotherapy efficacy (see Strupp, 1986). Pragmatism would be most powerful if we can find a way to avoid what often happens when philosophical critiques make their way into psychology: an extended period where the position simply is used to refute an increasingly vacuous image of some allegedly outmoded practice in the past. Although the means by which pragmatic goals are to be achieved are quite loose and open, there appears to be justification for the usage of well-formed scientific methods, as long as they are treated as appropriately nondefinitive.

There is another perspective from philosophy that has potentially profound implications for the entire territory we have traversed thus far in this chapter. This is the perspective of transcendental realism, promulgated primarily in the works of Roy Bhaskar and a few others.

Critical and Transcendental Realism

Manicas and Secord (1983) introduced what they called the "new philosophy of science" to U.S. psychology. In contrast to the longstanding trend in philosophy emphasizing the ascendancy of ideas and the problem of uncertainty, this work emphasized the scientific importance of fundamental assumptions about reality, however difficult these assumptions ultimately might be to verify. Bhaskar (1978, 1979) referred to this position as *transcendental realism*, as contrasted with Western philosophy's tendency toward *transcendental idealism*, or as Bhaskar put it explicitly, *super idealism*. Bhaskar made a frontal attack on the overemphasis on uncertainty found in philosophy that is not dissimilar to that found among positivist philosophers like Ayer (1952), nor that made by Rorty and other pragmatists. However, Bhaskar's strategy was different in its emphasis on the long-neglected problem of ontology (the nature of being) as opposed to epistemology (the nature of knowledge). In so doing, he was able to incorporate both the apparent historical facts of the creation of knowledge in science and the problem of the social construction of reality, particularly as they pertain to the social sciences.

Reality for Bhaskar is transcendent and knowable, but never completely so. On the one hand, traditional positivistic science, in promoting empiricism, has confused the reality of sensory experience with the totality of scientific reality. Thereby, science has confused the atomistic experience of events (that which is seen, e.g., the patient's depressed affect) with whole events (that which is assumed but not seen, e.g., the patient's affect with a loved one), with classes of similar events (e.g., general characteristics of depressed patients with loved ones), or with theories about an underlying order in reality that transcend empirical events and that are only accessible as mental constructions, not as observations (e.g., problems in the serotonergic system create depressed affect). Thus, outcomes of experiments are generalized freely to all like situations and the processes presumed to operate in specific experimental outcomes are freely promoted as general laws.

On the other hand, antipositivistic, or super idealist, philosophers have confused the powerful need for theory with the totality of reality, thereby making an implicit equation between knowledge of reality and reality itself—which Bhaskar termed the *epistemic fallacy*. This equation asserts the ascendancy of ideas over experiences in the generation of scientific knowledge, as in Kuhn. However, Bhaskar argued that in recognizing the link between theory and observation, as they commonly do, idealist philosophers are unable to account for the extraordinarily effective science we actually seem to have. That is, science seems to work so well, it must be describing something external to the ideas used in the description. In effect, the confusion of ideas and observations undermines the original belief in the ascendancy of ideas.

Bhaskar asked what the world must be like for science, as we know it, to be possible. It must have qualities that endure despite our changing perspectives, which he termed *intransitive* properties, and properties that change as knowledge and culture changes, which he termed *transitive* properties. The intransitive refers to a world that transcends our knowing; the transitive refers to that knowing itself. One implication of Bhaskar's position is that we need a humble understanding of reality in which we recognize that it will function quite independent of our ability to understand it, and indeed our ability to ever understand it. Hence, the assumption of a transcendent ontology on which epistemology operates fallibly.

The power of this position is that it allows us to pursue our naive dream of truth and to make commitments to levels of certainty in our explorations, while at the same time keeping us honest about the ultimate incompleteness of our knowledge. This attitude is especially powerful in the social sciences, where Bhaskar believed real social structures operate within historically situated contexts to make culture and knowledge what they are, which in turn affects the nature of these real underlying structures. Thus, the social construction of reality is possible, yet it is not purely social in that, at any given point in time, ideas can be seen to butt up against palpable realities of both physical and social nature. At the same time, these realities themselves are in the process of modification across time as social construction processes operate.

Implications of Transcendental Realism for Local Clinical Science

We believe that some version of *transcendental realism* or *fallibilist realism* (see also D. R. Peterson & R. L. Peterson, in press) is useful for scientific inquiry, particularly space and time localized inquiry. Inquiry ultimately is about asking questions, opening oneself to evidence, and making commitments based on what one has observed. These tasks are relevant to any world of inquiry, be it socially constructed, pragmatic, or subject to positivistic principles of verification. The problem of the relative significance to be assigned to good ideas, empirical information, and consensus-generating operations remains to be solved. However, in keeping with our pedagogical stance, we leave it to the reader to decide for him- or herself which specific position is preferred through additional reading. For our purposes, the realist perspective most adequately describes our interest in pulling the threads of method and purpose out of philosophical inquiry for application in the local clinical realm. Among other things, the realist perspective underscores the need to be sensitive to the culture of science as well as to the empirical realities that science seeks to understand.

A Defense of Psychological Science as Practiced

The local clinical science perspective forces us to look at exactly how focused and helpful, or not, philosophical thinking can be in the professional sphere. For the most part, we would have to say that it has helped to keep debate and questioning alive but, in so doing, it has hovered far from the practical realities of professional life—and, indeed, the philosophers themselves never have sought to make their work useful for we practical types. At the same time, we can say that philosophically minded psychologists like Cronbach and Meehl, Koch, Lamiell, Meehl, Miller, Rychlak, and numerous others have given us much food for thought in the design of methods for psychological science. Furthermore, methodologists such as Campbell and Stanley (1963), Cook and Campbell (1979), and Cronbach (1957, 1975a, 1982) actually have identified ways we can use questions about certainty and doubt to enhance our ability to ask and to answer scientific questions (Chapter 4). That scientific questions have not always been answered successfully in local inquiry seems as much a function of the lack of reasonable attempt as any fundamental flaws of the underlying perspective, as is recently suggested (e.g., Gergen, 1992).

Nevertheless, there is a tendency in psychological science that deserves severe criticism, namely, the tendency to act as if our own clinical and scientific preferences (e.g., for psychodynamic approaches, family system approaches, or approaches based in experimental traditions) are the only correct forms of practice, despite the lack of meaningful support for such displays of confidence (e.g., as evidenced in the pervasive negative commentary about rival theoretical perspectives that infects professional conversations). The cost of such commitments to certainty has been high. Too often it has led to the suppression of other ways of approaching scientific inquiry that could have helped long ago (e.g., qualitative research methods), and too often it has led us down overly narrow paths in one generation that simply beg for revision in the next, thereby weakening the possibility for any scientific continuity we might have had (see Boneau, 1992). We believe it is time to move beyond these unjustifiable prejudices and tendencies toward overstatement and, happily, recent philosophy of science is helping us to do so.

If we look carefully at science, and adopt an open, careful, and scholarly stance toward recent scientific history and toward scientific professional practice, we can say that, despite its imperfections, science has kept our thinking moving across the century. This movement has been our greatest asset in learning whatever we have learned through the efforts of science (Stricker, 1992).

Let us now look more concretely at how philosophy is relevant to professional inquiry.

EXTRAPOLATING PHILOSOPHICAL TRAJECTORIES
FOR INQUIRY TO LOCAL INQUIRY

Our discussion of philosophy of science suggested three overlapping trajectories important for any inquiry: the empirical, the paradigmatic, and the sociocultural. Pragmatism suggests that our actions and our understanding are intimately related and, consistent with the intuitions of clinicians, that there is a strong aspect of science that finds its justification in effective action. The new realism offers something even more exciting: an image of a transcendent reality that extends beyond the grasp of even our best conceptualizations and that holds out the possibility for renewed scientific exploration of the most well-trodden clinical territory. Finally, even our own science, which can seem so alien and distant from practice requirements, offers useful frameworks for understanding clinical situations if we look beyond the politics and often stultifying rhetoric of scientific certainty (see also Chapter 9). Clearly, philosophy has much to offer practitioners in bringing the compelling aspects of our work out of the back rooms of science.

The Philosophical Trajectories for Inquiry Framework

The framework we propose involves the conceptual crossing of the local information settings described in the last chapter with the trajectories for inquiry from philosophy. In this way, interesting questions can be raised that focus attention on particular qualities of the local clinical situation. To begin the presentation of the framework, consider some basic questions associated with the settings of local information and the philosophical analysis trajectories taken separately.

Some Questions Attending the Examination of Local Information Settings

Recall that the four local settings of information identified in the last chapter are: the local as an instance of a general formulation or category, local cultures, the locally unique, and the space-time local.

Local Information as the Instantiation of a Particular General Formulation. How does a scientific finding or theory inform our understanding of a particular clinical situation? For example, what are the implications of a particular position for the impressionistic scenario of seeing the young man on the walkway? Is there a general theory, say of nonverbal communication and emotional expression, that might be relevant? If so, how? If not, with what implication?

Local Cultures. The social constructionist perspective, and clinical experience, tells us that one thing is certain in local clinical inquiry: Everyone involved will have an opinion about what is going on. What are the implications of the realities of multiple beliefs and perspectives on local interactions? Are we necessarily lost in an

ever-moving sea of relativism? Philosophers definitely have had problems with
relativism. How can we hope to handle it as psychologists and as local clinical
scientists? Is there any meaningful way we can turn the problem of relativism to our
favor? What are the philosophical and scientific implications of our attempts to do so?

Locally Unique Information. How might we become aware of such information, and with what implication for our inquiry? If we are bound to paradigmatic
restrictions, does this necessarily imply that localized discovery is not possible, that
we can never break out of our paradigmatic blinders? What would such a breaking out
process be like? Can philosophical perspective be helpful here?

Space-Time Local Information. Imagine yourself to be the clinician in the
example of the young man. What was that look in the young man's eyes that was so
compelling? Was it in any meaningful sense the awareness and attention you might
have thought it was? What exactly about the observation made it seem that way? Is
this like the problem of the page number, forever ambiguous as we try to be certain
about what we are asking one another to believe about an empirically given phenomenon? Or is this moment different somehow? You might say: "It was my observation,
localized in a moment in space and time?" What exactly was it and what are the limits
on my ability to grasp what it was? Who decides these limits, and once they are
decided, does it mean I can never approach certainty? If I feel I know something about
what happened, what do I make of it?

Raising questions about the nature of local knowledge seems to cut to the heart of
the problem of how one knows something, and what it is that is known. Philosophical
perspectives push these issues still further.

Some Questions Attending the Examination of the Philosophical Trajectories

Table 3.1 summarizes how the three trajectories from philosophy of science that
we have discussed raise questions for inquiry. Note that the major feature of these
trajectories is that they point to problems in need of exploration and analysis in the
process of the inquiry. Precise methods to accomplish this exploration and analysis
are not specified, and indeed it is unlikely that they can be. Rather, the trajectories
represent directions to pursue, by whatever methods are appropriate and available,
that promise to offer new, potentially compelling perspectives on a problem.

The Full Framework Described

Table 3.2 presents a full model for using the philosophical trajectories to explore
a local clinical situation. It outlines the kinds of questions raised and information to be
sought when the four settings of locally specified information are crossed with the
philosophical trajectories. The 12 cells resulting from this conceptual crossing represent different possibilities for reflection and critique of what one knows about a

TABLE 3.1

Definitions of Philosophical Trajectories for Local Clinical Scientific Inquiry

Trajectory	Definition
a. Positivistic/empirical trajectory for analysis	Involves forms of physical, event, or personal experiential evidence (information) that can be identified in as specific and commonsense a manner as possible. It tends toward the ideal observational language of traditional logical empiricism, viz., that which is available to the senses. But it is not subject to the same constraints or restrictions, because it necessarily includes hypothetical entities and linkages that are both observable in principle, though perhaps not in practice, and fundamentally unobservable though effectively "real" [cf. Polanyi's (1967/1992) discussion of perception]. Reliability and validity are issues defined in terms of the realistic constraints of the inquiry. This trajectory seeks to identify information both positively, by recognition of a specific observational event, and negatively, by recognition of a nonevent.
b. Idealistic/paradigmatic trajectory for analysis	This trajectory also might be called an epistemic trajectory. It involves theory, research, common sense, personal experience, general world knowledge, and implicit and explicit forms of guidance provided by experts in one's area of endeavor (some of which may never be written down). It also involves manners and traditions of linking theoretical beliefs to applications and action. It also involves the ways ideas, or what we might call subsidiary meanings following Polanyi (1958, 1967/1992), are realized in direct experience of an object or event. This trajectory tends toward an idealized implementation of the logical and theoretical languages of traditional logical empiricism, and an idealized implementation of a paradigmatic approach to the problem (e.g., perfect application of a cognitive-social learning approach to psychotherapy). Consensus about the adequacy of the implementation within the peer culture (disciplinary matrix) is central to the adequacy of action along this trajectory. This trajectory seeks to identify such theory as it applies to the local clinical situation, again, both positively and negatively as in (a) above.
c. Sociohistorical/ constructionist trajectory for analysis	Involves culture, politics, economics, trends, critiques, and personal self-interests (both overt and covert) that may affect an understanding of the local clinical situation. It further involves a kind of self-conscious historiography for understanding how particular views evolve in a sociocultural milieu in which one is embedded, and how one has come to use them as tools for phenomenal access to reality. It is a reflexive recognition of embeddedness within a social matrix. This trajectory tends toward enlightened (or enlightening) self-awareness, and toward modifications of formulations and their implicational structure based on this awareness. It tends toward the identifications of the typifications and relevancies (Chapter 7) that undergird particular forms of theory and inquiry from a sociocultural perspective. The ability to communicate across sociocultural boundaries about similarities and differences without necessarily compromising one's own reality is a major indicator of adequacy of analysis along this trajectory. This trajectory seeks to identify social limits and constraints on the generality and meaning of a formulation and to deal with them in an enlightened manner. This trajectory necessarily takes one into the realm of moral/ethical questions both as manifestations and as absences. However, it recognizes that such issues are subject to the same contraints on certainty as are other forms of analysis, and they are incorporated into the overall formulation accordingly—that is, in a way that is consistent with the picture emergent in the overall analysis.

TABLE 3.2

Philosophical Trajectories Extrapolation Model Representing the Type of Information to Be Sought in Local Clinical Inquiry

Local information	Trajectory for analysis		
	Positivistic/empirical	Idealist/paradigmatic	Sociocultural/constructionist
Instantiation of general	Search for exemplars, or "windows" to higher-level category. Low-level, concrete, observational windows particularly relevant here. Trajectory moves toward empirical, specific, concrete, and universally recognizable.	Identification of how specific scientific and disciplinary ideas are mapped onto empirical observations and taken-for-granted realities. Recognition of how mapping involves more or less precision depending on particular inquiry.	Identification of the ways sociocultural and active construction processes and biases affect recognition or theoretical instantiations in the particular case. May involve a social (critical) analysis of the sources of legitimation of the theory, particularly as pertains to the local situation.
Local culture	Search for observable, or directly given, evidence of how local culture construes conditions pertaining to instantiation of theory.	Identification of explicit or implicit implicational structure(s) of primary paradigm as it interacts with a local cultural "paradigm." A way of balancing and integrating paradigms, and of bounding the inquiry, is sought.	Involves larger sociocultural issues involved in the application of a general professional paradigm in a particular local cultural context. Culture, gender, ethnicity, race, religion, and class are frames of reference that have particular relevance here. Locally intact subcultures can be very small, as in families or particular close relationships.

Unique	Identification of observable particulars of the case not fully identified by theory and integration into conceptualization.	Identification of ways paradigmatic implementation excludes certain material, renders it irrelevant, error, or unimportant. Questions involve commonsense or alternative-paradigmatic search for information that either clarifies and endorses implementation of primary paradigm (or at least doesn't question it), or raises possibility for alternative schema.	Sociocultural assertions pertaining to identification of unique characteristics of a situation are identified and evaluated. Evidence pertaining to support of a sociocultural perspective is identified.
Space-time specific	Identification and analysis of the particular observational circumstances that lead to an assumption of reliability of an observation. Four-dimensional space-time model is metaphor for analyzing observation–event–experience confluence.	Involves reflexive scrutiny and analysis of space-time specific cases of paradigmatic recognition in the situation, and identification of space-time specifics of the process of linking these to taxonomic and inferential conceptualizations.	Sociocultural influence and context for all space-time specific analyses are identified and questioned. Also, space-time specific identifications of cultural influences are identified and scrutinized for limits of reliability, when considered as given in a space-time specific context (e.g., postmodern *Zeitgeist* may lead to heightened relevance of certain sociocultural influences and diminishment of others).

particular situation based on input from a variety of sources including science, practice traditions, local observations and inquiry, expert opinion, personal experience, and common sense (Chapter 8). Filling in the cells of the model for a particular situation facilitates problem definition and analysis with respect to some major issues in the science–practice integration, as localized to a particular situation. It pushes one's thinking into the aerial perspective we have been discussing. It requires the practitioner to take a broader view of the contours of an inquiry without diminishing what seems to be known in science and practice traditions, nor what might be gained from other forms of analysis such as historical, critical, or political. It also suggests that the whole picture necessarily is larger than any disciplinary or perspective-based interest can support. In this way perhaps, it represents the realities of practice for the entire profession, better than do simplistic notions about applied science or theoretical allegiance (D. R. Peterson, 1995; Schön, 1983; Chapter 9). The local clinical scientist will have to choose his or her commitments carefully, with full recognition of, and responsibility for, the consequences of selecting among the many views of the clinical situation that exist in our discipline.

An Example

Table 3.3 illustrates an analysis of a particularly vexing problem in recent psychotherapeutic work, that of the "reality" of repressed memories (e.g., Loftus, 1993; Trierweiler & Donovan, 1994). Specifically, Table 3.3 shows how bits of information associated with a hypothetical case of possible repressed memory can be classified according to the extrapolation model. Professionals will recognize that real clinical cases will have much more information for the professional's consideration than can be represented here but, at the same time, often formulations hinge on even less than is depicted. We have included enough information here so that the reader can perhaps get a feel for the ways information might be identified and categorized to enhance understanding. For example, if a clinician were insightful enough to actually collect the information for the unique local information setting, and were to notice the conjunction between the patient's fondness for wearing black—which might be revealed in an offhand comment—and a potential religious stricture on black clothing (see Table 3.3), then a conversation about religious matters might be appropriate. This model and others described in Chapter 9 can be used to facilitate a Sherlock Holmes type of inquiry (Chapter 8), which is a good model for naturalistic inquiry in the practice context (Truzzi, 1983).

Note that this approach does not solve the many problems surrounding the repressed memory issue, either in the literature or in a particular clinical case. However, it does flesh out and expand awareness of numerous possible influences and questions that have a legitimate place in contemporary professional inquiry (see also Chapter 9). It also makes clear the kinds of intellectually rigorous scientific and clinical questions that are being avoided when a professional makes commitments to simplistic, overgeneralized positions without extensive analysis (e.g., all memories are necessarily true as remembered, or no memories have truth value because all are constructed, or any of the variations in between). Note also that this framework encourages the examination of the actual reports of a memory, and the circumstances surrounding these reports. For example, in Table 3.3 the clinician's changing understanding of memory, or political preferences, may be as influential in decisions about particular memories as is any patient report. We suspect that if all of the allegedly repressed memories identified by clinicians in recent times were analyzed this intensively, a substantial number would no longer support this hypothesis and those that did would be better justified.

Tables 3.2 and 3.3 require careful study, and we encourage readers to add information we have missed, and to expand the problem space to better suit a local clinical problem of interest to them. Even better, we invite readers to bring such analyses into interactions with supervisors and colleagues. Not all cells will be filled in any given inquiry. However, reflection on the type of information that might be available, or required, in a particular cell in any given circumstance, can help a clinician choose how to proceed in the inquiry. Additionally, this type of reflection can help clinicians determine exactly how published scientific results might fit into particular local circumstances. For example, evidence that males in their 30s tend to be involved in reflection on their values and on making decisions about their goals for the future (Levinson, Darrow, Klein, Levinson, & McKee, 1978) might be useful in analyzing a particular male patient's doubts about marriage. Hidden concerns about the possibilities of achieving valued goals (e.g., achieving success in the eyes of his family), excluded from repetitive and problematic conversations with his partner about his commitment to the relationship, may be part of the locally unique patterns in the man's life. These may have empirical implication in the content and tone of actual conversations, paradigmatic implication in fitting with emerging adult development literature (e.g., Levinson et al., 1978), and sociocultural implication in grasping fundamental values and background issues from which the goal aspirations might originate. Whenever the clinician cannot fill in a cell of the model because of a lack of information, then a possible direction for inquiry emerges.

CONCLUSION

This model is but one of many possible extrapolation devices that could be constructed from philosophical inquiry. For example, a particularly exciting device for precise thinking, logic, is yet to be tapped by professionals in local clinical inquiry. We will discuss basic logic in a later chapter. The range of other possibilities seems limited only by our creativity and openness to as yet unseen possibilities. But let us repeat that this model is not, and should not be considered, definitive even in accomplishing its central goal of showing how extrapolation from large themes in philosophical inquiry is possible. It is a preliminary tool for exploration of an event or

TABLE 3.3

Some Examples of Information that Might Be Considered in the Application of the Philosophical Trajectories Extrapolation Framework to the Identification of a Repressed Memory

Local information	Trajectory for analysis		
	Positivistic/empirical	Idealist/paradigmatic	Sociocultural/constructionist
Instantiation of general	Client shows distress in discussing memory, details are vague, inquiry into memory strained and difficult or prohibited by client's anxiety. Client expresses strong sense of remembering something that had not been remembered before. Memory blocks occur—client forgets what they were trying to do in thinking about the memory.	Paradigmatic model of repressed memory requires that there be no sense of having thought about the memory before, and that unconscious conflict makes the remembering difficult or impossible, even as the client tries to do so. Conflict might be revealed in dreams, or by other indirect means. Remembering should happen in context of gradual, deepening insight into personal feelings and drives previously defensively removed from consciousness.	In the past 15 years research on population rates of various forms of abuse raises awareness of its possible psychological impact, thus reviving trauma theory. A sociocultural milieu examining the effects of oppressive forces in society leads to the proliferation of victim and trauma theories in many areas of inquiry. Popular books modify and expand the definition of constructs like repression, either revealing what had previously not been seen, or redefining what has always been known but attended to differently. Previously accepted authorities, who established the definition of the construct, are discredited, or interpreted to be biased for sociopolitical reasons. Clinician comes to redefine emphasis in identifying examples of repressed memory to be more inclusive than in the past, and focus on traumatic aspects of the repressed more prominently than in the past.
Local culture	In particular case, client reports being deeply religious and heavily engaged in an effort to avoid sin and temptation. Also reports having no say about how things were done at home, and that doors were always open to adults. Client is hesitant to talk about any aspect of sexuality, or any strong emotion.	Repression theory requires an inability to retrieve a memory even if actively attempting to do so. This is different than difficulty a person from a strongly religious family might have in reporting a conflictual memory to a therapist. Examination of how religious beliefs interact with treatment inquiry is needed.	In general, theories based on aggregated results raise questions about other assumptions made in relation to a particular culture, or sociocultural category. For example, a clinician might assume that sexuality cannot be healthy if it cannot be discussed in therapy even if the client is from a religious family. Healthy sexuality may be defined differently in a particular subculture.

	Formal and informal evidence in the media that abused individuals are more prone to become abusers themselves, leads to presumption that anyone who has been "abused" will become an "abuser" without taking local conditions, both previous and current, into account. Individual presents as a member of a group seen to be disempowered in the prevailing society. Society views individuals having characteristics such as this client's as having an active role in determining their life course, or of having little role. Black clothes are frowned on in particular religious groups, except when individual is in mourning. *Zietgeist* suggests that individuals should be different from their family of origin so freethinking is encouraged and admired.		An increasingly educated society becomes unwilling to accept theories of psychological problems that implicitly suggest blame or inadequacy at some level. Theories that suggest that self-interest underlies the creation of such blame theories are convincingly communicated. It becomes difficult even to frame a blame theory in the profession, and previously accepted theory is interpreted as blaming and leads to censure by colleagues.
Unique	Memory thought to be a repressed memory seems to contain information about a room that is not identifiable to the client. Client claims no knowledge of time when repressed event might have occurred. Client is conflicted about a current romantic relationship. Client recently read a book about the effects of trauma on current psychological functioning. Individual seems to have considerable skill in dealing with children. Client likes to dress in black. Client has trouble remembering childhood in general.	Repression theory does not necessarily identify how current interpersonal conditions, or qualities of memory in the general case, should affect a clinician's judgment about the fact of the repression. Indeed, the phenomenon is rarely discussed separate from an extended discussion of the case, in the original literature positing the phenomenon. Question of which unique circumstances pertain to the clinician's judgment in this case is prominent.	
Space-time specific	First mention of memory came at the beginning of a session. Therapist unable to identify when the book about trauma was mentioned. Momentary doubt about the memory rejected as unsupportive of the client. Therapist experiences believing the memory immediately and is hard put to identify the basis for the belief.		Therapist, after several years of doubting the generality of trauma theory and not dealing with it much in professional work, has recently become convinced that it needs additional attention. Therapist had mentioned this change of thinking recently to a colleague, some weeks after this client revealed the memory alleged to be repressed.

problem, and an aid in tightening and clearly articulating standards for evidence for particular formulations in local contexts.

It becomes apparent from all of this that the notion of extrapolation is a complicated and intellectually demanding approach to problem solving. Even if one were to take this model as definitive—and we have no intention for it be taken that way—we are a long way from having well-formed methods of executing the analyses implied by each of the cells in Table 3.2, and for deciding when our work in imagination and in interaction with the local clinical situation has advanced sufficiently to justify some level of certainty about our conceptualization. The goal here is not to specify the end point of an analysis, but rather to encourage a sophisticated process to get us to whatever end we can manage within the exigencies of real local clinical situations. The model implies that coming to grips with a reasonable level of uncertainty is inherent in our work as professional scientists.

This model is primarily a tool for reflecting on knowledge from observation and direct experience, from professional culture, and from science, among numerous other sources. It makes clear that mastery of a particular approach to clinical work does not, in itself, constitute grounds for certainty about problem solving in specific situations. Indeed, if we examine various approaches, via the model, we will find them strong in some areas, and strikingly weak in others (e.g., DSM-IV categories tend to emphasize symptom observations at the expense of sociocultural contexts). The more difficult it is to fill in the cells, or to find models in our formal learning to help us do so, the more apparent it becomes that many professional and scientific theories have led us away from this sort of locally relevant formulation. This information deficit seems particularly salient around the identification of phenomena at a space-time local level of specificity. At this stage in our development, it seems we can do little more than attempt a good-faith approximation of this level of inquiry. We hope that future theoretical formulations, which are better linked to space-time processes, will aid this effort (e.g., see Trierweiler & Donovan, 1994).

The local clinical scientist, as a professional measuring instrument, needs to be affected by whatever structure exists in nature without being overwhelmed, forced into too narrow strains of certainty, or too loosely connected with the enduring properties of events in space-time. This is the philosophical part of the open scientific attitude we have been talking about: It is an openness that recognizes how even most rigid experimental design can inform one's thinking in the local context. This is the next part of our journey.

4

Issues in Research Design

[The investigatory process] starts upon the supposition that when you have
eliminated all which is impossible, that whatever remains, however
improbable, must be the truth. It may well be that several explanations
remain, in which case one tries test after test until one or other of them has a
convincing amount of support.
—DOYLE, quoted in TRUZZI (1983, p. 67)

In its widest sense, the experimental method signifies opposition to fixed
ends, to system-making and changelessness; it signifies a refusal to divorce
thought from action. It stands for provisionalism and tentativeness, the
reliance upon working hypotheses rather than upon immutable principles. In
this way, science is by no means limited to the professional scientist; it
represents an attitude that can function in any area of experience, an attitude
of free and effective intelligence. The extension of such a temper would
indeed be the "unified science" that is being sought in many circles.
—GEIGER (1941/1992, p. 20)

Imagine that the discipline of professional psychology was so advanced that problem
solving was simply a matter of collecting the facts, identifying the relationships
among these facts, producing an orderly account of the problem, and implementing
corrective measures to solve it. Imagine further that the tools of professional inquiry
and healing were definitive: that they were beyond refutation either from within the
profession or from without. The relationship of the art and science of professional
practice with the public would be positive—something like the idealized physician of
the 1950s. Expertise would be granted without question; success would be assumed
unless somehow the winds of fate blew one's problems beyond the reach of the
profession, in which case the only gripe could be with fate, never with the professional.

Professional psychology seeks this ideal, but matters are considerably more
complicated than this charming, and obviously antiquated, portrayal. We are a society
of doubters and, as we move into the next century, professionals increasingly are
being called on to justify their practices. Early in their training students often
experience a pang of anxiety when they find out that professional life and status has
never been as simple and secure as they might wish it to be. How should a profession
address questions raised by an increasingly aware public? Do they not reduce to a
question about how well we can accomplish what we claim to accomplish, and then to

our ability to communicate this skill to the public? Isn't it a bit like the problem of certainty of knowledge we confronted in the last chapter? Restating this problem in terms of effectiveness: If our approach to a problem was uniformly and indisputably effective, would we not establish the grounds for the kind of professional respectability described above? Of course we know that rarely does any professional achieve this level of efficacy, even with years of experience—even plumbers and other craftspersons rarely approach the theoretical ideal. As the social constructionists might suggest, society, via credentialing and the like, grants us permission to be experts even though our skills might fall short of perfection. The generosity of this social groundgiving depends on the politics of the times. Still, our claim to professional status depends ultimately on our ability to accomplish what we claim to accomplish. The Boulder conferees were well aware of this bottom line and organized psychology has focused much of its scientific energy on demonstrating the efficacy of psychotherapy and other psychological interventions. To this end, they have drawn on the power of science to reduce ambiguity and to generate consensus to the extent this is possible.

The power of science is centered in an ever-changing corpus of scientific research methodologies. The research design tradition has been concerned primarily with arranging scientific events, often called *experiments*, in an effort to generate consensus about the nature of phenomena by ruling out alternative explanations or descriptions. If there is a scientific method, then its account lies in the lore surrounding research design. It is the pragmatic expression of the hopeful enthusiasm of logical empiricism; it is the hope that questions about what is known can be settled by way of an approach to problem solving that anyone could implement, rather than a dependence on authority or rhetorical skill. It epitomizes centuries of effort to bring ideas out of the realm of the abstract into the realm of the natural and everyday.

Our task in this chapter is to explore some of the conceptual bases of traditional research design, to understand how it has been thought to work. The goal here, and in the next chapters, is to use scientific methodological thinking as a basis for the development of strategies for inquiry and analysis in the local clinical situation. Therefore, we will emphasize the hows and whys of particular methodological issues. We will discuss the overarching issues in establishing scientific belief, in problem generation and hypothesis formation, in the problem of induction, in the basics of causal inference in science, and in contemporary formulations of research design. We then will pull the entire logic together and offer some strategies for using research design thinking as a scheme for critical analysis of a local clinical problem.

In contrast to the more free-ranging ways of philosophy, science operates based on two influences on our thinking about the world. These are (1) logic, in the sense of an argument structured such that the conclusions seem to follow necessarily from a set of premises, and (2) empirical observation, in the sense that one becomes convinced of the truth of a proposition based on one's ability to see it operating in the world. These are the "logical" and "positivistic" parts of logical positivist science. They do not lose their power to convince simply because philosophers have raised doubts about them as a singular foundation for producing knowledge. Rather, they will continue to play a prominent role in a pragmatic science and they continue to affect us often in subtle and unconscious ways. Consider, for example, the pervasive concern expressed in our culture by the courts about how the media can affect public perception of criminal trials simply by its power to show events in particular ways. Science attempts to harness this same power of direct revelation by arranging experiments in such a way that logic and empirical observation come together to illuminate a particular problem, so as to reduce the number of alternative conclusions one can draw from what is revealed.

Let us look again at the question of how we know something to be true. In so doing, we will see directly how the mechanisms of scientific research design spring from the sensibility of philosophy and logic. Peirce (1877/1955), the pragmatist philosopher, provided a reflective account of how matters of inquiry have developed in the Western world, which we discuss next.

THE FIXATION OF BELIEF

Think for a moment how you come to believe something. This thought, when directed toward a particular belief or toward questions of which of several beliefs concerning a particular situation might be the best, is the beginning of scientific inquiry. This is true both for general and for local science. We will emphasize the latter here, both because of our interest in professional scientific inquiry and because the methods and culture of general science often can make this foundational question less relevant than it otherwise might be. We can, for example, test and develop beliefs already existing in science without pursuing their origins simply by pursuing problems as elaborated in the scientific literature. This is legitimate scientific practice, however constrained it might be from a scholarly perspective. Local science, in contrast, depends on the persistent conscious focus on basic questions about belief, particularly when elements of local practice do not fit well-elaborated practice models.

Peirce suggested that questions about belief arise, on the one hand, out of a personal experience of a tension between the sensation of believing and the sensation of doubt, and on the other hand, out of the social problem of settling matters of disagreement. Peirce elaborated four so-called *methods* for fixing beliefs. These give us a sense of some of the issues we face in seriously examining our own beliefs about matters pertaining to professional practice.

The Method of Tenacity

The method of *tenacity* describes a lazy position; it is a choice to believe something simply because one wants to believe it. The "truth" of the proposition resides in the steadfastness of the belief. If we choose to believe that "children never lie about abuse," or that "women can never perform as well as men in track and field," then there is essentially no need ever to test one's thinking because there can be no doubt. By the same token, one can never learn that one is wrong. Unfortunately, numerous beliefs one finds being voiced in professional work, particularly those based on unstated political positions, often simply are based on tenacity. This has been a perennial problem in clinical case conferences (Meehl, 1973).

The Method of Authority

Peirce's second method, the method of *authority* is as common in our highly communicative society as is the method of tenacity. Here we accept what an authority tells us to accept. Authority often is tied to particular demonstrations of competence of expertise. Psychologists strive to demonstrate expertise in healing psychological problems. Although authority is stronger than tenacity, in that it has the potential for public settlement of disagreements, there are no intrinsic guarantees that it will lead to greater understanding. Authorities can be flawed or stretched beyond reasonable applicability: Consider that the author of a good book or the director of a deeply moving film often is treated as expert on all matters of living.

In professional psychology, we quite naturally gravitate to those who have clear and compelling answers for our questions about practice: The therapist who authors a provocative book on treatment, or who is revered by students, can influence decades of practice, as did Freud in the field of psychoanalysis. The method of authority is not fundamentally flawed; indeed, it has great power in generating consensus and often leads to much benefit. We all depend on it, and will continue to do so however powerful science, or some other form of inquiry, becomes. However, in most cases, the acceptance of an authority, in itself, offers little basis for determining the range of its appropriate exercise. This only can come from the local clinical scientist's own critical evaluation of the authoritative position.

The Method of a Priori Belief

The third method, that of a priori beliefs, is also important to the local clinical scientist. This is something that is believed because it makes sense: It follows from what one already knows and believes. It is something between personal taste and inference that is based on one's knowledge of the world. It can work well for us when we stay within restricted domains of inquiry. For example, it is often reasonable to assume that a patient who has persistent problems with authority figures may, at some point, have problems with the therapist. Yet a priori thought also can have insidious effects on our ability to see beyond that which we think we know. A fascinating example of the power of a priori thinking in recent times has been the fall of the longstanding presumption that most gastric ulcers were the result of stress. The recent discovery of a bacterial cause for ulcers (Bishop, 1993)—which is as much a discovery of a new way of thinking about ulcers as it is a new observation–revealed sharply how very reasonable a priori assumptions can mislead one. Professional psychology is replete with a priori beliefs as rich, as varied, and undoubtedly as misleading as are the theories that guide our thinking. The question is how do we manage and critique these beliefs when they can be so taken for granted as to be barely discernible.

The Method of Science

Actually, critical evaluation is a perplexing task for all of the nonscientific methods of fixing belief that Peirce identified: They can come to us so directly and influence us so subtly that evaluating them requires great effort. In contrast, the process of specification and evaluation—and, by implication, a good deal of hard work—is built into Peirce's fourth method, the *scientific* position. This method concerns reducing a belief to its essential features and then finding a means to evaluate it that is external to one's wish to retain or reject it.

Peirce (1877/1955) compared the four beliefs as follows:

> If I adopt the method of tenacity, and shut myself out from all influences, whatever I think necessary to doing this, is necessary according to that method. So with the method of authority: the state may try to put down heresy by means which, from a scientific point of view, seem very ill-calculated to accomplish its purposes; but the only test *on that method* is what the state thinks; so that it cannot pursue the method wrongly. So with the a priori method. The very essence of it is to think what one is inclined to think. . . . But with the scientific method the case is different. I may start with known and observed facts to proceed to the unknown; and yet the rules which I follow in doing so may not be such as investigation would approve. The test of whether I am truly following the method is not an immediate appeal to my feelings and purposes, but, on the contrary, itself involves the application of the method. Hence it is that bad reasoning as well as good reasoning is possible, and this fact is the practical side of logic. (pp. 19–21)

Method is of the essence for a pragmatic science. It is an active process of externalizing, and putting forth for public discourse, that which is believed. By putting greater emphasis on the methods for answering questions than on the existence of beliefs about what is true, science seeks to put both those beliefs and any given example of scientific work to continuing public test. Of course, this too can have unintended consequences; claims about the superiority of one's knowledge of method can be wielded as easily and as arbitrarily as can substantive truth claims. Social and intellectual sources of belief and theory can become so deemphasized that the inquiry can move almost imperceptibly away from the original question. But, for good or ill, scientific methodology spurs action and continual development of one's thinking, even if it cannot always guarantee bona fide progress.

Implementation of the scientific perspective depends on one having some grasp of alternative explanations for a phenomenon. Also, the phenomenon must be clearly identified and bounded as an inquiry begins. Standing in the midst of the clinical or scientific research situation, one must make some commitment to what is known and accepted in order to proceed. In science we often use the literature to aid this process, and often the same is expected of clinicians in professional psychology. However, the use of prior knowledge and theory, linked appropriately to local observation, is only the beginning of scientific inquiry, not the endpoint it often is portrayed to be (see also Chapter 9). All inquiry involves a creative process that, perhaps more than anything else, depends both on the attitude of openness and on one's clinical, scholarly, and observational skills (e.g., Kaplan, 1964; Peirce, 1955a).

GENERATING HYPOTHESES

[O]bserved facts relate exclusively to the particular circumstances that happened to exist when they were observed. They do not relate to any future occasions upon which we may be in doubt how we ought to act. They, therefore, do not, in themselves, contain any practical knowledge.

Such knowledge must involve additions to the facts observed. The making of those additions is an operation which we can control; and it is evidently a process during which error is liable to creep in.

Any proposition added to observed facts, tending to make them applicable in any way to other circumstances than those under which they were observed, may be called a hypothesis. (Peirce, 1950b, p. 150)

The Problem

Before we can move on to the logical basis of experimental thinking, we need a way of understanding how belief comes to be realized in inquiry. Science begins with the generation of ideas about the nature of reality that follow either from theory or from observation. These ideas are summarized as hypotheses; hypothetical statements about how reality operates under certain explicitly identifiable circumstances. This definition is less precise than that found in standard research methods textbooks, where the emphasis is explicitly on identifying the relationship between variables (e.g., Kerlinger, 1986). As we will discuss in the next chapter, because variability may be undefined in the local situation (e.g., Lamiell, 1987), local scientists must pay careful attention to how phenomena combine in particular situations to yield specific outcomes, which, in turn, have implication for events and phenomena that follow in time. Nevertheless, it is useful to consider the properties of a good scientific hypothesis as a model for what we might wish to achieve in the local clinical situation.

Successful local clinical inquiry requires that we both generate and then investigate good hypotheses. Professionals too often depend on formulations that support, however weakly, their theoretical predilections without looking very deeply at the adequacy of such thinking in the local clinical situation. Only a conscious effort to see matters in a different light will overcome this tendency. For example, what appears to be a patient's defensiveness may, with carefully directed questioning, turn out to be embarrassment about being in therapy rather than motivated avoidance of certain material. The hypothesis that extends one's methods into new territory (the questions in this example) is likely to yield the most useful information.

Hypotheses for the Local Clinical Scientist

An explanation of a scientific problem involves connecting facts to other facts. Why does the child exhibit anxiety and fear when going to school? Why does the young man always avoid women who may show romantic interest in him? Why is the teenager's night so filled with fearsome dreams?

Professionals will recognize each of these as only partial statements of a clinical problem. Yet any one could be the immediate reason that treatment is sought. Professionals initially will engage such problems by connecting them with constructs known, through science and professional tradition, to pertain to what the clinician observes and to the reports of the help seekers (Chapter 8). This is a process of selection and focus on certain information. At the same time, it is a diminishment of attention to other information that might have been the focus of the inquiry.

Cohen and Nagel (1934) discussed the following so-called *formal conditions* for scientific hypotheses, which are relevant to local inquiry.

Explicit Formulation

The hypothesis must be formulated so explicitly that deductions can be made from it that eventually might lead to a decision that it does or does not account adequately for the facts of the case. Even the most informal professional hypotheses have identifiable consequences when clearly elucidated. For example, a psychotherapy patient's religious amulet might lead to a hypothesis about the importance of religious beliefs in the individual's life, or about the possibility that these beliefs are related to conflicts reported by the patient. The behavior of a parent during a school-related consultation may suggest that he is not paying attention to the consultant's suggestions about how to handle a child's problem behavior. An organization may appear so overtly dysfunctional that a consultant is led to believe that some deeper value than that mentioned in the presenting problem is being protected, or a deeper conflict, which is perhaps more difficult to conceptualize from within, is being enacted. Such hypotheses can lead to fruitful inquiry. Sometimes they will be wrong, but sometimes they will uncover otherwise hidden information that can contribute to the professional's intervention. The process of thinking through and pursuing the consequences of such provisional hypotheses is virtually a no-lose form of inquiry, for, in local clinical inquiry, finding out that one is on the wrong track is often as useful as finding out that one is correct. Alternatively, the cost of jumping to conclusions, however compelling they may seem, can be a complete misunderstanding of the case and the limits on one's ability to affect it positively.

Relevance to the Question

The hypothesis should answer the question that initially led to the inquiry. For professionals, the lack of attention to this aspect of inquiry often is reflected in the transformation of a client's request into a formulation quite different from the question originally raised. In family work, for example, the *identified patient* and the problem identified with that individual often will not be the focus of the intervention, which often is framed in terms of larger issues in the family system. Clients can be alienated if we do not provide a logical argument as to how the systems-level formulation relates to the issues they originally raised. If the clinician is unable to make such linkages in convincing fashion, it suggests that he or she actually does not know how they might be made. If one changes the focus of the work, in keeping with high professional standards, a good hypothesis will address the original question, either directly or indirectly. The hypothesis offers the client a basis for deciding that it does indeed address the original problem, or alternatively, it provides a rationale for abandoning the client's original formulation in an effort to achieve greater benefit. Even a wrong hypothesis can lead to much fruitful inquiry, as long as it stays focused on the problem at hand. The inability to address the original question is one of the clearest signs in science that a hypothesis may be insufficient, however appealing it might be at the time.

Verifiable Consequences

The hypothesis must be formulated so as to imply verifiable consequences. That is to say, the hypothesis must suggest some predictable observations to follow at some future time. This notion can be overstated to imply that only those hypotheses that lead to clear predictions represent good science, and that prediction is always equivalent to explanation (see Manicas & Secord, 1983). Here, the actual attainment of accurate predictions is less important than the attempt to bring clarity to one's thinking and one's formulations by seeking verifiable prediction. Likewise, there is no implication that verification means physical observation, although this might be extremely useful in more cases than many professionals recognize. Rather, the goal is to attain a level of awareness of consistencies and inconsistencies between one's views and the unfolding realities of events outside of one's control. If, for example, a therapist experiences a client to be making progress in one area, but is oblivious to areas of deterioration that the client is hesitant to talk about—such as a calming of certain anxieties at the expense of ever-increasing dependency on the therapy itself— then there is a flaw in the relationship between formulation and prediction in the local clinical situation. In this context, prediction roughly is equivalent to enlightened awareness of how ideas and the realities of events work together, and in turn, how they interact with potential unknowns in ways that must be heeded by the local clinical scientist.

Simplicity

The last condition for a good hypothesis discussed by Cohen and Nagel is that, given a situation where there is more than one hypothesis to account for a situation, then the simplest one is the one to pursue. This takes us back to the Sherlock Holmes quotation that opened this chapter: Once one understands what cannot be true, by gradually ruling out alternative possibilities, then what remains must be true, however improbable it may seem at the time. Of course, as with all local clinical inquiry, there can be no certainty that one has eliminated all of the possibilities; it is entirely a matter of one's sense of having covered all of the bases. Experienced professionals will have a long list of examples of situations where clients will later—often much later—reveal a condition that strongly affected them, but that was unknown to the psychologist at an earlier time. For example, a period of heightened emotional lability might be revealed to be a time when the client was exploring a controversial romantic relationship. Or, a mysteriously terrible weekend—one that reveals to the client how really sick he or she is—belatedly is revealed to have been punctuated by a conflict-laden phone call from a relative. Skilled professionals always will have a route to pursue with a client, even through the most trying of times. Yet this same capacity to withstand uncertainty too easily can become the bane of simplicity of thought. Science and logic suggest it is far better to generate and pursue the simple and let the complicated and dramatic emerge by the force of its ability to account for the realities of things, than it is to start with the dramatic only to lose sight of the simple.

Managing the Relationship between Hypothesis and Observation

In considering these four components of good scientific hypotheses, professionals might say that this is all well and good, but these are idealizations. Life in the real world is too complicated and time is too pressing for such rules to provide any significant gain for professional thought. We agree with this concern, but not with the conclusion. Rules for good hypotheses provide a direction for expanding and pressing professional thought to higher levels. The relationship between a hypothesis and a particular observation is extremely important in the local clinical situation. Good hypotheses imply good observations—or the possibility of good observations—either because of the quality of the theory underlying the hypothesis or because of the structure of reality in the local clinical situation that theory and hypothesis bring to our attention. Goldfried (1991) suggested that the basis for integration of the various theories of psychotherapy lies in clinical strategies, midway between theories and techniques (see also Chapter 9). Good hypotheses operate at this level. If a hypothesis is well connected to the situation, there are always observations that go along with the hypothesis, and observations that should not be there if the hypothesis is viable.

Next we turn to some matters of logic that provide the groundwork for contemporary research design practices.

THE PROBLEM OF INDUCTION

In discussions of scientific methodology, we often hear about two types of logic that can be applied to the relationship between theory and empirical observation. These are deduction and induction. Deduction is top-down moving from theory to observation: Theory leads to a prediction about the nature of the observable world and we set up an experiment to test the theory. Induction is bottom-up: We look around the world until we begin to grasp how it is structured, and we then generate and, most importantly, test theories by extending them beyond our explorations. In the ideal, an experimental science is supposed to be deductive (or hypothetico-deductive; Hull, 1951), whereas a naturalistic science is inductive.

Cohen and Nagel (1934) pointed out that modern science often was considered to be more inductive than deductive. This makes sense to the extent scientists do indeed behave on the positivistic trajectory, in that multiple low-level—and presumed to be universally shared—observations yield hypothetical statements about the lawful properties of phenomena in the domain of inquiry. Such a bottom-up approach should be contrasted with a purely deductive science, where most of the action is in the theoretical realm, with an occasional prediction tested against a few choice observational circumstances. Cohen and Nagel suggested that, in any case, induction and deduction are highly related in science. This is because, by whatever course one comes to an observation, either by it having been deduced from theory or by it simply following as one explores the world, science will have the problem of determining the extent to which that particular observation corresponds sufficiently with the domain of all like observations. As long as one is in the empirical realm, the development of a scientific method depends on the ability of method to specify clearly how a set of observations supports a general conclusion about the nature of the world. Ultimately, this is a problem of induction, so our discussion must focus more on induction than deduction.

Intuitive Induction

Cohen and Nagel (1934) described two kinds of induction first discussed by Aristotle. The first is called *intuitive induction*. Certain aspects of reality seem to come to us directly, without any special mental inference on our part. Intuitive induction follows from experience, where object and event particulars are seen to combine into perceptual wholes (e.g., the tone of voice and rapidity of the exchange lead suddenly to the recognition that the couple is arguing rather than simply describing their reason for seeking therapy). Those wholes that are judged to be similar to one another are held to be categorically related (e.g., Rosch & Mervis, 1975). The notion that there could be a positivistic foundation for science depends on the apparent obviousness of certain types of observation, most notably in the physical realm. Indeed, it is this sense that empirical realities come to us directly and universally that has given the positivist position the power it has had over the years. Intuitive induction is presumed to be noninferential in that there is no proposition to be tested, but rather only similarities or invariances in observation that are directly given in experience. Kuhn (1977) called this direct apprehension of the nature of an object or event *ostension* (in Chapter 2 we raised the possibility of thinking about these in terms of the concepts of *apperception* or *apprehension*), and used the example of explaining the concept of swan to a young child simply by pointing to the groups of large birds out on a lake. The vision of the swan carries the meaning of the category, which the child will learn with time.

For experienced professionals, the power of intuition to yield fruitful hunches cannot be denied. There is a very real sense that, with experience, certain phenomena, like transference, which might once have been elusive, become more directly available to one's perceptual apparatus. Still, even if such intuitions are taken to be universal—and not all would agree they are, even at the most mundane level—there remains a problem in science of what to make of them. In received view science, these observations gradually shade into increasingly abstract, inferential categorizations of objects and events (Cronbach & Meehl, 1955). This shading, in turn, forms the basis for more cognitive or paradigmatic accounts of the inductive process. The problem with this type of induction, particularly as it pertains to professional science, is in determining when the intuition no longer is in contact with what is essentially consensual in science. Obviously, the diagnostic categories of DSM-IV are not given directly in experience, yet with sufficient experience with particular types of cases, it can seem as though some diagnostic categories are all too real.

The overlearned perceptions of the professional can also complicate communication with other professionals and, even more, with one's scientist colleagues. It can be difficult to convey how complicated patterns in cases can seem so directly observational when these colleagues do not share the same experience base. The subtle shift in a client's attitude or faint smile that signals improvement to a therapist, may be difficult to describe to another who has not experienced prior sessions. This is simply a fact of professional life. Increasingly sophisticated recognitions are available to those who gain experience, and this seems to be true in any area requiring observationlike expertise, be it in the sciences or the arts (e.g., Ericsson & Charness, 1994).

Inferential Induction

Even if one stays with the traditional scientific view of purely observable phenomena—such as manifested in a response to a questionnaire or a behavioral observation—there remains a second type of inductive problem in science. This is called *inferential induction*, or the *induction of probable inference*. It is a problem of generalizing from the scientist's experience. How can we know that observations of a given set of cases allow us to draw conclusions that then can be applied to a new set of cases? The problem can be characterized best by looking at the extreme situation where all of the objects of interest can be observed directly—what Cohen and Nagel refer to as *perfect induction*. Thus, a school psychologist might notice that, in a particular school, all of the children having problems in reading also demonstrate problems in gross motor coordination. The inference that there is a correlation between the two types of problems is justified in this group because all of the cases are represented. Generalizing to other schools, however, may not be justified because cases may be found there that do not exhibit the relationship. Again, this is perhaps easier to observe in the physical sciences, where once a rock is reasonably well classified, it can be treated pretty much like any other rock, with little controversy about the treatment ensuing. Not so with humans and human systems.

This second variety of induction is what primarily is referred to when we speak of the *problem of induction* in science. Given a classic example, such as the assertion that "all ravens are black," we can never be sure that we will not find a raven that is not black if we continue to extend our search to birds as yet unobserved. Thus, the universality of our assertion cannot be certain—a definite problem for the aspirations of a positivist science. By implication, this means that a career's worth of clinical practice, even with a great diversity of cases, may not expose one to a sufficiently broad range of population possibilities that one's generalizations about clinical work—based on one's experience—could stand up to scientific scrutiny. Unfortunately, professionals attend too little to such aspects of logic and rational discourse.

A major part of research design methodology has been created to deal with this second type of inductive problem. Cohen and Nagel noted that it is basic to scientific thinking that we not allow this problem to be as insurmountable as it seems to be in the abstract. They suggested that there are two situations where inductive inference might be justified: (1) when the universe of the generalization is relatively homogeneous, therefore supporting the assumption that one object or event in the domain of discourse is like any other; and (2) when the scientific problem is well understood, and the generalization is taking place within a nexus of other, perhaps better studied and understood, relationships among phenomena, thus enhancing the probability that an inference is justified. Achieving a "fair" or "representative" sample is critical to ensuring that these conditions are satisfied (see Chapter 5).

If, as professionals, we believe each new case is completely unique, then any general statement will be in doubt, or at least treated as though it is not as important as the uniqueness. Alternatively, if we allow that there are homogeneities across cases that are meaningful, then it is reasonable to draw more general conclusions. The question then focuses on the conditions under which generalization is appropriate (Cronbach, 1975a, 1982). Obviously, the credibility of this induction by probable inference depends on our ability to create a sense that no surprises are lurking out there in the population of interest. The better the sample, the more sound the inference is, as the logic goes. Alternatively, this also can be a trap of a priori thinking, where generalization seems appropriate (or inappropriate), but we actually might be incorrect.

CAUSALITY: A PREMISE OF THE EXPERIMENTAL METHOD

The goal of experimental design is to create events and event sequences where antecedent conditions clearly can be identified and controlled, and outcomes carefully can be measured. Science assumes nature to be orderly and composed of cause–effect relationships between objects and events. The task for the scientist is to discover order via: (1) direct observation of properties that coexist in objects or events, (2) observation of invariance and change over a span of time, or (3) the extension to particular circumstances of mathematical and general theoretical statements that describe order among phenomena. Having identified a scientific question of interest (e.g., why is depression characterized by a loss of interest in things previously found enjoyable?), the task is to arrange experiments in such a way that conclusions necessarily follow from the outcome of the research. Historically, the central objective of this logic has been to facilitate the search for cause–effect relationships. Therefore, to grasp fully how research design traditions have developed as they have, we must look at traditional thinking about causality.

Some Basic Ideas about Causality

For any possible cause, there exist four possible relationships between the cause and an effect of interest: The cause can be observed or made to exist and the effect can follow in time; the cause can be observed or made to exist and the effect can not follow in time; the cause can be not observed or not made to exist and the effect can follow in time; or the cause can be not observed or not made to exist and the effect can not follow in time. Because science ultimately is interested in identifying cause–effect relationships, experiments are designed to eliminate potential causes from consideration to the extent they do not show consistent and orderly relationships with the effects of interest. For example, in a classic elementary school experiment, plants are shown to require light for health and growth by equalizing all other conditions of soil, water, fertilizer, and temperature while varying the amount of light to which members of a particular species of plant are exposed.

Simple examples of cause and effect from our daily lives can seem so obvious as to merit little additional consideration. Yet the concept of cause is not a simple idea even though it is tied closely to our everyday notions of what understanding and explanation are supposed to be about (see Cook & Campbell, 1979). There is some evidence that we will impute causality naturally both to interactions among objects (Heider & Simmel, 1944; Michotte, 1946) and to those among people (Heider, 1958). Nonetheless, philosophers have shown how complicated it is to untangle the meaning of a concept such as causality if we look at it closely. Usually, scientists use the concept freely, as it helps them understand the object and event sequences in which they are interested, without much concern for broader definitional issues (see Cook & Campbell, 1979). Alternatively, some argue that using the concept is largely unnecessary as long as we concentrate on examining relationships among variables of scientific interest (e.g., Kerlinger, 1986). In considering localized phenomena, it is difficult to dismiss completely the concept, without replacing it with some proxy, such as the identification of so-called functional or contingent relationships between antecedent and consequent conditions in behavioral psychology.

There seem to be three basic ways we think about causality. First, there is the commonsense version of cause, where we seem simply to know—or to think we know—what causes what in our world. Usually these assumptions operate on information in the domain of direct, everyday experience, and it is a relatively rare event for them to be challenged. When they are challenged, as when we see how a magic trick actually works, we undergo a major transformation in our taken-for-granted thinking about a particular event. Second, there is the scientific sense of causality, related to common sense, and particularly relevant to material causes and effects. We discuss this in some detail below. Finally, there is a historical sense of cause, which contains aspects of both of the other two, but which deals with much more challenging, and often amorphous, information about the relationship between past—often distant past—events and more recent ones. Material evidence and broader knowledge are used to bring the causal narrative together. All three are important for professional work in psychology, they each present special problems, and they can stand up to varying degrees of formal scrutiny.

Below we look at the scientific attribution of causality and discuss how it relates to the other kinds we tend to take more for granted in our professional activities. We will pick up on issues related to commonsense and historical causality in the later chapters on qualitative methods (Chapter 7) and critical thinking (Chapter 8).

Hume's View of Causality

The modern scientific notion of causality is rooted in the thinking of Hume (see Cook & Campbell, 1979; Hume, 1748/1955). Hume described three conditions for judging causality: (1) contiguity between cause and effect, (2) temporal precedence of cause, and (3) constant conjunction where the cause is always present if the effect occurs.

Contiguity suggests cause and effect are proximal to one another: That is, there is some mechanism by which some instigatory property of the cause is transmitted to the effect. When considered in the clinical situation, this would suggest a need to examine how such proximity might exist in our causal attributions. Thus, if we believe early experience somehow is related to a client's current functioning, then attention to how the transmittal comes to be is in order. We often pass over such issues, acting as though the causal, or implicitly causal, attribution stands on its own. Yet this is clearly begging questions about the mechanisms of the transmission, and the circumstances under which they are and are not prominent.

For example, an individual who is treated in a demeaning manner by a parent may experience adulthood with low self-esteem. By what developmental process would this antecedent condition be responsible for our current observations of diminished self-esteem in the person? Are all such observations linked to this past, or are other plausible causal—or contributory—influences possible, such as economic experiences or simply bad luck? Do we have a theory that would allow us to distinguish various different influences, and distinguish differing observations we make of our client that might be more or less related to our primary causal hypothesis? Hume's insight about contiguity alerts us to the ultimate space-time interconnectedness of lives and events.

In an example from family therapy, we might posit that a systems-level dynamic is operative in the behavior problems of a child. The question is how. How, for example, is a problem in the relationship between the parents transmitted to the child within the system of interactions observed? Answering questions such as this could have major implications for the specific conduct of the therapy. When we speak of the local clinical scientist being ever aware of the rich texture of interconnectedness in the world, we are pointing to the insight that somehow causes and effects—or less strongly, antecedent and consequent conditions—somehow commune with one another in space and time. Thinking of the contiguity of causes is useful even if one ultimately rejects the mechanistic metaphor implicit in causal thinking. If what we observe is like a soccer ball being pushed along the grass, then we must seek the metaphorical equivalent to the point of contact with the foot that does the pushing. This will lead to fascinating and illuminating inquiry in many cases, even if we do not believe the contact point of the hypothetical cause in our clinical case is as singularly compelling a cause as is the foot of the soccer player. If nothing more, it will focus our attention on linkages that we may not understand fully given our existing knowledge of the case.

Attention to the property of *temporal precedence of causes* also can be useful in local clinical inquiry. Hume was suggesting that a defining property of causes is that they necessarily come before their imputed effects. If the effects do not follow from the cause, or they exist without the cause already being present, then the logical chain that ties causal reasoning together is disrupted, leading any theory grounded in this chain to be in doubt. In psychological research, the fit with this criterion makes certain variables, like age, always causal. In like fashion, we tend to take early life conditions as causal in relation to contemporary conditions, as in our self-esteem example.

Of course there are inevitable variations on this theme. For example, consider the belief that what professionals learn from clients about the past is modified by current conditions, as in the case of recent concerns about the authenticity of the events referenced in so-called repressed memories (e.g., Loftus, 1993; Ofshe & Waters, 1994). Another example is more general thinking about memory that suggests that early memories are as much a function of the persistent psychological conditions as actual events in the past (e.g., Bonanno, 1990), or existing mood conditions and the like (Bower, 1981). The point here is that, short of arranging conditions so we know that the imputed cause preceded the presumed effect, we really cannot know if temporal precedence has been satisfied.

Hume's third criterion for causality is *constant conjunction of events*. This implies an "if–then" clause that is operative when all other things are held constant or rendered insignificant to the events at hand. If all other possible effects are rendered irrelevant, then given the cause, the effect should follow. This is a primary and powerfully convincing fundamental to the logic of experimental design (see below). It carries the deeply held assumption that the world is fundamentally orderly. Therefore, if one produces the cause, or observes it as an event, then the effect must follow in an orderly world. This sort of thinking has allowed scientists to create experimental methods focused on producing conditions where several possible causal influences are minimized or eliminated in the hope of observing the influence of a few (see below). Even apart from experiments, perceived causality is a powerful influence on our thinking, as recently has been illustrated in cases where sexual abuse is asserted, even when there are doubts about the accuracy of the assertion. Individuals who otherwise would doubt experimental logic and the whole project of seeking causal relationships are often quite willing to accept certain kinds of causal attribution as definitive.

At this point many clinicians are probably saying to themselves that none of us really believe in these links this strongly given even the best of experimental results. In so doing, unfortunately, they are underscoring the problem in the science–practice bridge. If we take science seriously, we cannot pick and choose our understanding of causal linkages so freely, simply to fit our personal convenience, and expect to achieve increasingly compelling understanding of the clinical situations we confront. Our every action as professionals, our every assertion about the nature of our work and our understanding of a particular case, is laden with causal inference and implication, whether we choose to present it that way or not. We may never know which formulations are definitive, or even if definitive formulations are possible. Still, because there is an essential skepticism in scientific thinking—albeit one that holds the promise of solutions to the puzzles we formulate—it requires that we retain some level of appropriate caution in drawing causal conclusions even when the formal and informal criteria we set for such judgments seem to be satisfied.

Causality and Research Design

There are several important assumptions implicit in this discussion of causality that have been translated into contemporary research design methodology. First, there is a sense that, in making an observation or designing an experiment, one has a window to all possible circumstances under which cause and effect might be observed. Second, there is an implicit idea that we can reduce phenomena to their essences and thereby access their true (or truer) nature. Even if we do not believe we have reduced a phenomenon to its essence, we still might accept the notion that we have pushed it to its limits, trying to find the minimum conditions for its existence. If, for example, an effect, E, which is thought to be brought about by two causes, A and B, via experiment can be shown to occur under conditions where one of the two causes, say B, is absent, then it will be difficult for us to continue to weight the two causes equally in our thinking about E. That is, of course, unless we can somehow discredit the experimental demonstration. This sort of thinking clearly is a powerful influence on professionals, in that we often draw on our own experience of particular clinical causes or situations as though they are representative of more general phenomena.

Third, we assume that the limits or boundaries that surround a phenomenon, as we perceive them, are the limits for the phenomenon in the general case (e.g., a particular measurement of depression is assumed to be an instance of the general problem of depression). We tend to do this immediately and without reflection. Fortunately, the world is orderly enough and our thinking effective enough that this does not prove to be a serious problem most of the time. Good experiments depend on this assumption, but in such a way that even the most careful scrutiny leaves one convinced that some aspect of the phenomenon thought to be examined in the experiment indeed was examined. Thereby, experiments are presumed to have some more lasting status than more informal presentations. Fourth, well-executed experiments are assumed to offer the grounds for higher-level theoretical arguments. Even critiques of science draw on experimental results on occasion. Similarly, as we professionals discuss our case formulations, we act as though the phenomena observed are exemplars of the higher-level theoretical categories we are familiar with and use. The possibility that these beliefs would not stand up to more careful examination is rarely considered. Of course, it is also true that there are a great many published experiments that would not be accorded this status.

Each of the assumptions just discussed entails a sense of linkage between local and general observation and manipulation; the sense that the world is an orderly place where there are few surprises for the careful scientist (Chapter 6). Bhaskar (1978) questioned this fundamental notion that our direct, empirical observations, however true they may be in their own right (e.g., reliable), necessarily yield accurate representations of the events they are presumed to describe (observations are not necessarily equivalent to events in space and time), and, therefore, that they are instances of the larger theoretical systems that guide our thinking (Chapters 3 and 5) (e.g., the observed sad eyes may or may not reflect an ongoing depressed affect, which, in turn, may or may not reflect an instance of clinical depression). This linkage assumption may hold up fairly well in certain domains of the physical world where object and event boundaries can be quite well delimited and modified as needed to correspond better to an emerging understanding of a larger whole (e.g., crystals of various colors can eventually be identified as quartz; or ideas about the characteristics of particular plant species can change as new information emerges). However, the links between local observation and the properties of actual phenomena of interest in the social and psychological worlds tend to be much more tenuous (e.g., a behavioral outcome is presumed to be a manifestation of unconscious cognitive processing by some, an affective expression by others). The impalpability of many of the things that interest us will continue to be a problem for our science (Rychlak, 1981).

RESEARCH DESIGN

Experimental design embodies a set of logical tools and strategies for examining phenomena in greater detail, and with greater precision, than they might otherwise be examined. Interestingly for our focus on local clinical science, the logic of research design originated in the nineteenth century when science was still more natural philosophy than the complex social and political institution we know today. As such, the focus of method was as much on how to think about phenomena and how to advance an inquiry as on the particular operations needed to achieve an acceptable result. These methodological strategies were particularly focused on the problem of how to render cause–effect relationships observable. This is accomplished by eliminating the influence of anything presumed not to be involved in the cause–effect relationship, thereby identifying the conditions under which the relationship will be observed and those under which it will not.

Early empiricists such as Francis Bacon, who is credited with the standard notion of the scientific method, and John Stuart Mill, whose work we discuss next, played a major role in specifying the logic of experimental science.

Historical Roots of Research Design: Canons for Experimental Thought

Mill attempted to elaborate the conditions under which observation and logic might come together in a set of methods that, he hoped, would ensure the truth value of experiments. This was in keeping with the empiricist wish that science be driven by method rather than by the happenstance of revelation for particular scientists. Mill believed that such a canon would serve both purposes of guiding discovery in science and of allowing for experimental verification of scientific hypotheses. To this end, he designed a set of five "methods" presumed to specify the conditions under which a cause–effect relationship might be inferred. Although it is generally accepted that Mill's proposal fails as a definitive canon, his logic is fundamental to all modern experimental design taught in our textbooks. In particular, his work provides insight to the root logic for the seemingly modern innovation, the control group.

The Method of Agreement

The Method of Agreement suggests that when we can identify two instances of a phenomenon that share only one other circumstance, then that circumstance is either a cause or an effect of the phenomenon. Suppose we observe two families with conduct-disordered children, but the circumstances otherwise are markedly different. If later we learn that both families have experienced a period of serious marital conflict, by the logic described by the Method of Agreement, we will be prone to draw causal linkages between the conduct disorder and the marital conflict. In itself, this method is flawed in that there must be some prior basis for assuming other, as yet unknown, influences can be ruled out. Such reason seldom exists in even the most rigorous areas of psychological research.

The Method of Difference

The Method of Difference effectively describes the logic of the control group: If the phenomenon occurs in one situation, but not in another, and both situations differ in only one other circumstance, then that differing circumstance is the cause, or the effect, or at least an important part of the phenomenon observed. In contemporary research designs, experimental and control groups are assumed to be identical, except that the experimental group receives a treatment and the control group does not. Phenomena, like improved health, are viewed as causally related to treatments to the extent that experimental groups yield improvements whereas control groups do not. Any complexities in research methodology are usually problem-related attempts to achieve conditions of similarity and difference according to some variant of this logic. Again, as we can never be sure we have achieved perfect similarity save for the treatments administered and outcomes observed (and there are practical problems even here), this logic is imperfect. Still, the logic is useful for eliminating potential causes that are thought to bring about an outcome, but that are discredited when put to this sort of test—as when claims of the superiority of a therapeutic approach do not hold up in controlled studies.

The Joint Method of Agreement and Difference

The Joint Method of Agreement and Difference suggests that we should look for two or more cases with the presence of the phenomenon of interest, say improved mental health, and only one other feature in common, say a particular therapy, and contrast that with two or more cases where the phenomenon does not occur and that have nothing else in common save the absence of the circumstance (e.g., the therapy). Although this combination really does not add any power to the logic of either method taken separately, it illustrates a logic implicit in studying groups—as opposed to individuals—as is common in contemporary research designs. We say a treatment works when we have groups (multiple independent cases) in which only the treatment and the outcome are observed, and we compare then with groups (multiple independent cases) where nothing is in common save not receiving the treatment and presumably not achieving the outcome.

The Method of Residues

The Method of Residues involves direct elimination of all conditions that already are known to affect a phenomenon, so that whatever remains of the phenomenon is the result of the remaining conditions. This is a direct statement of the well-known "process of elimination" we often hear about in making logical arguments.

For example, this sort of thinking is involved in the notion of psychogenic causes for unusual psychiatric conditions such as glove anesthesia, where an exhaustive attempt is made to find a physical cause to no avail, and, moreover, it even can be determined that neurological structures would not support the described lack of sensation. Like Sherlock Holmes, the logic says that once we have determined what cannot be true, then whatever remains must be. But again, the problem is in deciding when there are no other, as yet unrecognized, possibilities not covered in our understanding of what remains as the residue of the inquiry.

The Method of Concomitant Variation

The Method of Concomitant Variation describes what is commonly referred to in modern parlance as correlational relationship. It states that when two phenomena vary together in some manner, one is either the cause or the effect of the other, or is connected with it by some as yet unknown causal function. This method requires measurement so as to observe the covariation, and the direction of causality must be determined by observations and theory other than that entailed in the method itself (correlation is discussed in Chapters 5, 6, and 9).

The Value of Mill's Methodology

These methods suggest the use of some basic thought operations that are essential to scientific inquiry—even in the local context—in domains of phenomena relating to our professional objectives. These are:

- Searching for similarities (invariances) or agreement
- Searching for dissimilarity (variance) or disagreement
- Searching for instructive combinations of the two
- Eliminating possible influences in the search for a necessary and sufficient residue
- Seeking covariations among phenomena that we previously had not recognized

A major problem with each of these methods is the difficulty that can exist in determining when all things are similar or different from one another, and knowing that the things observed to covary are the only factors involved in the observed relationship. In experimentation this is always a problem, even under the most controlled conditions, and it is even more of a problem in the natural world of the local clinical scientist.

Striking advances were made in the literature on research design by pushing scientific logic, like that of Mill's, into a set of methodological rules for scientific conduct (e.g., Campbell & Stanley, 1963; Cook & Campbell, 1979; Cronbach & Meehl, 1955; Runkel & McGrath, 1972; Underwood, 1957; to name a few). Let us turn now to some of this more specific and operational work to examine the critical questions it raises for inquiry in the local context.

Contemporary Practices

The translation of the logic of science into a body of methodological practices for psychologists took a giant step forward in the publication of a monograph by Campbell and Stanley (1963). Although there were other excellent works available at the time (e.g., Underwood, 1957), Campbell and Stanley's focus on the specifics of designing research studies in the general case, and on the level of strength of the findings resulting from different designs, gave researchers a direct guide for applying scientific principles in a variety of contexts. Campbell and Stanley specifically sought to encourage more careful research in educational and other applied settings in the hope of improved practices in those settings. Unfortunately, in so doing, they inadvertently raised the notion of a true experiment (which we discuss below) to such an idealized level that they helped to encourage a generation of psychologists to insist on experimental studies in scientific work, and thereby, they helped to set the stage for the professional break with traditional training that was described in Chapter 1. This misrepresentation was corrected some years later by Cook and Campbell (1979), where greater emphasis was placed on improving one's product, while recognizing the real-world limits on the possibility for definitive experimental designs.

Campbell and Stanley (1963) showed some ways that time, classification of groups, and manipulations of variables can be used to strengthen one's conclusions about experimental outcomes. Their work embodied all of the assumptions of order and continuity of traditional science, and took advantage of the types of thinking outlined in Mill's work to create a system that counters, if it does not solve, the problem of induction—in the sense of moving to higher-level conclusions based on successive observations at a lower, more particularistic level. As we examine this material, note that Campbell and Stanley's presentation assumed that research would be conducted with aggregates rather than with individuals and, therefore, that it involves intrinsically statistical assumptions, which we discuss in the next two chapters.

Validity of Experiments

Campbell and Stanley identified two sets of validity considerations in determining the extent to which a design achieves its objectives of approximating truth. *Internal validity* has to do with the overall integrity of the design itself in producing comparisons that actually approximate the ideals of comparison embodied in a logic like Mill's canon. *External validity* involves the extent to which the results of the study are generalizable to other relevant domains of applicability for the findings. Cook and Campbell (1979) added two more sets of validity considerations to round out the set and to address criticisms of the original formulation of Campbell and Stanley. These are *construct validity of putative causes*, following Cronbach and Meehl's (1955) classic article, and *statistical conclusion validity*. Next we briefly discuss each of these and their implications for localized inquiry.

Internal Validity. The internal validity of an experiment can be defined as the extent to which a set of comparisons between groups can be trusted to yield sound results, based on the degree to which the comparisons logically eliminate, or reveal, the impact of problematic influences other than those central to the experiment. In effect, Campbell and Stanley took on the problem of induction and addressed the weaknesses of design by identifying and directly controlling classes of hypotheses that are extraneous to the research problem of interest.

These extraneous phenomena usually are called *confounding variables.* If they cannot be ruled out by their measurement or elimination in a research design, the design is lethally flawed. From the standpoint of the experiment being a strong consensual test of the truth of a proposition, a lethal error means that one simply cannot know whether the results are a function of the accuracy of the scientific hypothesis or of a plausible rival hypothesis.

Clinicians may believe that a therapy works when simply measuring the patient's condition before and after the therapy and comparing the two measurements. However, science views such a finding as only suggestive, and not definitive, because it is possible that the change observed is related to something other than the treatment, such as spontaneous remission (e.g., Eysenck, 1952). If we set up an experiment in which one group of depressed patients receives a psychotherapy intervention and another does not, the internal validity question revolves around the extent to which the observed difference between the treated and untreated groups at the end of the study actually is related to the treatment as opposed to some other influence not identified in the design.

Usually any form of control group lends more credibility to a study than can be achieved without one. For example, if one worries about cases that simply are not tractable to treatment, it is highly unlikely that all such cases would be selected for the control group. Therefore, if change is observed in a treated group, but not in a reasonably similar and untreated control group, then one has a relatively stronger case for the effectiveness of the treatment than would be possible without the control group.

Campbell and Stanley identified eight possible threats that can affect internal validity and they used the extent to which these threats can be controlled in a particular research design to evaluate the design's overall internal validity. The threats to validity are: history, maturation, testing, instrumentation, statistical regression, experimental mortality, selection-maturation, and other possible interactions between the first seven. Because these design confounds raise interesting questions for local inquiry, we will discuss some of them in greater detail later in the chapter. Readers should consult Campbell and Stanley (1963) or Cook and Campbell (1979) for a complete discussion.

Threats to internal validity are handled by using group comparisons to answer questions about phenomena and about the operation of potential rival hypotheses in a great many differing research situations. Three basic operations are involved in generating these comparisons. First, comparisons can be strengthened if assignment to experimental groups is random, meaning that any given individual has equal chance of being assigned to a treatment or a control group. Statistical homogeneity between groups thus is achieved (Chapter 5), increasing the probability that the groups are comparable, and thereby reducing the probability that unknown influences are operative—such as a situation where people who would improve whether treated or not happen to be overrepresented in the treatment group for the entire course of a therapy. Second, events may be manipulated such that one group gets an intervention and another does not. Explicit manipulation ensures that the researcher is aware of exactly what happened to the participants within the time frame of the study. Third, individual results are aggregated so as to reduce the impact on the overall results of unpredictable differences in the ways individuals respond to a treatment. Particular cases may or may not improve for idiosyncratic reasons without damaging the over-all trend of the results. Moreover, aggregation improves the chances that relatively small experimental effects can be discerned over the noise created by individual differences.

Note how, in all of this, the overarching strategy is to identify how problems might flaw a design and then to proceed to rule them out by setting up appropriate conditions and comparisons among groups. This eliminative strategy not only is important in its own right for understanding how research design methodology works, but it also is a useful strategy for thinking through the integrity of a local inquiry, and the structure of one's data collection in the local clinical situation. Although a treatment episode is not a rigorous research project, one's understanding of such a local exchange is subject to the same logical considerations as a formal scientific inquiry (see below and Chapter 8).

External Validity.   External validity concerns the generalization of findings from a study to an appropriate domain of applicability. It may be exciting to find a therapy that works for depression in a particular community, but one would doubt one's findings, or at least one's understanding of them, if similar results could not be achieved in another community. There are two basic questions associated with external validity. First, can the experiment itself be repeated in a new circumstance that is within the domain of reasonably expected extension of the experimental finding (e.g., a universal learning principle should generalize to women even though initial experiments were conducted with men)? Second, do the results of the experiment generalize to a relevant nonexperimental context (e.g., does an experimental math training program generalize to the classroom)? Threats to external validity thus concern aspects of the experimental situation, such as careful testing, that may not correspond to the natural context.

Four factors were identified by Campbell and Stanley that might have delete-rious effect on external validity. These are: reactive or interaction effects of one's testing operation with the results of the study, interaction effects of selection bias and the experimental variable, reactive effects of the experimental arrangement itself, and multiple-treatment interference. We will only be able to discuss some of these below, so once again, readers are referred to Campbell and Stanley, or Cook and Campbell, for details.

In considering the generalizability of a research finding, the local clinical scientist will need to be concerned not only with the impact of the unique properties of the experimental context, but also with the unique properties of the local clinical situation. How is the local clinical situation similar to, and different from, the situation of the experiment? Cronbach (1975a, 1982) discussed the problem of generalizing from research settings to local contexts (Chapter 6). Professionals need to be on the lookout both for evidence that supports generalization and for evidence that might raise doubts about generalization.

Construct Validity of Putative Causes. Even if we design a study that has internal validity, and we believe that the variable presumed to be causal actually had a causal impact on the dependent variable, we cannot be sure that the causal mechanism works as we suppose it to work. Thus, experimenter effects (Rosenthal, 1976) or demand characteristics (Orne, 1962) of the situation can create outcomes that are inconsistent with a researcher's theory about what is happening. This domain of threats to experimental validity is grounded in Cronbach and Meehl's (1955) work on the general issue of construct validity in psychological measurement. Construct validity will be discussed in Chapter 6. Note here that, to the extent experimental arrangements do not address the construct validity question directly, other considerations, outside the experimental setting, are relevant to assessing how well this problem is handled. Often construct validity will depend on the quality of the theoretical framework surrounding and justifying the research design, and the plausibility of the linkages drawn between theoretical statements and particular operational realizations of those statements. As we will see, the same issues apply to the local clinical situation.

Statistical Conclusion Validity. Statistical conclusion validity primarily involves the problem of ruling out the hypothesis that any observed differences between experimental groups occurred simply by chance (Type I error), or conversely that an observed lack of difference between groups occurred by chance because the power of the statistical test was too low to ensure a statistically significant result if the predicted effect indeed is present (Type II error). This threat is handled by the standard statistical methods of increasing sample size, adjusting the acceptable probability of Type I error, improving the reliability of measurement devices, and so on. Given the amount of time spent in statistical significance testing, it is surprising to find that the logic of the test is perhaps the weakest in our science (e.g., Cohen, 1994) and, for psychological applications, the use of the test is among the most questionable things we do (e.g., Gigerenzer & Murray, 1987; Meehl, 1978). Although the test has a certain logical elegance, and appeals to our wish for certainty (or for the appearance of certainty), it has little direct implication for understanding local phenomena. Probabilities of events are relevant to describing groups, but random events are not random at the local level (a life-threatening illness, once present, is a fact to be managed, not a random outcome of some unspecified aggregate or universal property; there is no vulnerability or resilience—which are both aggregate properties—at the local level, just the facts of one's life and the things that come with those facts). We will discuss these issues more in the next chapter.

Falsifiability and Converging Operations

Two additional concepts are needed to round out this discussion of experimental methodology.

Falsifiability of a Theory.   In Chapter 3 we discussed how positivist positions were committed to a notion of empirical verification and how this proved to be a significant weakness. It is often assumed that, although any given observation may not itself be grounds for verifying a theory, a carefully wrought experiment, which rules out major rival hypotheses, might be. Experimental findings are often treated as though they verify particular viewpoints (e.g., that a treatment is effective for a particular condition). Unfortunately, this thinking is logically flawed insofar as the problem of induction remains, however successful and well conducted one's experiment is. This means that even a large number of successful experiments would not verify, in the strict sense, the theory that predicted their outcomes, however appealing that theory might become as a result of those experiments.

The philosopher Popper (1959) argued this point forcefully, eliminating verification as the experimental ideal for empirical science. In its place he established *falsifiability*. Arguing that there is no such thing as inductive verification, he noted that there does exist inductive falsification, as in finding the one white raven that falsifies the theory that all ravens are black. Thus, the goal of a science operating at its highest level, logically speaking, is to put theory to the test of falsification. The task is to find those conditions where the theory is most likely to fail, then to let it demonstrate empirically that it will succeed. In so doing, weak or nonfalsifiable theories, as psychoanalysis is often described to be (e.g., Grünbaum, 1983/1992), fall by the wayside, leaving only the strongest competitors in the science. The attempt to falsify theory operative in the local clinical situation is one of the strongest strategies a practitioner can implement, albeit an uncomfortable one if a favored theory fails (see Chapters 6 and 8).

Converging Operations.   Garner, Hake, and Eriksen (1956) discussed the idea of converging operations, a condition where two different theories lead to different outcome predictions for a single experiment. In this way, an experimental outcome can affirm one perspective while eliminating its rival. The problem of induction still applies to the affirmed theory, but the possibilities are reduced.

The converging operations strategy encourages the search for situations where two perspectives, which might yield different or opposite predictions, can be fruitfully pitted against one another. In particular, therapy outcome investigations have benefited from comparing different forms of treatment to one another in an approximation of converging operations.

Pitting incompatible perspectives against one another is a useful investigatory strategy for the local clinical scientist. For example, in marital cases it is often useful to assess the level of commitment in the couple by having them tell the story of their courtship. Depending on how this conversation unfolds, clues can emerge supporting the couple's fundamental love and commitment, thereby falsifying the hypotheses that they are already heading toward separation, or the converse. Although this example does not achieve the more definitive hopes of a completely convincing falsification of one theory and affirmation of another in the converging operations paradigm, it does show how this thinking can be used realistically, if somewhat more tentatively. Another example might be in assessing substance abuse by inquiring about auto accidents, accidental injuries, money difficulties, and the like. The outcome can falsify a more or less extreme version of the problem if substance abuse is present (e.g., few or no accidents suggesting a more constrained abuse than commonly found, as opposed to many), or it can raise interesting questions if substance abuse is not present (e.g., many accidents without substance abuse, or no accidents which puts the inquiry about substance usage on a different track).

Summary of the Logic of Experimental and Quasiexperimental Designs

We now have laid the groundwork for a summary statement of the basic logic of experimental design. This logic is the understory of modern science in psychology.

Experimental design starts with assumptions of order and continuity in nature, and the meaningfulness of causal or, less presumptuously speaking, functional relationships among variables. Certain conditions of similarity, dissimilarity, manipulation, and elimination of characteristics of phenomena are used to isolate causal relationships in closed systems (as discussed in Chapter 2). We assume that such closed, eliminative conditions represent a window to phenomena and relationships among phenomena that would not be available to observation were we not to arrange experimental conditions carefully. In addition, we assume that the actions associated with this experimental analysis of a problem do not significantly alter basic processes that actually occur in nature—a point of concern for Bhaskar (1978), Cronbach (1982), Manicas and Secord (1973), and others who have focused on external validity issues, and a point of support for those who argue for the ultimate validity of the experimental approach even in the face of ecological critiques (e.g., Berkowitz & Donnerstein, 1982).

Experimental units are designated to be groups in the hope of eliminating individual effects that might shroud basic lawful relationships (e.g., individual differences or random error). This is necessary particularly for effects that may not be dramatically apparent in the observations of individual cases. Group comparisons are created so as to isolate and observe the behavior of cause–effect relationships. In the ideal world, successive studies are designed to account for phenomena of interest in increasingly exacting causal terms. The ultimate goal is to achieve complete causal understanding of the roots of a phenomenon. Thus, for example, in the ideal experimental world, depression as a human phenomenon would be accounted for in all of its psychological, interpersonal, intrapsychic, and biological aspects. Even if a particular primary cause could be isolated—say a brain chemical—science would not necessarily stop until the operations of that cause on all other aspects of the condition are understood.

The Logical Importance of Randomization

As this grand scheme is to be accomplished by group comparisons, there must be some basis for clearly revealing the similarities and differences among the groups so that causal effects can be observed in a comprehensible fashion. Randomization is one remarkable device for achieving similarity among groups, which can, in turn, be manipulated to create meaningful differences for additional scrutiny. Within groups homogeneity is the background against which meaningful differences among groups are revealed. Randomization works because sufficiently large samples of cases randomly selected from a population tend to have the same statistical characteristics as the population, and therefore are considered representative of the population. Two representative samples from the same population are considered equivalent for purposes of experimental comparison, even though they might involve different people. In the logic of experimental design, with its focus on collections of individuals, the unique properties of individuals are less important than the representativeness of the sample.

Campbell and Stanley labeled designs with random assignment *true experiments* in recognition of the power of randomization to achieve representativeness and, therefore, equivalency among experimental groups. *Quasiexperiments*, in contrast, are those where all of the properties of design and careful comparison are operative, but random assignment is not possible or implemented, and therefore equivalency cannot be assumed. This latter point is important, for it is only the extent to which a design facilitates the assumption of equivalency that makes randomization, or any other aspect of good experimental design, convincing to the scientific community. Randomization can fail, and there is no way of knowing for sure that equivalency has been achieved on all of the relevant variables (Meehl, 1970). Operations like randomization only ensure that a method will tend toward statistical equivalency if it has been implemented correctly. With sufficiently large samples, or with successive replications of a controlled design, the probability of nonequivalence becomes increasingly small.

The final step in the logic is comparison of outcomes across time and between groups that differ in theoretically important ways, such as before–after, and treated–nontreated samples. Each design creates a set of conditions that imply that a causal, or more generally, independent variable has a particular effect on an outcome, or dependent variable. Conversely, if plausible rival variables, such as historical conditions, produce an outcome quite apart from a treatment (e.g., improved mood in a depression intervention study), then a good design will include possible comparisons that ensure the detection, or the elimination, of such effects. This is what is meant by achieving *control* with an experimental design. Research textbooks like Cook and Campbell (1979) or Kerlinger (1986) describe a remarkable array of designs that can be concocted from this basic logic.

EXTRAPOLATION TO LOCAL CLINICAL SCIENCE

Research design is highly developed, mature, and elegant logic for scientific work. It is subject to critiques of both a methodological and a substantive nature that we will discuss as we progress into other methodological domains in this book. Nonetheless, one must respect the advanced development and precision of the logic that has sprung from traditional scientific thought.

Direct Extrapolation as a Guide for Critical Thinking

We believe there are two broad aspects of this material instructive for the professional enterprise. First, there are the possibilities for direct application of scientific thinking to address professional questions, such as psychotherapy outcome, examination of the specifics of process in professional practices, and the examination of various forms of pathology. Even in local clinical situations there may be opportunities to arrange miniexperiments, which are more or less formal depending on the problem, where the benefits of comparison (similarity and dissimilarity), eliminative induction, and observation of causal influence can be exploited to benefit professional ends.

For example, a psychotherapist formally might examine the characteristics of her caseload, seek similarities and differences between cases, make judgments about the efficacy of the treatment in the caseload, and look for similarities and differences among the cases that might covary with the most and least successful cases. Formalizing this process as an exercise in professional development might yield information about how success is or is not achieved and thereby might set a direction for continuing education and development for the professional. It also might facilitate her ability to articulate what she does and how it works to others, and lead to hypotheses, testable in future work, about more or less subtle aspects of her approach. Obviously, randomization will not be possible in such work, and there will be limited possibilities for eliminating characteristics of cases that might lend confusion to particular questions in focus at a particular time, but, then, this is the nature of the local clinical situation. By extrapolating research thinking to that situation, we at least have a structure that operates around basic questions and that offers a framework for pursuing an inquiry. As an added benefit, such extrapolation could help professional practice move beyond the overarching structure of authority-based supervision, or exposure to experts, that currently is a primary mechanism for the propagation of professional skill. Local clinical scientific inquiry supplemental to a standard way of practicing could liberate the practitioner to find his or her own way—something he or she will do in the professional work in any case. Even more, this exploration could be articulated to colleagues and consensual decisions could be made about how to handle certain local clinical phenomena (e.g., the variety of ways poverty manifests itself and is interpreted within a clinic caseload).

Consider the more specific example of a case of depression. First, in recognizing the depression to begin with, the practitioner is engaging in a classification operation that is akin to the basic scientific operation of measurement that we will discuss in the next chapter. This is true even in situations where the clinician experiences the recognition as affective or empathic, as in cases where one suspects a masked depression exists.

How might research thinking be applied here? Consider the possibilities for control. How might a direct observation made in an intake session be related to an appropriate control situation? Clearly, we cannot clone the person to develop a perfect match, excluding only the depression, and then use this match as a comparison tool for examining the sources of the depression. Nonetheless, the exercise of thinking this through might be useful. In so doing, we might bring our general concepts of depressed and nondepressed to bear in our analysis, like the treatment and control groups in some actual studies. What are our notions about such groups, and how do these ideas actually coordinate with the scientific literature? Is this perhaps a basis for pursuing that literature in a way meaningful to our own local practice? But, apart from the cloned client metaphor, might we ask in another way what the patient is like when not depressed? Are there other times proximal to this when there was no depression, and how were things different then? These may be questions a clinician does or does not ask, but formalizing the extrapolation of research thinking to the local clinical situation provides a heuristic for justifying and extending such inquiry (see also Chapter 9). Obviously, unpacking the control-group metaphor in the local situation has enormous potential for stirring one's thinking in particular clinical instances.

Critical Questions about Phenomena Extrapolated from Research Design Thinking

Trierweiler and Stricker (1992) described another way that research thinking can be applied to local clinical science that is more directly related to standard thinking about research practices. This is to view the conceptual bases of research methodology as raising a set of critical questions for analysis, critique, and development of a local clinical inquiry. In Table 4.1 we have included and expanded Trierweiler and Stricker's list of questions raised by the various threats to the validity of experiments as discussed by Campbell and Stanley (1963) and Cook and Campbell (1979). Our approach is consistent with that of Cook and Campbell in their discussion of validity issues for quasiexperimental designs, where the power of randomization cannot be used to ensure equalizations of comparison groups. They suggest that, short of randomization, even considerations of internal validity are deductive, based on careful examination of the measurements and control existing in the particular circumstances of the research. Similarly, in the local clinical situation, careful specification of what is and is not known in a particular case can greatly facilitate deductions about the trustworthiness and accuracy of assumptions and conclusions applying to the case formulation. We have not included all of the issues that Cook and Campbell discussed, and the reader is urged to review these matters in greater detail. However, there should be enough in Table 4.1 for the reader to get a sense of how the search for critical questions in research thinking might work.

As Table 4.1 shows, contrary to the ethos of professional training that led to the separation of venues for professional and scientific training in our field, we propose a situation where research methodology is a framework for advanced scrutiny of any professional or scientific inquiry. This is particularly relevant to incisive exploration of the local clinical situation, using whatever tools are available, as opposed to bemoaning the lack of correspondence of such tools with some scientific ideal. This is not to say that a professional should not be skeptical about the yield from such tools, but only that the skepticism be applied in a fashion consistent with the realities of the clinical situation. Thus, when a clinician is confronted with an individual in pain and must work with that pain in an attempt to find out what is going on, good local science begins with that recognition and proceeds accordingly. Such empathic sensitivity and affective awareness is considered important and perhaps a significant intervention in its own right. However, it is not necessarily an endpoint in the inquiry, and it does not preclude the conscious introduction of additional scientific analysis, not necessarily focused on the pain itself, somewhere in the course of the inquiry. For example, the possibility that the pain and its expression may lead the patient to reveal some, but not other, information during therapy sessions could be of great significance to the treatment and must be considered in good scientific clinical inquiry in such a case (e.g., relationships that cause pain are mentioned, those that cause pleasure are not). Being cognizant of the insufficiency of the causal attributions that seem most apparent in the case (those following only from an internal method of tenacity, or authority based on one's standard preferences in working, or a priori beliefs untested in the local context), one can put one's beliefs to a stronger test that may confirm the original understanding or lead to something new. This is the critical and realistic consciousness that we believe is the essence of good local science.

Table 4.2 takes this a step further by showing how questions and directions for inquiry can be generated via the crossing of concerns about alternative hypotheses arising from research design traditions with the types of information available in the local clinical situation. Note how the focus on the individual case, and the particulars of local information, modify how particular competing effects should be concep-

TABLE 4.1

Examples of How Research Design Concerns Raise Important Critical Questions for the Local Clinical Scientist

Research concept	Scientific concern/research design solution	Critical question for the local clinical scientist/strategy for possible solution
		Questions based on threats to internal validity
1. History	A confounding event occurring during an experiment./Control group.	Are results of intervention due to some intervening effect unrelated to treatment, such as a job change or a change in marital status?/Inquiry into other concurrent influences on the clinical situation, interviews with significant others.
2. Maturation	Change due to the passage of time./Control group, randomization to equalize temporal influences, measurement of change.	Are maturational processes creating effects independent of the intervention? How is experience with the intervention affecting what currently is observed? Especially important in work with children, but also relevant to adults and social systems./ Developmental awareness, attention to the history of the professional relationship, assessment of change.
3. Instrumentation	Measuring instrument calibration can change from one measurement to the next./Control group.	How do standards for evaluation of an intervention change from one time to the next, including expectations for what is possible in the clinical situation? What intervention events might influence these standards? What are the implications for the intervention?
4. Statistical regression	Subjects in an extreme group often will change toward the mean purely as a result of a statistical artifact related to unreliability of measurement./Control group, improve measurement reliability, avoid selecting extremes of population.	Interventions virtually always deal with extreme groups. Are the effects observed statistically extreme for this client or for the populations the client "represents"? If so, what changes can be expected in the next measurement or observation?/ Recognize that one's observations may be temporally unreliable when extreme, avoid assumptions about temporal consistency of extreme characteristics until weight of evidence suggests no alternative.
5. Selection	Experimental subjects from a select group (e.g., volunteers) may limit the extent to which we can conclude that the observed results were due to the treatment./Control group, random assignment, measurement of possible confounding group characteristics.	Clients who seek treatment are a select group; those seeking a certain type of intervention even more select. Are observed effects due to special characteristics of these clients? Which characteristics and to what extent? How would the effectiveness of an intervention appear in an unselected sample?/What would a relevant control group be like? How does implicit selection process influence observed effects? Can interventions be modified to take such effects into account? Note which community subpopulations are selecting into one's intervention and how this impacts one's practices.
6. Mortality	A selection artifact may be created when participants drop out./Control group, randomization, identify dropouts and measure potential biases in resultant sample.	Dropouts are common in professional interventions. Too often they are taken for granted without careful consideration of the reasons they occurred./Carefully assess dropout situations, also periodically assess why clients stay with an intervention. If possible, identify community subpopulation characteristics that may contribute to dropping out, including both class and cultural diversity and attitudinal characteristics.

(continued)

TABLE 4.1 (*Continued*)

Research concept	Scientific concern/research design solution	Critical question for the local clinical scientist/strategy for possible solution
7. Ambiguity about direction of causal influence	When temporal precedence is unclear, as in many cross-sectional correlational studies, it can be difficult to determine which variable represents the cause and which the effect./Design of controlled true experiments where temporal precedence can be established.	This is a major problem in professional interventions, both in assessment of the causal influences on current status of a case and in determining the impact of interventions. Clients may offer narratives that assume causal influences that may be misleading. The temporal order of historical events may be confused and information left out. Current status may determine how the past is presented as much as the converse. Clients may influence the kind of interventions chosen by a professional, and lead the professional to believe interventions are more effective than they actually are. Conversely, interventions may also be presented as less impactful than seems to be true based on other evidence./There are no simple solutions other than careful verification of cause–effect attributions based on as many different information sources as possible, and the linkage of these different threads of information into a rich, internally consistent local theory of the case.
	Questions based on threats to eternal validity	
1. Interaction of selection and treatment	The relationship between a treatment and an outcome may be confined to the particular sample identified in the study./Expand samples to include as many different types of individuals as possible, make it easy for them to participate, randomization.	Interventions often are established in relationship to restricted samples of individuals. Understanding how an intervention works, or does not work, with different types of people is crucial to good practice./Recognize how one's mode(s) of professional intervention may combine with client characteristics to raise doubts about how case illustrations can be generalized. Conversely, establish a plausible basis for generalization by showing how similarities exist between extant and future populations for intervention.
2. Interaction of history and treatment	Historical events may serve to make a treatment effective within a particular time frame, but disallow generalization to future times./Replicate the experiment, show how similar conditions prevailed at other historical times similar to those observed in the present.	Constructionist theories suggest historical context is crucial to psychological intervention. Changing historical conditions may modify observed relationships between interventions and outcomes (e.g., longer-term work may be needed more in a traditional society to handle problems related to taboo topics such as sexuality than in a more open society; conversely, matters of discipline may be more readily handled in a more traditional context)./Seek exposure to diverse populations and contexts. Generalization of one's approach depends on a grasp of how it interacts

with historical conditions. Professionals must develop an openness to change and adaptation that is consistent with the historical context in which they operate. Adaptations should be both accommodative to the times and conservative depending on the nature of the changes and similarities existing in the population (e.g., children may not need any less adult attention in a world that expects them to achieve independence earlier than in a more contained sociohistorical context. This leads a professional to develop conceptualizations that adapt to the realities of the independence expectations while retaining a commitment to parental involvement and responsibility).

Questions based on threats to the construct validity of causal inferences

Threat		
1. Inadequate preoperational explication of constructs	Operationalization in an experiment needs to be directly linked to key properties of the theoretical constructs being examined./Explicate the conceptual and operational linkages in constructs in as much detail as possible.	Many professional operationalizations, such as the 50-minute hour—now the 40- or 45-minute hour—rarely are linked clearly to theoretical rationales of a particular intervention approach. Doing so may clarify how these arrangements can be made to enhance intervention, or to open up new strategies that might improve outcomes./Look at all operational strategies in a particular assessment and intervention domain to clarify construct–operation linkages.
2. Experimenter expectancy	Experimenters can communicate an expectation to subjects who then behave in a manner confirming the hypothesis of the experiment, but not because of the independent variable being studied./Design experiments so that experimenters are blind to desired outcomes.	Has the psychologist communicated an expectation to the client that may yield results consistent with that expectation? For example, it is not unusual to note differences in symbolism that appear in the dreams of clients in psychotherapy with therapists of different orientations./Be attentive to countertransference manifestations.
3. Hypothesis guessing within experimental conditions or demand characterstics	Subjects are not passive recipients of experimental procedures, but are active participants who think along with the experimenter, discern purposes, and often follow the demands of the experiment to behave in a certain manner./Design studies where demand characteristics are controlled or treated as an intrinsic aspect of measurement and the treatment.	Clients also are active participants. Are they following the thinking of the psychologist, discerning purposes and behaving in a manner consistent with the psychologist's expectations, regardless of the conditions surrounding the original problem? This may be one of the "common factors" in psychotherapy that help explain why vastly different approaches yield similar results./Recognize the power of persuasion as it contributes to the overall picture of psychological intervention (e.g., Frank, 1991). Work with the client to determine if conformity to therapist expectations is a desirable outcome—it may be if the therapist can conceive a desirable outcome (e.g., a child's improved school performance); it may not be if the therapist has no basis for such a conception (e.g., is this the man the patient should marry?).

TABLE 4.2
Some Examples of How Research Design Confounds Can Guide Thinking about the Local Clinical Situation

Local setting	History	Research design concern	
		Maturation	Selection
Local as instantiation of the general	Are events other than those identified in one's theoretical formulation responsible for the effects observed?	Are maturation processes, not identified or attended to in one's theoretical formulation, responsible for the observed effects?	Does this case accurately "sample" the population specified in one's theoretical formulation? If so, how? If not, with what implication?
Local culture	Are there events that might have special relevance in the client's local culture, but not identified in one's theoretical formulation, affecting observed effects?	Are maturation processes, not identified or attended to in one's theoretical formulation, interacting with, or having some special significance within, the client's local culture to produce the observed effects?	Does the local culture affect the extent to which the case is adequately represented by the major population associated with one's theoretical formulation? How and with what implications?
Locally unique	Are there particulars of the case that make certain historical events more impactful than they might otherwise be, and thereby affect the accuracy of a theoretical formulation?	Are there particulars of the manifestations of maturation processes existing in the case that affect the accuracy of a theoretical formulation?	Are there particulars of the case that affect the extent to which the case is adequately represented by the major population associated with one's theoretical formulation? How and with what implication?
Space-time specific	What exact sequence of observation/experiences lead you to notice certain effects? How do they point inductively or deductively to a theoretical formulation? Are there circumstances that rival the theory in yielding the same observational moments and their sequence in time?	Exactly how do maturational processes and those identified with one's theory converge on the exact space-time sequence of observations one has identified? Are there maturational circumstances that rival the theory in yielding the same observational moments and their sequence in time?	Exactly how do selection processes and those identified with one's theory converge on the exact space-time sequence of observations one has identified? Are there selection circumstances that rival the theory in yielding the same observational moments and their sequence in time?

tualized. The reader is invited to study Campbell and Stanley, Cook and Campbell, or some other research text to expand Table 4.2 to include other possible confounding influences. Clearly, even the most obvious case for scientific practice, that of determining that the case is an instance of a higher-level scientific classification or law, is ambiguous when the full logic of scientific analysis is considered carefully.

CONCLUSION

The logic of research is complex. Although highly developed in some respects, work still is needed in developing logical strategies for analyzing specific situations (Chapter 8). It is important for local clinical scientists to understand that traditional research designs do not provide our science with definitive knowledge, rhetoric to this effect notwithstanding. Research design is nonetheless a powerful methodological tradition that will move an inquiry forward if properly implemented, even if that movement is the discovery that favored ideas do not work as well as originally thought. To avoid this type of logical thought, because it is difficult to implement or because it does not come naturally to one's preferred style of work, is to ensure that an inquiry will not be pushed beyond the opinions of authorities and that there will be no independent means to develop, clarify, or contradict these opinions. We believe that efforts to eludicate the nature of logic in the different settings of local information can bridge the gap between the general, definitive, skeptical, and aggregate extremities of traditional research design and the need for specificity, flexibility, openness, and individuality in the local clinical situation.

Next we explore the role quantification and the theory of data play in scientific analysis in general and local contexts.

Issues in Quantitative Analysis
Foundations

> Measurement provides a precision of differentiation and definition in
> observation that can be had in no other way; mathematics provides the
> necessary means of carrying measurements through a logical development to
> their consequences without loss of their precision.
> —BORING (1929, pp. 14–15)

All professions have tools. For the psychological scientist, few have had the dominating importance of statistics. Statistical findings are often equated with reality. In this chapter, we discuss why this is true. We also will try to illuminate why practitioners tend to have a love–hate relationship with this tool of the scientific trade. We will show that the scientifically minded professional neither should be dominated by statistical versions of reality nor should ignore them. Standing in the local clinical situation, the professional is surrounded by aggregate realities as well as individual ones. These are more or less local, depending on how one bounds the inquiry. Some are revealed in direct empirical observations, others are hidden from any palpable scrutiny. Scientific research can greatly facilitate our ability to access and draw on these realities in our local formulations. By the same token, this same research can be overemphasized and distorting, creating constructions of uniformity (Kiesler, 1966) that may have no basis in local or even extended realities.

In the following we discuss some fundamentals of quantification in psychology, some fundamentals of statistical thought and measurement theory, and the use of extrapolations from quantitative thought and methods in the local clinical situation. As always, our selections in this chapter are incomplete, designed more to offer a perspective about the root logic of quantification than to provide a comprehensive portrayal. We define terminology as thoroughly and nontechnically as possible, but we must request the reader's forbearance if the discussion deals with unfamiliar material. Some background in basic quantitative applications will be necessary to appreciate fully the issues we raise here, although we suspect much can be gained even without such background. We believe this critical-pedagogical approach delves into some issues that have been underground too long in our field. They are complex, and this presentation must be considered but a beginning. Nonetheless, we hope readers will agree that the perspective engendered by the local clinical scientist model puts an interesting twist on some taken-for-granted aspects of scientific methodology.

THE STATISTICAL IMAGINATION

Statistics deal with the mathematical conceptualization, summarization, comparison, and analysis of collections or aggregates. These collections can consist of anything that can be measured; that is, anything to which a numerical designation can be meaningfully assigned. Thus, we can speak of collections of people, objects, groups of objects, events, situations, environments, and so on. It is not customary for us to think in terms of collections of objects in daily life, save in a few technical areas such as business and finance. We are especially unlikely to think in terms of aggregates in our face-to-face dealings with other people—although recently there is a trend to define inappropriately the characteristics of others in terms of group characteristics, which is in part a misapplication of the statistical thinking found widely in the media with polls, surveys, and so on (see Paulos, 1995). It is unlikely that we would invent statistical thinking ourselves, or in our work as practicing psychologists, had it not been handed down to us from other scientific disciplines, and had it not demonstrated some historical usefulness in the inquiry into human psychological phenomena. The traditional logic and usage of statistics to serve scientific ends comes to us as a product of the past two or three centuries of scientific work. As with all of the methods we will discuss, statistical tools were invented by ingenious individuals to serve certain ends, often in advancing scientific inquiry. In another sense, statistics can be seen as a branch of applied mathematics.

The point about it being unlikely that we would invent statistics is important: Consistently, in the history of statistical applications, theories based on simple single observations, or small numbers of observations—such as might be available to a professional over a lifetime of practice—become questionable when larger numbers of observations are combined.

For example, the strong link between cigarette smoking and cancer, which is taken for granted today, was denied or ignored for decades. We now attend to the link largely because years of accumulating statistical evidence, along with changing social conditions, could not be denied. At the individual level, each of us knew someone who had smoked and also seemed ill, but often there was someone who had smoked for years who seemed very healthy. Stories of individuals who have lived to their 90s and 100s while smoking heavily can be found in the news media on occasion even today. Yet, data suggesting that smoking and illness are linked have been available for quite some time. Tufte (1983) showed a powerful graphical display of the relationship between lung cancer deaths in 1950 and cigarette consumption in 1930 for several industrialized countries (p. 47). This graphic was based on data already published in 1955! The correlation plotted was .73, considerably larger than those typically found in psychological research.

This example illustrates how data can speak for themselves, even quite loudly, but it takes time for us to learn to listen. Why? Undoubtedly because we are not by nature statistical thinkers and observers (Gigerenzer, 1996; Gigerenzer & Murray, 1987; Tversky & Kahneman, 1971), and because a leap of imagination is involved in grasping how to apply statistical thinking to local problems. We turn now to some thoughts on the nature of that imagination.

FUNDAMENTALS OF QUANTIFICATION

Statistics are quantitative interpretations of observations that need to be examined as carefully as observations in any other theory of inquiry. Statistics are not esoteric tools simply to be accepted like bitter medicine from distant but wiser authorities. Certainly they can be complex, but our interest in statistics is entirely dependent on their ability to advance the interests of scientific inquiry. Let us repeat that: Statistics are only as good as their ability to enlighten our awareness and understanding of our world. Although their designers were truly brilliant logicians, there is no magic in the logic of statistics, nor in the numerical representations of data that they yield. Like so many of the valuable lessons of research methodology discussed in this book, statistics simply will not give up their secrets without effort on the part of the student—and we are all students in such pursuits. Statistical tools, as used in psychological research, are relevant to the interests of practitioners to the extent they describe the logic and justification of scientific generalization, and can shed light on how scientific findings can rationally be applied to the local clinical situation.

Why Quantify?

Some feel that quantification has been overemphasized in our field, but from a larger scientific perspective it is hard to say it has been overrated. If science is about operations that aid the process of generating consensual formulations of the nature of things, then few steps facilitate this end as effectively as does the operation of quantifying phenomena of interest. Properly implemented, quantification allows for precision in specification of phenomena and communication about them that would otherwise be impossible. Even more, quantification brings a discourse into the powerful conceptual and transformative structure of mathematics. Torgerson (1958) identified the properties of quantification as order, distance, and origin (zero point). Physical systems seem to have these properties intrinsically, and therefore quantification can be a highly useful way of abstractly representing such systems. This compatibility with the symbolic and transformative properties of mathematics is one reason behaviorists have tried to materialize psychological phenomena by focusing on physical behavior. Still, even if phenomena are not so palpable, benefit can be derived from the extension of the numerical metaphor to more abstract phenomena to the extent such extension is done carefully. If phenomena correspond well to the properties of numbers and mathematical operations, and if the quantification is done with sensitivity to the relationships between a phenomenon and its quantitative measurement, then advances in the empirical examination of the phenomenon are usually in the offing (e.g., Likert scaling; see Dawis, 1987).

Of course, phenomena do not always correspond well to basic mathematical operations, and it can be surprisingly difficult to determine when quantification has been properly implemented. Many have argued that it is a naive enamor with quantification, pressing science to focus only on the study of things quantifiable rather than things theoretically important, that has been a major problem in the advancement of psychological science (e.g., Lincoln & Guba, 1985; Manicas & Secord, 1983; Polkinghorne, 1983; Rychlak, 1981). Alternatively, one could say that it is not the quantification itself that is the problem, but rather the lack of a theoretically sound understanding of the reasons for doing so that have created these problems. We discuss qualitative approaches to research that have arisen out of this basic dissatisfaction in a later chapter. Here it is important to concentrate on the formidable power of quantification and the striking correspondence that seems to exist between properties of quantity in science and empirical observations, which continue to amaze even seasoned scientists and mathematicians (e.g., Penrose, 1989). The recognition that, when this link is working, the study of properties of numerical representations can actually lead to direct insights about the nature of other, usually physical, realities explains the enthusiasm with which psychological scientists have pursued these ends.

What Is/Are Data?

The term *data* entails two distinct meanings. The first meaning is as an overarching concept describing the empirical evidence used to draw scientific conclusions. To speak of data is to bring the entire notion of scientific inquiry and all it entails into the conversation. We collect data, broadly defined, so as to produce a body of evidence from which to generate interpretations of phenomena of interest, such as a psychiatric diagnosis. Usually this evidence is based on the transformation, or codification, of observations into a particular form, such as a diagnostic category, that summarizes it and makes it available to support various conclusions a scientist might draw.

A second meaning of *data* is as the plural for *datum*, which refers to a specific instance of an observation transformed, or reduced, for scientific analysis. This more specific and technical meaning, which entails tasks basic to any scientific research project, such as coding and data entry into a computer, is extremely important for grasping how quantification operates in science, and it specifies an aspect of scientific operations that is important for qualitative and professional inquiry as well.

It is hard to believe that so basic a notion, which is part of the taken-for-granted landscape of quantitative science, could be as complicated as it is. Yet, the theory of data is a very complex, mathematical topic that extends well beyond the scope of this presentation, as was brilliantly established by Coombs (1964) and interpreted by Runkel and McGrath (1972). At the same time, it is so fundamental that some basic ideas need to be discussed in suggesting extrapolations from quantitative science for a local clinical science.

First, note that it is easy to confuse the notion of observation in science with the notion of data. They are not equivalent and should not be treated as such, as they often are in informal conversation. Observation refers to the act of gathering information, as in watching an event, or making a numerical scale available for a respondent's report about an experience. In the latter example, the observation is the mark on the form containing the scale. Depending on the medium or mechanism for the observation, it can be very precise (as in gathering an answer to a specific question) or broad and laden with nonspecific meaning and implication (as in watching how family members interact in a family therapy session). Observation is a point of direct contact with empirical reality; the creation of data is an interpretive step beyond. Recall that in Chapter 2 we described four versions of observation that Shakow (1976) posited to be relevant to the clinical psychologist (objective, subjective, participant, and self); these differing observational modalities invite different contacts with empirical reality and different interpretations may follow.

A datum is an abstraction that operationalizes a relation between two categories or objects. The datum of a numerical scale designation is the relation presumed by the scientist to exist between the stimulus to which it refers, such as an attitude statement or a description of marital satisfaction, and the person making the designation. The *observed* numerical scale designation, then, is presumed to reflect the strength of relation existing between the two *object* points of the inquiry (e.g., person and stimulus, two persons, two stimuli, two events, two constructs). Runkel and McGrath (1972) stated the general definition as follows:

> A datum is a relation on a pair of points. More fully, a datum is a relation on a pair of points (or pair of distances) that serves to interpret an observation. (p. 257)

The points referred to here can be anything. Runkel and McGrath discussed actors, stimuli, contexts, and so on, but any category of information that is meaningfully identifiable to a scientist would apply. What is important is that interpretation of an observation involves identification of a relation.

Any statement interpreting an observation is a datum of sorts. Saying "that is a swan," as in an example discussed by Kuhn (1974), is to identify a relation between the large bird seen on the lake and the linguistic category described by the word *swan*. "The patient exhibited severe depression," is a similar interpretive statement. Traditional science has endeavored to make these basic data generating operations as precise and replicable as possible, but they are interpretations in any case. Consequently, the step of moving from direct observation to data is (1) occurring in all inquiry, whether we are aware of it or not, and (2) is always interpretive, and therefore subject to error, or at least it is not definitive, in accurately representing the empirical. This means that a given observation might support a great variety of data relationships a scientist might identify, and that the scientist must decide which are most fruitful. Runkel and McGrath suggested that observation limits what data might be possible, but will not necessarily suggest which data specifications are the best ones. Data definitions are, thus, subject to the creativity of the scientist and the theory that guides the research. In this way, recent versions of traditional science, which have moved beyond the strict positivist notions of verification, are closer to constructionist thinking than they might superficially appear to be.

Depending on the tools used to identify data-level designations (such as sorting, direct numerical estimation, collections of items on additive scales), they can be viewed as one of two types of relations: *dominance*, where one thing exceeds another or not, or *proximity*, where a hypothetical distance is seen to exist between the two points in the inquiry. Highly similar items might be represented with a short distance, whereas highly dissimilar items would be represented by a greater distance.

Coombs's (1964) *Theory of Data* classified the information value of such relations. The reader should see that book, or Runkel and McGrath (1972), for a description of this interesting methodological theory. For our purposes, this theory identifies some fundamental ways that objects are linked to constructs of interest and compared with one another. The classification identifies four broad types of data: (1) single stimulus, as when a single score for an individual is directly identified relative to some stimulus, such as a group norm (e.g., the patient exceeds the criterion for depression); (2) stimulus comparison, as when some quality of two stimuli from the same set is directly compared (e.g., patient A is more severely disturbed than patient B); (3) preferences, such as when an individual makes a preference (distance) choice between two objects (e.g., clinician X likes doing outreach work in the schools better than working in an office); and (4) similarities, such as when a respondent compares relationships (distances) between pairs of objects from the same set (e.g., two members of a friendship group show a more intimate relationship with one another than does any other pairing of members).

Runkel and McGrath (1972) outlined the assumptions required for translating observations into data, as construed in Coombs's theory. First, as we have discussed, a datum is viewed as a relation between pairs of points (note the invocation of a geometric metaphor here). Second, there is an assumption of at least one dimension of interest. Arraying points on a dimension is fundamental to quantitative thinking in taking advantage of the properties of order, distance, and origin existing in the number system. Third is the assumption that all cases in the domain of interest must be classified by the system—no points are allowed to be indeterminate. In effect, for the classification to work well, scientists must seek exhaustiveness in classifying possibilities. Of course, exhaustiveness can be achieved by reducing the size or comprehensiveness of the domain of interest thereby reducing indeterminacy of the data generation process. Some of the complaints about oversimplification in quantitative science (see Chapter 7) might be about the extent to which the domain of admissible phenomena in scientific psychology has been reduced to eliminate the indeterminacy of complex or impalpable phenomena in the service of quantifying the more material or palpable, as in physicalistic behavior. If one is seeking to use cutpoints in one's quantification, that is, to use dominance data (e.g., one thing exceeds another or a cutpoint), then we must also assume there is, fourth, a positive direction on the dimension, more or less, and fifth, that the dimension is monotonic, which is to say, having more of the quality described by the dimension will never put you below some cutpoint you have already surpassed (e.g., you can never get so sick you suddenly become healthy).

Although a complete treatment of the implications of this thinking is beyond the scope of this presentation, a brief example may help illustrate how Coombs's theory can inform professional thought and practice. Remarkably, this abstract formulation raises questions and guides thought even about the simplest aspects of professional inquiry.

Consider a diagnostic interview where a clinician is attempting to determine if the patient experiences early morning awakening, a symptom of depression. The inquiry might begin with a general question such as "How has your sleep been?" The patient might answer "Not good." *Observing* this response in effect suggests a location for the patient on a dimension of good–bad sleep. It suggests that a cut-point, at least as defined by the patient, for "good" has not been achieved. It may suggest that the patient is more proximal to sleep patterns of patients who have early morning awakening than those who do not. Note how, from his own perspective, this latter proximity relationship is not part of the patient's description of his sleep. Only the clinician will interpret at this level because only she is drawing on the comparative observation for interpretation. The clinician needs to know how this response, and its implicit cutpoint, relates to the formal diagnostic criterion cutpoint, usually as specified in the history of the clinician's training and experience. Obviously the clinician must collect more information, or observations, that determine which data are the most supportive of a yes or no answer to the question about early morning awakening. A patient who reveals that "not good" sleep means only 7 to 8 hours as opposed to the 10 preferred, is different from one who reports only getting 3 or 4 hours of sleep. This is because we have normative cutpoints operating in our assumptions about what is being said (another relation), and this will affect our observation and data collection accordingly. The patient who describes that a passion for old movies often keeps her awake is different from one who is sleeping 7 hours but finds herself roaming the house in the night thinking about her job. Either might ultimately be classified by the clinician as having early morning awakening, or not, but the data path supporting the decision—which is obviously interpretive even though the classification systems surrounding it could be quite structured—is different for each. Each step can be said to depend on a link between an observation and an interpretation, which is an act of specifying an interpretive relation. If we consider the clinician herself as a data generating instrument, then her calibration with some general strategy, such as a formal measure of depression like the Beck Depression Inventory, becomes relevant. The different types of data outlined by Coombs and by Runkel and McGrath can be a guide to analyzing these details. Although we cannot look at every question we ask in such detail, we can perhaps benefit from looking more closely at our evidence generation process as the identification of relations between points in a problem space. At a minimum, such exploration will clarify how constructs are being linked to observations in the local clinical situation (Chapter 8).

Variables and Values on Variables

If the study of groups and quantification has gone hand in hand, and if such study reduces the impact of idiosyncratic effects of observations on overall research outcomes (Chapter 4), then the idea of studying variables follows readily. Instead of looking for similarities and differences on individual exemplars of scientific constructs, we can look at groups of exemplars, arrayed on quantitative continua, and thereby reduce the likelihood that we will be led astray by misleading observations unique to a particular case. A variable is an abstraction, usually captured in a symbol such as "X," that refers to a quantity that can vary within a collection of observations. This captures the basic idea, which is essential to scientific observation, that we learn about nature via comparisons among the elements of our inquiry. When there are no differences, then it is difficult to say anything about what is going on that makes a difference. Keep in mind that this notion of varying always requires a collection of observations, and it is never defined within a single observation.

It is important to distinguish the variable from a value on a variable. Often, when we measure something, we are interested in how it compares with something else. Take temperature, for example. If the world were always 75 °F, then we would probably never have created a measurement system for outdoor temperature. Of course, we have an interest in today's specific temperature—apparently a single observation—so we can decide whether or not to wear a jacket and the like. Nonetheless, this interest is mostly defined by how it relates to other days so that we might adjust conditions accordingly. At least this is the thinking found in statistically based science. In the next chapter we will discuss work by Lamiell (1987) that suggests some other ways of construing these matters that are highly relevant to local clinical science and that makes things a bit more complicated. Great care must be taken to keep the idea of a variable, and its values in a particular instance, separate in one's thinking. As we will discuss below, this is one place where the aggregate and the individual can be thought to meet with important implications.

Basic Mathematical Operations

There are two basic mathematical (arithmetic) operations that underlie virtually all statistical devices. It is essential to have an intuitive sense of these operations for one to truly grasp how statistical tools accomplish the operational goals we attribute to them.

The Arithmetic Average

Anytime you divide the sum of a set of numerical designations by the number of designations in the set, you calculate an average, formally called a *mean* in dealing with populations and samples (see below). The major interpretation of this operation is always as a summary tending toward the middle of the distribution of measured elements. Given proper foundations like the symmetry and bell shape of a normal distribution, an average will tend to be a good numerical description of a group—although it is not always the best one—and, as such, it provides one way of characterizing how a group or shared quality can be thought to be distributed across the cases. The idea that there exists a general quality shared with some variability across all relevant cases is essential to general science considered as a statistical science. One must assume that a particular characterization of a set of cases as belonging together is adequate before numerical designations are assigned. Usually this is not a major problem. Thus, each month one's electric bill can vary up or down by some amount, and one can certainly keep track of each unique number and characterize a given year by a set of 12 monthly amounts. But it may be easier to characterize the year by the average amount, thereby facilitating comparisons with other years, and providing a useful summary of one's general usage.

Anytime one averages, the group quality is described in summary fashion. This is because the average responds to the magnitude of scores in the group and their frequency. The summing of scores for the numerator of an average in effect creates the total score value of the set; the dividing by the number of scores effectively distributes this total value across all of the scores in the set. Thus, the average of a sample can be compared with the average of other samples, which, in turn, can be compared with the population value, if that number is known. Or, one can average the averages of numerous samples, thereby getting an excellent estimate of the true population value. It can sometimes be confusing in statistical thinking about how this averaging operation is being used. We average scores from samples, but we also average deviations of scores from samples' means, products of deviations of scores from distributions of two different variables, and so on. For our purpose here the important point is that we are always summarizing groupness when we average. Never do we describe individualness, even though we might well be talking to an individual with a score on a given variable that is very much like the group average. When studying statistics, keep in mind that any division by N in any formula represents an average of scores as given in some specified group or subgroup context.

The Proportion

A second basic operation is the idea of proportion. Many statistical devices are interpretable because they are proportions, or derivations from proportions. *Webster's* defines a proportion as "the relation of one part to another or to the whole with respect to magnitude, quantity, or degree." A proportion is most interpretable when considered as a representation of a part-whole relationship.[1] Thus, two trees are of equal height when the proportion of their individual heights, that is, tree A's height divided by tree B's height, or vice versa, is 1.0. Anytime you divide a smaller number by a larger one, you make such a quantitative comparison and you will get the proportion of the smaller number in relation to the larger one on a scale of zero to one. Multiply

[1]Some distinguish proportion from the concept of *ratio*, with the former referring to part–whole representations and the latter to a more general designation of relationship in quantity between two values. Commonly, the two ideas are treated as equivalent. We use the broader designation for the term *proportion* here to emphasize that, in many statistical applications, the intent is to make decisions based on a quantitative comparison between a given value and a relevant standard, such as error variance, even in circumstances where part–whole relationships are not at issue.

that proportion by 100 and you get the percentage, which is just another way of representing the part–whole relationship described by a proportional representation. This simple idea is extremely important in the way it carries a quantitative representation of the idea of comparison: We compare the small number to the larger and generate a number that represents this comparison with precision. Statistical inference is based on such comparisons. Thus, we ask if differences in means between two groups are relatively large in relation to differences existing among people within the two groups, or we talk about proportions of variance accounted as a way of saying how we think an observed relationship between two variables works in the real world—one variable is presumed to produce or describe, as in a causal relationship, differences observed on another variable.

For example, verbal aptitude might be used to account for differences observed on a set of reading scores we have collected. In talking about variance accounted for, we might consider the reading score differences as a whole to be described, and differences related to verbal aptitude as a part for comparison. To the extent the differences correspond to one another—meaning the variables covary—the verbal aptitude measure can be said to "account" for some proportion of the variance of the reading scores. This is the thinking that goes into the ideas of correlation and of coefficient of determination, which is the square of the correlation coefficient, that one will find in basic statistics books (these are discussed in greater detail below).

Whenever we consider making comparisons in this way, it is useful to think of the numerator as the thing being considered and the denominator the standard for comparison. Thus, our whole yearly income is the standard against which to consider the amount going to taxes. In psychological research, the variance reflecting the combination of individual differences and measurement errors (within-group variance) is often the standard against which to compare between-group differences (i.e., the between-group variance; e.g., with treatment and no-treatment control groups, the F statistic in the analysis of variance is the between-treatment-group variance divided by the within-group variance, the latter of which is often called *error*). In the formula for the Pearson product-moment correlation coefficient, the observed covariation between two variables is compared with a representation of the covariation that would be observed if the correlation were perfect (i.e., 1.0) in the population. Do not be confused because such comparisons do not always run from zero to one; just the most easily interpretable ones will do so. Sometimes proportional comparisons require larger numbers to be divided by smaller numbers, and the result can be many times larger than one. For example, an F test, which is the proportion of between-group variance to within-group variance, will usually need to be considerably larger than one to be statistically significant as conventionally specified (viz., $p < .05$). When a researcher talks about comparisons of some kind, as in size of relationship, variance "accounted for," or even "statistical significance," there is usually a simple proportional comparison going on somewhere. Local inquiry requires an assessment of the descriptive adequacy of the particular comparisons implicit in the research described as they pertain to local observations. We will elaborate this point later.

Other Mathematical Operations

Basic statistics are powerful because they describe very simple ideas of summary and comparison with great precision. As long as our assumptions about the importance of populations and the value of samples in describing them hold, we can draw on the power of mathematics to facilitate the conduct of empirical research.

In addition to the arithmetic average and the proportion, keep in mind the meaning of some more fundamental ideas of arithmetic—which we actually use to generate averages and proportions, and that you probably take for granted.

1. The operation of addition involves bringing things together, in effect, a quantitative blending of elements in the inquiry where elements are metaphorically linked to one another.
2. Subtraction is an operation of taking things apart—a quantitative separation.
3. Multiplication is another type of blending where one quantitative representation magnifies another; multiplication captures the idea of two things interacting with one another.
4. Division is the process of comparing two quantitative elements, or of distributing the properties of one across the elements of the other, as in the case of the average.

These basic metaphors, as realized in the formulas for averages and proportions, provide the logical basis for using statistics in research applications. To the extent assumptions and their application are adequate, they can be very useful and difficult to argue with—the link between smoking and cancer is getting increasingly difficult to dismiss, though some still try. To the extent the assumptions and the ideas they are presumed to describe are not well linked, arguments and doubts abound even in the best of statistical worlds. These are matters critical to the local clinical scientist, because even if research results are adequate in the general case, as defined statistically, there is no assurance the conclusions drawn from them will apply simply and directly to the individual case, particularly in the open systems of practice. We will discuss how these issues pertain to specific situations later. Before doing so, we need to consider how linkages are made between observations and quantities in the fundamental operation of measurement.

Measurement

Much of the above discussion about data actually is about the scientific operation of measurement. Measurement occurs in any situation where numbers are assigned to objects or events of interest to the observer. This allows the observer to use the power of the number system to organize and analyze information. But this operation is not simply about numbers, for any classification, or any statement that assigns some meaning to an observation, object, or event, has properties that are implicitly quantitative, or at least mathematical in the logical sense. Therefore, if people say something is "good" for them, they are including this object in the set of things that are "good," implying that it is not bad—by the logic of conventional usage of language and one's set of categorizations—and they are implying that it is better than something not good, but not as good as something that is wonderful. This is generally true. To say a person is conscientious is to imply that characteristic is applicable to him, and that he has that characteristic to some extent. This characterization could be made in terms of magnitude, or simply involve a categorical identification; at a minimum, we are making a logical set classification in making such attributions (Chapter 8). Thus, we are mathematizing our experience in more or less primitive ways all of the time. The same is true when the categories being used are numbers, and this is why numerical coding is so useful as a way of assigning meaning systematically to the observations. The coding process creates operational linkages between codes that carry particular meanings and particular observations. This is the formal process of turning observations into data that are then considered as research variables.

It is important to note that measurements refer to properties of objects, rather than to the objects themselves (see Torgerson, 1958). Thus, the definition of the property being measured is important. Definitions can be *constitutive*, or framed in terms of verbal description as in a dictionary definition, or *operational*, meaning that the operations of the measurement actually define the property being measured, as in counting. Torgerson suggested that sometimes numerical measurements are more intrinsically reflective of the properties being described than at other times. He called the situation where both the constitutive and operational aspects of the definitions of a property are entailed in the numerical assignment, *fundamental measurement*. Examples of fundamental measurement are length, volume, and weight. Consider how both verbal and operational definitions are entailed in the measurement of these properties. He referred to another situation that is closer to much measurement in psychology as *measurement by fiat*. This measurement depends on a presumed, usually definitional, relationship between a concept and an observation, which is the data–observation link Coombs talked about. Thus, by fiat, answers to certain digit-span items are presumed to relate to the construct of memory. Note here how the operational aspects of the measurement do not completely capture the construct being measured, and indeed, numerous operational and constitutive possibilities exist for such a construct. We will discuss these distinctions further in the next chapter where we elaborate some of the theory of validating constructs in science.

Levels of Measurement

There are four levels of quantitative measurement (Cattell, 1944; Nunnally, 1967; Torgerson, 1958) that actually overlap with more qualitative information in an interesting way as we discuss later. These levels of measurement suggest the extent to which efforts at quantification of observations are drawing on properties of the number system. Higher levels of measurement draw on more properties and thereby admit a greater range of approaches to using quantification to organize and interpret the data.

Nominal. A number is used to assign a name or a descriptive category to an observation with no implication of order or any other property of the number system as we move from one number to another. This is basically using numbers as names. An example of this typical in research is the classification of religious preference (e.g., Catholic, Jewish, Protestant, Hindu, Islamic) where there is no implication of order or value suggested by the numerical assignment, although the sets of members belonging to each group are identified. Another example is the number assigned to the jerseys of sports players. They may come to have important symbolic meaning—and even be retired—but there is nothing in the number itself, apart from its coordination with a particular player, that gives it meaning.

Ordinal. Ordinal measurement uses both the naming and the ordering property of numbers. Thus, ranks and street addresses involve ordinal information. There is no necessary implication as to how far the distance between two addresses might be, but we do know that 209 is farther down the street than 207.

Interval. With interval measurement we truly get into the precision of quantification with the implication that the numbers describe not only rank, but also the measurement interval separating two objects; that is, how much greater or lesser the numbers and the objects to which they are assigned are presumed to be in relation to one another. If an individual is assigned an 8 on a scale of 10, he is two units less than the top score but two units greater than he would be if he were assigned a 6. This may seem simple, but we rarely consider the implications of accepting interval representation of phenomena. Adding, subtracting, and averaging scores are meaningful operations with interval-level data.

Temperature is a good example of an interval scale in that degree units are presumed to be equal in magnitude across the scale, and we must create measurement devices (thermometers) that exhibit this property within some reasonable range of errors. Note, however, that the interval difference described by a measurement device capable of registering equal units across a numerical scale, may not correspond to subjective experience of the construct measured. For example, the difference in temperature between 90 and 70 °F, or between 50 and 30 °F, may feel greater to many than the difference between 70 and 50 °F.

Ratio. The final and most powerful level of measurement is called ratio. It involves equal intervals, but there is also a *true* zero point known to exist on the scale. Temperature has a zero identified with the freezing of water, but only when we get to the theoretical level of absolute zero, where all molecular motion stops, do we have a nonarbitrary zero designation below which no measurement is meaningful. So, functionally, temperature in everyday usage has no true zero. [Water freezing can be used as a reference point, which is very important statistically, because we need to specify reference points on a distribution of numbers so as to draw comparisons among measurements. Indeed, we often use the arithmetic average (mean) to serve this reference function—see below.]

Usually, we do not have a true zero in psychological measurement, even though assumptions of equal intervals are reasonable. There is no true zero in intelligence measurement, for example—what would a score of zero mean? The existence of a true zero allows us to say how one measurement is proportionally related to some other measurement on the scale. So, the number 50 can be considered to be two-thirds of the number 75, because zero is truly zero on a simple scale of counting—say of coins in one's pocket. Consider that if negative coins were possible (credit card debt might serve this purpose), then the proportional relationship just described would be incorrect and there would be no foundational reference for deriving such proportions. We do not often have ratio scale measurement in psychology except when counting. But it is useful to understand that this is part of the measurement system and a useful possibility when it can be implemented. Proportions can be used for understanding relationships between scores because of the clarity of the foundational reference point given by a true zero. Our intuitive notions of height, for example, are grounded in this way, and this may be why a given height—say the 5' 11" individual we have seen or the person 15' tall we have not seen—can seem to be so directly comprehensible to us without any direct comparative operation.

Problems in Confusing Levels of Measurement

Great confusion can arise when these distinctions among measurements are ignored or forgotten. In the social sciences, we cannot use quantification with the same precision as in the physical sciences, because we typically do not have ratio scales or simple unambiguous measurement devices of universal applicability (e.g., all yardsticks work about equally well in all measurement circumstances; it is uncertain whether all good cognitive aptitude measures do the same). The very idea of quantity differs in significant ways between the social sciences and the physical sciences. In the social sciences, it designates a matter of degree or proximity relative to a relatively vague reference point, more than a direct empirical representation of a phenomenon (measurement by fiat). Early in our training, for example, we learn that intelligence test scores cannot be treated as simple direct representations of mental aptitude. In the physical sciences, quantity is intrinsic to the material described, often a comprehensive description of that material for most purposes, and is measurable via comparison with meaningful zero points or simple reference objects, themselves obviously reflecting the quality of interest (fundamental measurement). Consider that there can be no Bureau of Weights and Measures that contains objects defining measurement scales for personality characteristics, like extroversion, as there is for measures of mass, volume, and the like.

As we will see below and in the next chapter, there are ways of working around these problems in psychological research that have important implication for bridging the gap between our quantitative science and the local clinical situation.

FUNDAMENTALS OF STATISTICAL THINKING

We have been discussing the general problem of quantification in psychology. Now we will discuss how statistical concepts and tools are used to achieve and work with quantified observations. In reading this material, keep in mind that (1) the scientific goal of quantification and (2) the use of statistical tools are complementary but not equivalent endeavors in our science.

Discussions of statistics present the roots of statistical thinking in a variety of ways. Hayes (1981), for example, presented the more abstract mathematical formulations of probability and set theory as the foundational material and then applied these concepts to thinking about populations and sampling. Kerlinger (1986) took a similar tack in presenting the link between statistical and research design thinking. Others have started with simple properties of quantification, such as frequency distributions, or basic ideas about measurement (e.g., McNemar, 1969). Any of these approaches work, and readers might have found still others in their work with statistics. Actually, most readers probably do not recall exactly how their statistics book started. Like many mathematical topics, statistics are often presented with a kind of "this is the way it is, and no further justification is required" attitude that can actually inhibit one's grasp of how they operate as tools for scientific inquiry. It is true that statistics can stand alone as a mathematical discipline having to do with quantification of collections of entities, but the local clinical scientist can ill afford simply to take this academic material for granted in applying scientific thinking to real-world scenarios. This is why we need to spend this time working on the basic definitions of concepts such as population (see below).

Overview of the Basic Logic

The basic logic of statistical research runs as follows:

- Science is interested in general properties of an orderly nature. Therefore, it is useful to study the operation of these generalities directly by focusing our examination on collections of observations rather than on single observations.
- Statistics concerns the mathematics of collections. Probability and sampling theory, through what must be considered the magic of order in nature and its representation in abstract mathematical formulations (e.g., the law of large numbers—see below), suggest that if we draw adequate samples from a population of interest to us scientifically, the statistical properties of the sample will, most of the time, closely mirror those of the population.

- An adequate sample is a representative one; one wherein the range of relevant properties, those measured and not measured, are represented in the sample in the same proportions as they can be found in the much larger population. Randomized sampling is the means to this end. This mathematical correspondence between a good sample and a population, which can be readily demonstrated, justifies the examination of samples of manageable magnitude in an effort to understand populations that cannot be studied directly, with the looming proviso that bigger is virtually always better—up to a few thousand cases where returns from adding additional cases diminish rapidly, even in studying extremely large populations.
- On this view, the scientific task is to draw samples on variables of interest and study their statistical properties as related by inference to the population, which cannot be directly accessed but which is inferred to exist objectively as a context for the inquiry. The population, thus, is of the essence in evaluating the applicability of a research finding.

Consider now some of the assumptions involved in implementing this thinking.

Combining Observations

Statistical thinking begins with the acceptance of an assumption that observations can be meaningfully combined. This assumption, which is critically important to the entire enterprise of statistical research, is related to the problem of induction described in the previous chapter. There it was noted that we must be able to assume that successive observations are sufficiently homogeneous in important ways for their combination to be meaningful. How do we determine that observations are homogeneous? There is no easy answer to this question, and it points to the very positivist roots of our wish to have an empirical science.

Stigler (1986) discussed how this idea of combining the similar has not always been accepted in the sciences. Rather than viewing aggregation as a means for mitigating the effects of error, as we do today, it was often feared that combining observations would increase the impact of successive errors. Many psychologists and social scientists continue to have these doubts. Stigler suggested that the social sciences, not having the organizing framework of a Newtonian physics or even the control engendered by the invention of the experimental method in psychology, were particularly slow to accept the notion that combination could be fruitful.

This question about the wisdom of combining observations cuts to the heart of the problem that the professional psychologist faces in incorporating and adapting contemporary psychological science to local inquiry: Commercing with a world of complex individuals, questions arise about the appropriateness and meaning of combining observations across many individuals. Alternatively, the psychological scientist, working mostly with information in the form of aggregated summaries, finds it difficult to grasp how the professional can be so resistant to the implications of statistical findings. Science has amply demonstrated that there are some gains to be had in allowing observations to combine, and today there is no reason to question the assumption that such combination can serve to reduce error—or what might better be characterized as the impacts of ancillary differences on certain phenomena of interest—as opposed to magnify it. However, there is too little dialogue in the field about how the combination of observations in various circumstances, which is essential to the application of statistical methods, affects the acceptability of research findings within particular substantive domains and contexts for inquiry.

If we assume that all cases in a given domain are unique, or that the similarities across cases are not important, then there is little basis for combining successive observations and we would have to forgo the use of statistical tools. This has been long argued with respect to personality psychology, where there is good reason to question the extent to which characteristics·identifiable in aggregates actually capture the phenomena we associate with personality (e.g., Allport, 1967; Lamiell, 1987). Conversely, and more in line with what science in psychology has actually been like over the past few decades, there is the problem of assuming similarity without careful specification of its limits. If professionals are to use statistically based science, then we need ways of thinking about the relationship between the individual and the aggregate, the unique and the normative, that do not currently exist in the psychological literature (Chapter 6).

Defining Populations and Samples

The problem of defining populations in statistical research has received too little attention. A typical introductory textbook will spend virtually no time on this issue. Yet, the assumptions we make about populations are central to any conclusions drawn in the conduct of statistical measurement and analysis. The population is literally the universe of discourse for an inquiry; it is the domain to which one's findings are presumed to apply.

Hayes (1981) discussed how populations primarily are defined by the way they are sampled. This is an extension of thinking about operational definition; we know what the scientist means by the operations she applied in generating a sample. Of course, this action does not ensure that all is going as intended. True randomness, for example, as a means to the end of generating true representativeness in a sample, requires that all members of the populations have an equal opportunity for entry into the sample. This is almost never possible, and indeed, we almost never have the requisite list of all members of the population from which to draw the sample. Moreover, scientific research is usually concerned not only with the current sample and population, but with all future, and indeed all possible, like samples. Because we work with human populations, there are also issues about consent to participate in a study, the participant's interpretations of the experimental procedure, and the sampling of volunteers versus nonvolunteers that impact population definition.

The substantive value of research often hinges on the definition of a population.

For example, race, which is often discussed in the United States, would seem to be a clear way of designating differences between subpopulations within a geographic boundary. However, it turns out to be of questionable value when considered on a world scale (Yee, Fairchild, Weizmann, & Wyatt, 1993). Perhaps this is a case where similarities and differences, thought to exist based on a too localized observation or a premature generalization, break down when the universe of discourse is expanded. Do we really believe that our findings from statistical studies, even with large samples, actually apply to all of humanity? If so, what is the basis for such belief? Alternatively, as the discussion of the importance of culture and ethnicity increases, perhaps more differences will be found than a combinatory statistical study would suggest, even to the point where comparisons are meaningless. Making matters even more complex, the variables being studied influence the conditions under which more or less individual differences would be acceptable—attitudes, for example, are more likely to differ in important ways across cases than are some (not all) cortical functions. Thus, there is a theoretical component, too often ignored, in population studies that cannot be avoided.

It must be kept in mind just how little the statistics themselves say about these issues. Any collective to which numbers have been assigned will have means, variances, and so on; these numbers only become meaningful when placed in perspective through their definition in the theoretical basis for the study. There is some discussion in the recent psychological literature about the nature of population definitions, particularly with respect to the impact of culture on psychological phenomena (e.g., Hughes, Seidman, & Williams, 1993), and of the nature of psychiatric disorder, caseness, and so on (Jackson & Truax, 1991; Wing, Mann, Leff, & Nixon, 1978). More theory and research concerning these matters would be useful.

Clearly sample definition is an act of social construction, and an obvious point of interpretation in scientific approaches. Researchers typically try to base sample definitions on characteristics that are as obvious, observable, and general as possible. It is hard to argue with a psychological study in which the sample consists of individuals in a geographic area who can execute the data collection demands of the project and who might share other fairly obvious characteristics such as gender, race, age, and so on. These characteristics are empirical and positivistic, in the sense that we would rarely question that another could reliably identify them, and therefore, we tend to accept the implicit population definitions given in descriptions of a research sample. Moreover, we tend to accept other implicit, commonsense properties of a sample without their even being mentioned; for example, we would rarely question whether the study involved living or dead individuals, but would assume the living unless otherwise stated. Unfortunately, obviousness also is the pitfall in trying to remain only with noncontroversial sample definitions: If probably unimportant matters can be taken for granted, such as living versus deceased subjects, then it is undoubtedly true that some important ones may also be hidden in our sample specifications. For example, gender and ethnicity have often been ignored in the name of general psychological principles (Hughes et al., 1993).

The main advice to take away from this discussion is to ask a question often and with great care: What population does this sample come from? This question might draw out a number of important consequences ranging from issues of special experiences of different genders, races, and cultures, and even more for the local clinical scientist, the special samples implicit in the particulars of individual lives. For example, what of being poor but extremely physically attractive; or highly intelligent, but through the misfortunes of life also being extremely chaotic in persona and manner. Certainly, these are not representatives of populations one will readily find discussed in a journal article, but even mentioning these ideas begins to suggest hypotheses about the generic aspects of experience driven by these characteristics. This is truly inductive thinking from the ground up; the rules of populations and sampling can make us aware of the issues involved and provide schemes for thinking about what we might wish to know in light of our end of helping in the local clinical situation. By the same token, the local clinical scientist must exercise caution in generalizing from the very select and limited samples found in professional practices to any wider population.

In summary, some general statements we can make about the problem of population definition are as follows:

1. There exists a tendency in population definition toward normative definitions at a high level of abstraction, pulling for elements of generality, or prototypicality in the theoretical construct(s) comprising the definition. Usually there is an attempt to generate definitions that are directly given if possible, or empirically verifiable by some accepted (reliable and valid) means.

2. Population definition is an act of observation and scientific construction. This is where statistical studies link to the induction problems outlined earlier, and to the epistemological concerns and solutions of received view science.

3. As such, population definition is an act of inductive imagination (Chapter 4); asking a question about the nature of the population is a major step in grasping the adequacy and limits of scientific studies, and in opening one's mind to possibilities yet to be fully grasped in the natural realm.

4. Because of the practical limitations of scientific inquiry, population definition will necessarily involve the assertion of some characteristics and the ignoring, or negation, of others (Chapter 8). It is easy for scientists to fall into the methodological trap of drawing on implicit "like me" or "not like me" representations of populations, and to be unduly influenced by implicit theories. Science, both general and local, needs to do better than this by discussing issues of population definition and sampling rationale more thoroughly (Hughes et al., 1993). Local clinical scientists should make special efforts to evaluate such possibilities in their reflections on a case.

5. Much traditional research (and assessment) is oriented toward finding theoretically important and interesting general characteristics and specifying their distribution in identifiable populations. Practical conclusions of

dubious scientific credibility often follow too readily from inadequate, and incomplete population observations (e.g., coffee is good, coffee is bad, coffee does not matter!). This is a serious danger in any research that carries the mantle of scientific legitimacy, and local clinical scientists must be prepared to manage the public's appetite for certainty and simplicity that is often inappropriately fed by incomplete population studies (Paulos, 1995).

6. Population thinking is a special case of categorical logic (Chapter 8) that is related to the comparison logic discussed in Chapter 4. Similarities within and between populations can be compared. Likewise, it is assumed that samples drawn from populations are relatively more homogeneous than those drawn across populations. This may not be a valid assumption in many circumstances.

7. Population thinking can serve to reduce the influence of certain errors of logic, such as the representativeness heuristic (Kahneman, Slovic, & Tversky, 1982). Professionals often want to study issues of great specificity and power in explaining particular cases, but then they are prone to act as if specific and relatively rare issues should apply to all. Statistical thinking provides a frame for considering the tenability of such hypotheses in one's thought and reflection.

To this point we have discussed some basic assumptions in statistical logic. Next we describe how actual procedures work and how they might impact the work of the local clinical scientist.

Describing Populations and Samples

Means and Variances

Introductory statistics books often start with descriptions of means and variances and then quickly move on to other topics. Yet, from the standpoint of understanding how statistical variables might actually represent substantively interesting psychological phenomena, these simple statistical devices are of enormous importance. The local clinical scientist must have a thorough understanding of their meaning.

What the Mean Means.   Hayes (1981) described several interpretations for the mean that are useful to keep in mind for extrapolations from aggregate findings to the local clinical situation. These are essentially interpretive metaphors for linking statistical findings to substantive concerns. First, the mean can be thought of as a measure of the "center of gravity" of a distribution (p. 148). This suggests that it captures the bottom line that is common to all, and toward which all would fall (or rise) excepting for circumstances that create variation around the mean. This is clearly illustrated in thinking about genetic influences on human structure and functioning. Given consistent environmental conditions, a single gene for, say, height (assuming height were governed by a single gene) should manifest itself in a uniform manner.

Because environmental and surrounding genetic conditions are not uniform, the average may be the best way to glimpse this singular genetic influence. If conditions change, on average, this average height might change. It may be, for example, that humans are taller today because the average level of nutrition available for human consumption has increased on a world scale, even though there are people with more than they need and other people with far too little locally. Note how, in a case such as this where everyone has height and everyone eats, the problem of characterizing the population as a whole and the use of the mean as a descriptive summary seem intrinsically suited to one another. This may not be so clear in some psychological studies. For example, the assertion that everyone has a level of extroversion, which we imply to be true in measuring it, does not have the same empirical status as the assertion that everyone eats, even though the actual data for a test of extroversion may perform just fine from a statistical perspective. Note how, in this example, we are revisiting the problem of deciding when it is appropriate to combine cases and around what dimensions such a combination should be considered.

A second interpretation for the mean is as a "best guess" for scores in a distribution. This works especially well when the distribution is normal and the variance of the distribution is small. A good strategy for guessing the age of an individual in a classroom is to guess the mean age for the population of students from which the classroom is a natural sample. Given a normal distribution, the mean corresponds with the most frequent score, the mode. Therefore, the probability that any given individual will be at or near the mean (we are quite tolerant about age guesses being close) is high.

Third, the mean of a sample can be seen as a representation of the population mean. Thus, a representatively selected sample mean will frequently be close to the actual population value if the latter were measurable. If we could gather the ages of every U.S. citizen, we could calculate the average age. This is what is estimated by our sampling procedures for age. The same would be true if we were measuring self-esteem. Alternatively, we can view a sample mean as an indicator of the *expected value* of the population. In so doing, we are suggesting that it represents the average of the means we would obtain across infinite successive samplings of size N, say 2000, in the U.S. population. This way of looking at the mean suggests that there is a constraint on representatively sampled means that will limit the extent to which they can stray from a specific value that exists in the population. This constraint is called the *law of large numbers*, which basically states that with increasingly large random samples, the probability that a sample mean will diverge greatly from the expected value for the infinite samples within the population will be decreasingly slight.

Finally, we can think of the mean as the origin for the variance of a sample. This interpretation of the mean emphasizes how the mean is a relatively stable anchor around which differences among scores in a distribution can be characterized.

Indexing Difference with the Variance.   Sets of scores can be characterized in terms of the property of central tendency as described by the mean, but they also exhibit spread across the measurement scale. If the scores on a particular test can range from zero to 100 with a mean of 50, it is possible that a distribution for a particular group can be tightly packed around the mean, with virtually no scores at the high and low end of possible scores, or they can be spread out across the entire possible measurement scale. The mean value, in itself, cannot reveal which characterization is accurate; means only tell us about elevation of scores on a numerical scale, not how scores spread out across the measurement scale. This spread is most typically described by the *variance* statistic, or its square root, the *standard deviation*.

If X is a raw score in a sample and X' is the sample mean, then the variance statistic is conceptually defined by a comparison between each score and the mean ($X - X'$), which is called a *deviation score* (note that subtraction is a mathematical realization of the idea of comparison). These are squared, which weights large differences more than small ones and gets rid of negative values resulting from the comparison of Xs below the mean, and then summed, which conceptually collects them together. Finally, this *sum of squared deviations* is divided by N, the sample size. In effect, we have produced the average of the squared deviations from the mean when we calculate this variance statistic. Because it is based on squared deviations, it is a difficult number to interpret even though it is quite a precise description of the group property of spread in a particular set of scores. To aid interpretation, we take the square root of this value to get the *standard deviation* (SD), viz., a characterization of the typical deviation from the mean as defined by the mathematical operation of averaging. Note that other characterizations might be possible—we could, for example, talk about the most common or modal deviation from the mean—but we use the SD because it happens to be a reasonably precise and useful representation of spread in many cases.

Scientific research in psychology and the social sciences is thought to be the study of variance (e.g., Kerlinger, 1986). We can thank Darwin (1859/1968) and later Galton (1869/1965; Lamiell, 1995) for identifying variation itself as something to be studied in the context of the taxonomic classification and evolution of species, including humans. The act of assigning a number to an observation and subsequently of combining such measurements into distributions of scores, directly represents the similarities and differences existing among observed elements in the population. We are measuring the differences existing in the scores by anchoring our examination around a stable group characteristic like the sample mean. In so doing, we gain a basis for comparison within the group, and at a higher level, across groups. Simple notions from statistics, particularly the concept of *variance*, are directly linked to the philosophical position that all learning comes from the awareness of difference in our experience of the world, be it in physical perception (e.g., the edge of a table; Gibson, 1966) or in the attribution of motive (Bateson, 1972; Heider, 1958). The variance statistic gives us an aggregate representation of differences that exist within a sample, and that are inferred to exist in the population. It is a summary of those differences between scores in the same sense that the mean is the summary of the scores themselves. Thus, we can use it to characterize differences within and between groups.

As an aside, note that the theory of natural selection that Darwin (1859/1968) argued for so convincingly is intrinsically linked to the observation of variation. Indeed, it was variation itself that the theory of natural selection was designed to explain. Only later did variation, systematized in the variance statistic, become a method for studying something else, such as being a means of classifying groups of individuals on common properties, such as personality traits, or for examining correlational relationships among diverse classifications (variables). An interesting subtheme in the *Origin of Species* was Darwin's argument with a group he called the *systematists*, whom he described as wishing to ignore small differences—what he termed *individual difference*—as being unimportant to the larger taxonomic task of natural science. Darwin, in contrast, argued that even the tiny differences are of the essence because of what they reveal about propagation of characteristics across generations. He drew heavily on the observations of animal breeders, who were already highly advanced manipulators of these small differences in Darwin's time, to support his arguments. The point here, as we discuss later, is that the tension between broad systematic classification and the virtually infinite variation one finds in direct contact with individuals is a longstanding tension in science and of the essence in working with statistical versus nonstatistical characterizations of reality. Additionally, it is apparent that the theory of natural selection is so linked to the process of generating variation that the study of variance, in exploring the theory, would mean something quite different than in many of the contexts in which variance is used as a methodological device today. To the extent there exist incongruities between substantive theoretical questions and descriptive statistical tools, there are problems in linking scientific statistical studies to the local clinical situation, as we discuss in the next chapter.

Variances can be usefully compared between groups with different characteristics to answer scientific questions. In analysis of variance (ANOVA) we compare the variance calculated between groups of interest, say an experimental and a control group, with the variance found within groups. The within-group variance is presumed to represent errors with respect to the group analysis. This variance consists of true random errors of measurement and individual differences. If the comparison is statistically significant (defined by convention as a probability that the comparison would occur by chance with a probability of .05 or less under conditions where the null hypothesis were true), we reject the null hypothesis that they are the same and accept that they are different. From a substantive standpoint, we are saying that the difference between the groups would occur sufficiently infrequently under chance conditions that we are willing to allow that they may reflect conditions other than chance, such as a treatment actually having an effect (see also the discussion of randomness below).

For our purposes, note that it is through the comparison of variances that this system gains its substantive significance. In effect, the model suggests that group differences—as reflected in differences between means—must be large relative to differences among individuals within the groups, adjusted for sample size. Nothing is said about the actual size or theoretical significance of difference. So-called "point predictions" about the expected size of differences to be observed, based on theoretical deduction, are virtually nonexistent in psychology (Meehl, 1978). Thus, small effects, as measured on the original scale, can be statistically significant with large sample sizes, or if individual differences and error are small. Alternatively, effects must be relatively larger with small samples or large individual differences and error. Depending on how one looks at this, it can lead to worries about any trivial effect being significant, particularly with large samples, where the null hypothesis may always be rejected (e.g., Bakan, 1966; Cohen, 1994), or about the extent to which small samples make it impossible for the significance test to represent true difference even though, for substantive reasons, the null hypothesis is known to be false (Schmidt, 1992). These problems merit careful study, for nothing is as it appears to be at face value in this system; in particular, statistical significance does not in any way imply theoretical significance. Only data analyses that actually incorporate effect sizes, often represented in terms of standard deviation units of difference between groups, will allow one to interpret such effects (see Schmidt, 1992). The implication for the local clinical scientist is that there is a need to know how much change should be expected from an intervention, on average, not simply whether the effect was significant or not, and after having that information, observing how much impact can actually be attributed to the local situation, and drawing conclusions accordingly.

Examining Relationships among Variables: Correlations and Group Differences

There are two basic ways data are looked at in traditional research. Both concern the study of variance, which Kerlinger (1986) suggested is central to scientific work, and both are about the study of relationships between variables—which boils down to the study of variance shared by two variables, or more specifically, *covariance*.

Let us begin with something simple like the relationship between height and weight. Recall that, in traditional research, we are always studying aggregates, and therefore we are seeking phenomena that apply to all, or at least to many people, and scientists doubt that the study of the individual would actually answer the relevant questions in a coherent way. We collect many people together and begin by observing their heights and weights, and develop operations, such as a tape measure and a bathroom scale, to assign numbers to our observations.

The pairs of numbers for each person are called ordered pairs because when we put all of the measurements together we have pairs for each individual ordered by their attachment to that individual—call height X and weight Y. We are interested in the relationship between X and Y, so one thing we can do is to string all of the numbers out and ask if certain things are happening. What would we want to know about these numbers? Thinking in terms of high and low numbers (height and weight are both ratio scales), we can ask if high and low numbers go together across ordered pairs. More specifically, is the ordering of the high and low numbers the same if they are determined separately on each variable? If they are similar, and we have drawn an adequate statistical sample, then we can say that there is or is not a relationship between height and weight in our data. Pearson invented a more specific way to accomplish this with the product-moment correlation coefficient. This accomplishes the same thing as eyeballing our data but in a more precise manner, by allowing us to calculate a value running from minus one to plus one that indicates the kind of relationship existing between the two variables, defined in terms of both rank (ordinal) and interval properties of the data.

Although we cannot get into detail about how the correlation works here, we can outline what it tells us about our data—our ordered pairs of values on variables of interest. It starts with the relative position of each score on a variable relative to the means for all scores on the set for that variable. Then it answers a question about the extent to which that relative position is the same for the first member of the ordered pair (call it X) as it is for the second member (call it Y). Thus, using the height–weight example, if the number for the first person is relatively high on the height variable (X), meaning above the mean, is it also relatively high on the weight variable (Y), meaning above the mean for all of the weight scores? If so, and the correspondence holds across the range of scores for each variable such that high Xs correspond to high Ys and low Xs with low Ys, then we will observe a high positive correlation across all of the pairs of numbers. If the opposite is observed, where high X scores tend to be paired with low Y scores and vice versa, then we will observe a high negative correlation. If nothing systematic can be observed about the relative magnitudes on each variable across successive ordered pairs, then we will observe a correlation tending toward zero, which indicates no relationship between the variables.

The correlation should be studied carefully to be understood intuitively. Basically, it is the average cross product of the z scores, which are the raw scores on each variable expressed as a proportion of the standard deviation of that variable. A z score of 2.5 indicates a score residing 2.5 standard deviations above the mean, a z score of -1.75 is a score 1.75 SDs below the mean. If we multiply the X z scores by the Y z scores, which is what we mean by cross (X to Y) and product (multiply), then, by the rules of multiplication, positives times positive will yield positives, and negative times negatives will also yield positives. Averaging these products (i.e., dividing by the number of ordered pairs) will yield a relatively high positive number, which is our correlation. Alternatively, a high positive z times a high negative z will result in a high negative number. If this pattern holds across the ordered pairs we will sum many negative cross products and average to a high negative correlation. Positives and negatives will balance out when we get a correlation close to zero. All variations in between are possible.

There is a certain elegance to using the mean as a reference point, so that the operation of multiplication gets positive and negative values to amplify one another or to cancel themselves out mathematically, thus yielding the highly interpretable—or so it seems—Pearson product-moment correlation coefficient (typically referred to as r). This shows how correlation, as an average (and a proportion when we consider how raw scores become z scores), can only be defined across a set of scores where mean and standard deviation have been calculated to act as reference points for describing what is happening within and between the variables being correlated.

These substantive facts of the correlation, which are more important than some of the statistical facts taught in textbooks, should be studied carefully by practitioners to achieve a thorough grasp of what a scientific statement of correlation is actually saying. The correlation refers to shared variation between two variables, not some direct theoretical statement asserting a causal, structural, or functional link between them. Nor is it saying anything directly about percentage of cases likely to show certain scores on one variable given their scores on another variable. In this sense, the formal statistical relations identified in a correlation coefficient are on a different logical level than the specifically measured (quantified) relations between objects and events identified in Coombs's theory of data. It is important not to confuse these levels. Direct causal, structural, or functional links might indeed exist between the two correlated variables, but there is nothing in the correlation that guarantees this. Rather, these links are based on the theory the scientist applies, the development of which may be assisted by observing correlations among variables in various relevant contexts (Chapter 6). Also, statements about correlation never are meaningful for individuals; they would be so only if there were additional theory and observation saying that somehow the correlation directly reflects more specific intrinsic linkages between values on variables observed to actually occur within individuals. Thus, for example, height and weight have a reasonably high positive correlation in the population, and we can grasp that body mass, weight, is structurally related to metric extension in space, of which height is one measure. Correlation still does not exist within the tall individual who weighs more than others, because correlation requires multiple ordered pairs, but we take the structural mechanism of the correlation to be self-evident even at the level of the individual, both because of the absolute properties of the original measurements (see discussion of *fundamental measurement* above) and because it makes sense to allow that the covariation is indeed distributed across all ordered pairs in the set.

Still, even with these very concrete circumstances, there are important implications for the local clinical scientist. If we observe a short person who is very heavy, or a tall person who is very light, our observations are running counter to the central message of what is known to be true in the population. Such cases regularly occur in correlations that are less than perfect (Lamiell, 1987). This exemplifies, at a very mundane level, the extraordinary problems the local clinical scientist faces in grasping how to interpret a particular case in light both of direct observation and of scientific assertions about the nature of reality.

This may make us prone to generate theories that contain illusory correlations (e.g., Chapman & Chapman, 1969). Consider a relationship between self-esteem and depression. If we observe the relationship, say an inverse one, in the population, then the question is are we seeing a phenomenon in our individual that directly mirrors the mechanisms underpinning the aggregated observations in the population? Research may show that low self-esteem tends to correspond to high levels of depression, but as is typical in psychological research, the correlation might not be very high. If we observe, via formal assessment or otherwise, low self-esteem and level of depression in our individual, we still have no way of knowing that what we are observing involves the same mechanisms found in the larger population. This understanding would need to depend on other information, perhaps direct observations of the mechanism underlying the correlation via some other measurement, e.g., a study showing that the people with low self-esteem have trouble making friends and this depresses their mood. If we observe high self-esteem and high depression, the resulting ambiguity is in no way addressed by the population study, without some arbitrary decision about which to give precedence. Thus, we may look more carefully and find that an assessment of high self-esteem was incorrect, or conversely, we may wonder about the variability in ordered pairs that exists in population studies—which is never presented in quantitative research reports (e.g., what range of depression scores correspond with self-esteem scores within a given range). If we simply take for granted that the two go together, based on a priori belief or research data, we may not look more closely to see how elements of high self-esteem may be strangely linked to elements of high depression, and in wearing the blinders of this thinking, we may miss important properties unique to this individual—which would comprise an element of the variability existing in the population that is not well represented in summary population studies (Cronbach, 1975a).

Population values do allow for varying degrees of prediction across cases in the sense that predicting the ordered pair of measurements for the next case in a series of cases will conform to the central message of a reasonably strong correlation more frequently than not. Thus, such correlations may have operational policy implications relative to sets of cases and may give the impression of predicting the individual. However, short of a strong theory that substantively explains the necessary link between two measurements, such as in the height and weight example, the correlation, in itself, does not offer information about the individual case. The local clinical scientist, in bridging the local and the aggregate, must be interested in actual conjunctions of measurements in the particular case, as well as correlations that exist across many cases (Chapter 8). Unfortunately for our efforts to develop local translations of aggregate findings, these two interests are not equivalent.

These issues are complex and have important implications for the bridge between research findings and practice. Therefore, we revisit the problem of localizing the interpretation of correlations below and in Chapters 6 and 8.

The Study of Group Differences

Correlation is a way to study relationships between variables. Another way to study such relationships is to examine group differences. This is most useful when discrete groups are clearly definable, such as in a situation where we can give treatment A to one group and treatment B to another and then examine the relative efficacy of the two treatments by comparing the groups on a relevant dependent variable, such as level of depression. This is an example of experimental manipulation as described in Chapter 4. Naturally occurring grouping variables, such as sex, can also be examined for their relation to other variables, such as attitudes or interests.

We describe the issue of determining the statistical difference among groups on a dependent variable below. Before doing so, it is important to note that correlational and group difference strategies actually accomplish similar things in some cases, like looking at the same mountain from different perspectives (see also Chapter 6).

If we were studying the relationship between family discord and social skills in children, we might generate a continuous measure of family discord and correlate it with a continuous measure of social skills. Alternatively, we may become interested in distinguishing families with actual physical abuse going on from those where there is no evidence of physical abuse. If our measure of discord has physical contact scaled as an increasingly intense level of family discord, then we might divide the groups around that portion of the discord scale and examine mean difference on our social skill variable. In general this is not a good practice because some of the power of our correlational analysis can be lost in the splitting of a continuous variable into a discrete one, but this example illustrates how the two approaches are similar.

Cronbach (1957, 1975a) referred to the correlational and group differences approaches as the two disciplines of scientific psychology. We discuss this distinction in the next chapter.

To summarize, quantitative research logic depends on our ability to index relationships among variables defined as ordered pairs of scores collected across many people. Similarly, in studying differences we are studying relationships among variables defined as discrete classifications as related to dependent continuous variables. Correlation and group differences, in the sense of analysis of variance, are highly related mathematically and actually combined in a broader methodological strategy entitled the *general linear model* (Wilkinson, Hill, & Vang, 1992). Interestingly, one will hear of univariate and multivariate statistics of great variety, but no matter how complex they become, they depend on the basic ideas of correlation and group difference we have discussed above.

Statistical Inference and the Problem of Randomness

Unlike many other forms of thought, statistical thinking has a concept of error built into it, and even a way to handle the problem that error presents. This is because the notion of sampling from a population always presents the possibility that the sample is biased or distorted. This concern about whether or not properties of a sample represent the operation of chance or some more substantively interesting process is the essence of the problem of statistical conclusion validity discussed in the last chapter. From a realist standpoint, one can draw correct or incorrect statistical conclusions, and therefore, some method is needed for handling this problem. The key is to ask a question about the extent to which an observed result could have happened by chance or not.

Statistical inference involves procedures for deciding the extent to which a sample value, say a mean, should be interpreted as being a result of chance or something else, such as an experimental manipulation. This is the standard test of statistical significance. The observed value in a sample is considered against the value that would be expected by chance, the so-called null hypothesis (two group means are equal, a correlation between two variables is zero, and so on). If certain probability conditions are met, then the chance interpretation is ruled out in the particular case; if not, then chance is not ruled out.

Although this is quite an interesting model of reality for dealing with the vagaries of sampling, and it seems to endorse certain conservative values—for example, we are not going to say something is acting (as opposed to not acting) unless certain conditions of care and effect size are present within a given sample—it offers no assurances that one is making the correct choice. One can rule out the null hypothesis when it should not be ruled out (Type I error), or accept it when it should not be accepted (Type II error). Statistical inference procedures only offer a policy for proceeding; not a guarantee of accuracy or success.

As already mentioned, questions have been raised about this entire procedure and its potential deleterious impact on scientific advancement (Bakan, 1966; Cohen, 1994; Lykken, 1968; Schmidt, 1992). Although space does not permit a thorough discussion of the details here, the successes and problems associated with statistical inference raise concerns for the local clinical scientist.

First, we have already discussed how population definitions might be important in interpreting extensions of scientific findings to local circumstances. The concern about randomness in the selection process applies even in cases where population definitions are acceptable. At best, the typical sampling procedures are approximations of the ideal captured in the statistical inference model. To the extent sampling is not purely random, we are already moving outside the model (Gigerenzer & Murray, 1987). The model may be "robust" to these flaws in the aggregate, but sampling errors can play havoc on generalizations of aggregate findings to more localized groupings of cases, as when an individual is considered to be a member of what turns out to be the wrong population (e.g., a misdiagnosis). Moreover, when effects actually exist in the world, making the null hypothesis irrelevant in the first place (see Schmidt, 1992), great confusion can result in applying the significance testing model as framed in the abstract. Of course, the problem is that we usually have no way of knowing whether or not an effect actually exists, and the inferential problem does not go away because our methods, or implementations of them, are flawed.

Second, randomness has a clear definition in population sampling. That definition does not necessarily translate into an explanation at the local level. There are many events of life that are taken as random, but we must be careful about judging something to be random in a single case. Even if it is random from a broader perspective, an auto accident or a mugging will rarely be interpreted that way by the individuals involved, and even if it is, the distant emotional implications of that interpretation may not accompany it. We simply have no methodological device for handling randomness at the local level. Therefore, we must grasp how events, having random and nonrandom interpretations in the aggregate, operate within the local sphere—even to deciding explicitly the extent to which the randomness concept is applicable or has any meaning at all in a particular case.

At the same time, we must not ignore the implications for local circumstances that events recognized to be random in the aggregate may have. For example, auto accidents occur with some probability in different environments and are an unrelenting fact of life in automobiles. However irrational we may believe it to be, an individual can decide to avoid travel so as to rule out the probability of an accident. If that probability were to increase enough, none of us would drive. In areas where rates of auto accidents are high, this can become a fact of existence there—usually overestimated as with crime or any other event that can affect our thinking drastically. Understanding this aspect of local climate and culture can be very important for the local clinical scientist in understanding how individuals relate to their milieu.

Third, what we take to be random in our own experience as professionals may not be from a larger perspective. Thus, our caseloads are rarely random samples from a larger population. More likely they are subpopulations with characteristics relative to the whole that we may not be fully cognizant of. Critical thinking requires that we evaluate our direct experience in terms of its generalizability. The tendency to generalize our experience to other domains, such as the caseloads of our colleagues, must be tempered by recognition of limits on the validity of such thinking (Chapter 8).

We have now discussed the logic of some basic statistical operations as they pertain to description of population phenomena. Next we explore the logic of using applied statistics to generate and evaluate linkages between theory and aggregate data. This logic is referred to generically as *measurement theory*.

BASICS OF MEASUREMENT THEORY

Measurement theory (Allen & Yen, 1979; Nunnally, 1967) uses principles of quantification and applied statistics to generate useful tools for linking phenomena in the world to the number system. Stevens (1951) suggested that measurement is "the assignment of numerals to objects or events according to rules" (cited in Kerlinger, 1986, p. 391). As might be inferred from our earlier mention of Coombs's theory of data, we believe that this seemingly simple operation of linking phenomena to numbers is more complicated than it often appears, with striking consequences for the local clinical scientist. Kerlinger (1986) described the logic of measurement in terms of a mapping of a set of numbers onto a set of objects relevant to the research (this mapping could also be between words and objects as we shall see in the next chapter in the section on coding). The idea of *mapping* involves the generation of a one-to-one correspondence, or assignment, between the numbers and the objects of interest, be they people, words, events, or whatever. This is accomplished according to some rule, which is often implicit in circumstances where the mapping is thought to be obvious.

In having a couple fill out numerical scales describing their marital satisfaction, for example, we are allowing the research participants to accomplish the mapping directly, by using the scale to describe their answers to our various questions. An individual who responds "four" on a five-point scale describing satisfaction with the amount of time the couple spends together talking is suggesting a high, but not the highest, level of satisfaction. As Kerlinger suggested, the ultimate goal of such a mapping, which is bolstered by exploring self-report in the case of a satisfaction variable, is to have the mapping represent the reality of the situation, to the extent this is possible, given the properties of the number system (order, interval, and origin). Thus, the response of "four" should suggest greater satisfaction than a response of "three," were it possible to know the true "amount" of satisfaction for that individual. This degree of similarity between numbers and objects of interest, which Kerlinger referred to as *isomorphism*, can operate according to any of the levels of measurement described earlier. Thus, we could have isomorphism according to ranks, but not the interval properties of the numbers, and so on. Having some coherent understanding of this number–observed property link is actually how one determines the level of measurement one is working with.

In any set of measurements, it is possible for some of them to map reality correctly whereas others do not. One hopes to have more accurate representations than inaccurate ones. This depends on the precision, or reliability, of the measurement, which we discuss next. The important point is to recognize that it is the presumption of an isomorphism between properties of numbers and objects that makes the measurement meaningful. In effect, if the participant reports "four" accurately, then we must work with the numbers in ways that reflect this accuracy. Alternatively, if the report of "four" is somewhat arbitrary or an incomplete or imperfect representation of the actual condition being measured, as when it could just as easily have been "three" because the person could not make up his mind, but clearly could never have been "five," then, ideally, we would have some way to handle this level of uncertainty (this is a circumstance where grasping the reality may require an understanding of fuzzy logic; e.g., Zimmermann, 1996). Although there are no absolute ways of evaluating the degree of isomorphism between properties of numbers and situations in the real world, methods have been developed that use properties of aggregates of numbers to address this relationship indirectly.

Reliability

Reliability is the accuracy, dependability, or trustworthiness of a measurement (Cronbach, 1984; Kerlinger, 1986). The technical problem for science has been how to generate a precise quantitative characterization of this dependability. Although several approaches to this problem exist today, the basic notions about how this is accomplished in the reliability coefficient are captured in the logic of what has been termed *Classical True-Score Theory* (e.g., Allen & Yen, 1979; Nunnally, 1967). This theory consists of a set of assumptions and their extension into actual applied statistical realization in quantitative data. It is a wonderful example of how relatively abstract mathematical precision, and known properties of aggregates, can be used to generate helpful characterizations of data in the real world.

The assumptions of Classical True-Score Theory are:

1. *An observed score (X) on a test is an additive combination of a True Score (T) component for the individual and an Error (E) component. That is, X = T + E.* For example, if an individual receives a score of 84 out of 100 on an achievement test, that value might result both from the person's skill on the items (the True Score portion) and from guesses (one way of conceptualizing the Error component).

2. *Errors are assumed to be random.* Presumably, *T* is only a function of one's skill on the test. Errors, however, are not a function of anything; they are assumed to be random. In effect, this says they do not correlate with anything within a particular set of scores and are generated purely by chance. Assume a person only knew the answers to 82 items on the achievement test. This would be his True Score (*T*). If we were all-knowing about this particular testing, we would know that he guessed three items correctly that he had no knowledge about, and mistakenly circled an incorrect response on an item for which he did know the correct answer. These errors combine to give an observed score of 84, two points above the *T* in this case.

3. *The expected value of X is T.* What if we could give this individual the same test an infinite number of times without any given testing influencing the ones that follow? Because errors are random, some tests would have slightly increased scores, whereas others would have slightly decreased scores. A great many would be exactly at *T*. Thus, the mean of the infinite tests should reflect the balancing of tests where the score was elevated against those where it was depressed. Because, strictly speaking, we can never give the "same" test more than once (in the space-time local sense), we refer to the tests as *parallel*, meaning the *T* and the variance of the errors (i.e., the spread of errors on either side of the *T*s) are always the same across the successive testing.

If these assumptions are reasonable, we can make them work in scientific inquiry.

The Reliability Coefficient

We cannot give a person an infinite number of tests, and we are not all-knowing about the True Score and errors on any given test. We have only the observed scores, typically for a number of people. Statistics can indirectly index the extent to which a test is (or better, can be) an accurate reflection of a person's True Score.

Consider the ideal case where a number of people make no errors. Then the observed scores (X) would in fact *be* the True Scores, and the difference we observe among people would reflect true individual differences on whatever the test is measuring. If we gave the same people a second error-free, parallel test, we would observe the same scores. If we intercorrelated these two sets of observed scores, the correlation would be 1.0, because the pairs of z scores for each individual would be identical.

In some physical science measurement, this idealization is close to reality; it rarely is in psychological measurement. Where there are errors, the correlation on parallel tests must be less than one, because only the T components of the test can intercorrelate, errors being random. The two sets of scores should be close, however, because the hypothetical Ts are presumed to be equivalent on parallel tests. Therefore, the correlation should be high, if not perfect. Most importantly, because errors are random and cannot correlate with anything else, including other errors, we can assume that the correlation between two parallel tests actually reflects variance shared between the T components captured in each imperfect (error-ridden) testing. This correlation, then, is the reliability coefficient.

There is more to it than this: Other forms of reliability than the test–retest we have used as an example here answer somewhat different questions (e.g., internal consistency across items, interrater agreement across observers, cross-situational consistency), and there are other calculations based on somewhat different, often more specific assumptions (e.g., Cronbach's alpha; Cronbach, 1984). But the important thing here for the local clinical scientist is how aggregate phenomena are used to estimate dependability of measurements at the individual level. The larger the reliability in the aggregate, the less error there is assumed to be across the many individual testings. The standard error of measurement, which is based on the reliability (more error, lower reliability, more average error to distribute), is an averaged value distributing some of this aggregate error to each individual in the set of scores—in effect, it is a best guess for the dependability of the testing. Confidence intervals based on the standard error reflect the dependability of measurement as defined in the aggregate. Because errors are random, they should distribute themselves normally around the average, or true score, for each individual.

Note that some portion of the specificity of scores, which we have suggested is of interest to the local clinical scientist in examining the space-time specific level of local information, would be considered an element of error variance in this formulation. This has major implications for the local clinical scientist in integrating the substance of aggregated studies into practice, as we shall discuss later. Later, we also will discuss how there is reason to doubt the logic of applying the aggregate so freely in certain scientific domains, such as personality. For now, we should appreciate the elegance of the logic by which reasonable aggregate assumptions can reveal qualities and relationships (some of which should be the manifestations of enduring order in nature) of collectivities that would otherwise remain hidden to us. Once assumptions about group memberships are accepted and scores are aggregated, reasonable guesses can be made at the individual level.

Validity

Validity is even more relevant to the idea of a score reflecting some underlying reality than is reliability. Validity concerns the extent to which the variance of scores on a test reflects true differences in the property being observed among the units being studied (or, the amount of the true score variance that is related to the object being studied). The validity of a test is often characterized as the extent to which the test measures what it is supposed to measure. To reiterate something you probably have heard before and may have forgotten—or simply memorized without understanding—reliability must be established before validity can be established. In effect, if you cannot depend on the scores, they cannot tell you anything about the phenomenon that interests you. The reason is that a test must reflect enough systematic variation, so that it might correlate with itself in a reliability analysis such as the test–retest case, or it will not be able to show anything but chance correlations with something else of interest. A test cannot be more closely related to anything else than it is to itself.

Validity is indexed by the validity coefficient. This is a correlation between the test and some criterion which, according to theory, is presumed to be related to the construct measured by the test. Thus, a measure of depression might reasonably be checked against other measures of functioning, such as activity level, ability to attend to a difficult task, or quality of interpersonal relationships. The precise relationship between reliability and validity is specified in limits on the magnitude of the validity coefficient engendered by the magnitude of the reliability: The validity coefficient can be no larger than the square root of the reliability coefficient. In the validity coefficient and the *standard error of estimate*—a value that corresponds to the standard error of measurement in the reliability case and that reflects the precision with which scores on the test can predict scores on the criterion—we again see how aggregate data are used to judge measurement properties that ultimately bear on the individual case.

When we read in the literature that depressed individuals tend to make life difficult for those close to them (e.g., Coyne & Gotlib, 1983), we are, in effect, looking at a relationship reflective of the validity of the test of depression, and the scientific construct of depression, as well as learning something we may not have considered before. Additionally, if we bring this information into our practice, we should expect depressed individuals we confront to exhibit certain relationship issues with their loved ones. The accuracy of this prediction is estimated by a standard error of estimate, an average that can be calculated from the correlation observed in the research studies bearing on this issue.

There are three different methods designed for measuring the validity of a test—some would call them types of validity: content, criterion-related (concurrent and predictive), and construct validity. Content validity asks a question about how well a content domain has been sampled in the design of the test. For example, a test of achievement that concentrates only on traditional academic skills, leaving out, for example, the hard and planful work involved in successful childrearing or home maintenance, may be incompletely representing the notion of achievement as a human phenomenon. Criterion-related validity was discussed above: It is measured any time the test is correlated with some other measure that is thought to be a standard against which the test can be judged. Whether we refer to it as *concurrent* or *predictive* depends on the time that the other measure was administered. Because of the power of temporal precedence in affecting our sense of understanding, we tend to be particularly influenced by research suggesting that a test can predict criteria at some point in the future (predictive validity). Intelligence testing, following Binet, became so prominent because of its ability to predict later success in school, a goal not achieved by earlier versions of intelligence tests (e.g., Wissler, 1901/1965).

Construct validity is more complicated, and it is probably true that all other aspects of validity are special cases of the overall problem of construct validity. We discuss construct validity in some length in the next chapter, because of its importance as a general representation of science. Note that there are several other formulations of validity, which are actually special cases of the larger problem of construct validity, that involve different aspects of the overall problem of measurement in science, including convergent and discriminant validity (Campbell & Fiske, 1959), and various versions related to the ethics of the testing enterprise (Messick, 1980). These merit careful study by anyone wishing to understand the basic logic of measurement in psychology. All formulations of reliability and validity depend on a basic notion about the extent to which a measurement accurately reflects some underlying reality. Even when framed as an ethical issue, it can be seen that critiques of tests hinge on questions about what is included and excluded in the observations on which the measurements are based (Cronbach, 1975b; Messick, 1980). Also, they invariably depend on aggregate information in current formulations. There is remarkably little addressing the validity of measurements in the single case, apart from direct extrapolations from aggregate formulations. This will continue to be a major concern for the local clinical scientist.

In closing this discussion of formal measurement theory, note that, although we can estimate the reliability of a test, the test may have many validities, depending on the purpose for which it is being used (e.g., a Rorschach or an MMPI). It is rarely correct to ask if a test is valid generically, but rather, is it valid for a particular application? Similarly, rather than ask if a test is reliable or valid, it is better to ask about the extent to which it is reliable or valid for this application. Extending this thinking to the local clinical situation, the question becomes, given the demonstrated reliability or validity of a test for this application, presumably calculated in aggregate data, what is the range of possible measurement outcomes for the test in this circumstance? For example, a test that is generally reliable and valid at acceptable levels will still misclassify specific cases on occasion. The local clinical scientist needs to be ever alert for such possibilities and adjust interventions accordingly.

EXTRAPOLATIONS TO LOCAL CLINICAL SCIENCE

Consider now some possibilities for how quantitative thinking might relate to efforts to understand the local clinical situation. Then, in the next chapter, we will look at how this basic groundwork, which links interpretation to empirical observation, is related to scientific work in psychology in the classic works of Cronbach and Meehl (1955) and Lamiell (1981, 1987).

Observation Is Interpretive

Observations are not given to us in raw form, laying quietly in wait for our discovery. Nor are they completely created. Science, with its successes and failures, suggests that observations are a complex mix of structure that is effectively in the world and of perceptions and interpretations of structure that are in the head of the investigator. In their simplest form, they entail imputation of relations, as outlined above. These usually take the form of linguistic codifications that may be categorical, such as in a taxonomy, or propositional, as in a statement of a lawful relationship (Chapter 8), or narrative, as in the telling of an autobiographical story (Bruner, 1990).

Scaling and Measurement in Professional Thought

Often these relations, which are the data of our professional experience, will entail implicit quantitative implications. For example, consider one's sense of the level of pathology in observing a patient; or of skill, resourcefulness, or aptitude in assessing a child. With experience, these implicit assessments seem to come to us directly and are often implicit in our recognition of the specifics of the case. They could be measured more precisely with formal testing, as they often are. But often our guesses, based as they are in professionally informed experience, are quite accurate and testing only serves to confirm our formulations. Part of that experience involves exposure to the range and typicality of a quality (such as pathology) as it exists in a particular setting, and the ways outstanding features in our experience of a patient can be described using professional constructs. Of course, too often our guesses can be wrong or misleading, as only continual inquiry can reveal. Anytime such dimensional judgments are made, quantification is involved. We believe that, with experience, it is virtually impossible not to make such comparisons at some informal level. Even if one were to strive to avoid such thinking in the name of responding to the uniqueness of each individual case, certain patients will stand out relative to others in such a way as to force the issue.

Comparisons operating in our thinking might be with a norm or some other implicit standard, such as a local mode. In some cases it might even be meaningful to conceptualize a zero point. Is there, for example, a zero point for pathology? Or, is a norm, such as the average on any given dimension of pathology, effectively a zero point? These would seem to be questions relevant to deciding when something is nonpathological. We could rank order our caseloads on a variety of dimensions relevant to our work with them at any time. Doing this formally would probably be a useful ongoing tool for professional development. Even more, we could reflect on the extent to which nominal, ordinal, interval, or even ratio assumptions are being made in our thinking. Certain salient features of classifying cases, such as abused versus nonabused, may be treated as if interval-level measurement is involved simply in recognizing the category.

For example, a belief such as "given abuse there will be memory problems, or relationship deficits of particular types" may inappropriately lead to assumptions about magnitude of pathology that are less responsive to local observation and individual differences than would be desirable. If this thinking is dogmatically applied, it is as if the attribution of abuse moves the patient an unspecified interval distance into the realm of disturbance, without due heed to the possibility for variation both in the extent of the abuse, and its definition as such, and in the individual's response to events in the past. A problem of overgeneralized ordinality in thought arises when salient observations suggest, say, a high ranking on one dimension, such as avoidance of affect with the therapist, that is precipitously generalized to other situations or other dimensions, such as a presumption that similar highly ranked levels of avoidance exist in all relationships or in realms of creative expression (Chapter 8). Such assumptions are particularly pernicious to the extent they create a sense of false legitimacy and discourage the search for disconfirming evidence.

It is useful, via reflection, to get a conscious grasp on the quantitative, often dimensional, properties that can be implicit in one's thinking. For example, if in conducting a diagnostic interview with a patient, a clinician notices that questions about the past often are not answered directly, a number of interpretations are possible at several levels of abstraction. At first, the patient may seem evasive, noncooperative, or simply disorganized. This could become frustrating for the clinician, given the importance of anamnestic data. It may invite comparisons with other patients the clinician has seen, and representations of the patient in terms of higher-order categories associated with such patients in one's experience (the representativeness heuristic of Kahneman et al., 1982). In so doing, judgments of degree of severity, at least at an ordinal level, may follow quite readily. These judgments around the various symptoms identified by the clinician may sway him or her to make particular diagnostic decisions about the patient. In effect, the inability to get clear information about the past becomes an indicant of a symptom that then is woven into a local diagnostic theory. This is an example of instantiation of the general diagnostic category, as we outlined in the philosophical extrapolation model in Chapter 3 (see also Chapter 8).

On reflection, however, there are cases in which the direct recognition of the evasiveness and disorganization is not in itself a sufficient representation of a symptom, even though it is quite easily "scalable" on one's implicit dimensions for similar patients. For example, we have had several experiences in our own work where additional inquiry suggested that the difficulty in obtaining historical data was secondary to the interpersonal context within which the data were requested. Thus, an individual who may appear evasive may find reflection on the past to be difficult and anxiety provoking, and may actually be displaying the problematic behaviors and expressions that accompany his attempts to manage the situation of the inquiry, rather than the direct and indirect properties of the phenomenon seemingly observed by the professional. Recognition of such possibilities has, on several occasions, led us to modify a line of questioning, to seek answers to diagnostic questions in somewhat different ways, and to consider alternative and not obvious diagnoses. For example, we are aware of cases where patients who had been identified as character disordered, turned out to be better diagnosed with affective disorders (such as bipolar II) that have previously been completely unrecognized. These difficult-to-assess patients responded dramatically to lithium treatment when that possibility was seriously considered based on reinterpretation of data that were accessible, and plausible inference about data that were not (Chapter 8).

It requires imagination and effort, but each of the quantitative concepts we have discussed, and many more we have not, can be fruitfully applied to assist the analysis of problems in the local clinical situation. The job of the local clinical scientist is to understand this, and to be able to select tools with both direct and metaphoric value in assisting her thinking about existing data, and to implement the thinking in a plausible, logical fashion in an effort to advance understanding of the case and the context within which it unfolds. When base rates of particular disorders, forms of expression one encounters, and implications of particular patterns of behavior for daily functioning vary within different local contexts, the professional must adjust her thinking accordingly (Meehl & Rosen, 1955). Explicit awareness of how one is conceptualizing populations, averaging or estimating modal functioning, generating representations of spread, and managing the dialogue between the aggregate and the individual in establishing the reliability and validity of one's own work, can greatly facilitate thinking through numerous problems in the local clinical situation. In some cases, the actual collection of new, previously ignored, or unaccessed data may be possible. Where it is not, reflection, public discussion, and examination of indirect sources, such as local census data, or even exploration of the various characteristics of cases in one's own practice, may allow for valuable extrapolations.

Mathematical and Statistical Operations

Reflection on the quantitative aspects of professional thought suggests that we operate on data relations we experience in a variety of ways, adding them, weighting their importance for particular contexts, and considering them in light of implicit part–whole relations (e.g., when we consider how much a particular alcoholic patient might improve in the context of the alcoholic world in which he lives and works). Information that seems to be salient is added to a developing formulation. Rarely is information removed, even though new evidence might suggest that it should be. Removing an ongoing impression is difficult in any case. Anytime we note differences between events or people we work with, we are conducting an implicit subtraction that implies a judgment of magnitude of the difference. If we weight a piece of information such that it modifies the meaning of other successive pieces, as when a patient's conflict with her mother is seen to affect all other interactions with significant individuals, then we are carrying out an implicit multiplication that magnifies the impact of the maternal conflict. Reflecting on the mathematical-like operations implicit in our formulations can be particularly useful in assessing the adequacy of judgments of magnitude, distance (as in a marital relationship), and so on that we make in determining the properties of a case.

The idea of correlation can be confusing at the local level because, to the extent we are dealing with variables at all—and there is a clear sense in which we are not in the individual case—we are dealing with values on variables, not the variables themselves. It is important to distinguish deterministic relations (as in the soccer ball moved by a kick), or what we assume to be deterministic, from those that are more correlational and based on some sense of a relation holding in the aggregate sense of correlation. The correlation coefficient formally describes relationships between variables in collections of measured units. Such relationships may or may not be causal, and the correlation does not reveal which is true. As noted above, the correlation coefficient is undefined at the individual level.

Notions of cause and meaningful co-occurrence certainly seem a part of case formulations, but usually there is considerable unclarity about the details of what is actually thought to be true. Is the patient who describes going shopping after an argument with her mother suggesting the argument caused her to shop then, rather than at another time? Might the shopping trip have happened in any case? Do conflicts in relationships with parents cause the observed pervasive lack of confidence, merely set a context for it to manifest itself, or might the deficiency come from somewhere else, such as a patient's serious doubt about his sexual competence? As we suggested in Chapter 4, sidestepping direct causal statements while proceeding to interpret matters as if causality is assumed can be very misleading and eliminate the possibility of obtaining more decisive evidence. Local clinical scientists need to reflect on such matters to at least clarify which conjunctions (which would be values of variables in the larger frame of aggregated research) are presumed to be locally causal, and which are simply thought to coexist but not necessarily to be causally related. Coexisting conditions might set an important context for the operation of locally causal phenomena. Moreover, it is possible that phenomena correlationally but not causally related in the general case, are causally related in important ways in the local situation. For example, there might be a case where the stress of graduate school amplifies an individual's mild tendency to be obsessive about success which, in turn, leads to a level of depression and anxiety not previously experienced. A locally causal relation might exist between the obsessive tendency and depression that might not exist in another context, or in the general population. In this sense, the salient issue may involve person–environment fit (Pervin, 1980) rather than the operation of lawful relationships in populations. Clinicians who are clear about such beliefs will be in a better position to gather supportive or disconfirming evidence than they would be in simply depending on aggregate formulations or in avoiding causal speculations. On the other hand, to assume that all judgments about relatedness among characteristics observed locally need to be, or can be, affirmed in aggregate studies is to misinterpret the limits of correlational analysis seriously (Chapters 6 and 8).

Defining Locally Operative Populations

We might be more explicit about the population assumptions being made and the fit of the implicit normative description we might hold. Some individuals from the country, for example, are more like city people, and vice versa, than they are like the populations from which they originate. Some might be very average in many ways because they have important latent characteristics that have no clear context (population) within which these characteristics can express themselves. Consider, for example, the very smart person lost in an environment unable to mirror this ability in any direct way, or someone very humble and loving caught in a tense and driven career environment. Local clinical scientists need to consider the impact both of standard population definitions and differences, such as socioeconomic status, age cohort, race, and so on; and that of more subtle subpopulations that might provide meaning for individuals, either as sources of identity or as contexts within which to understand the individual's behavior and experience.

The Statistical Metaphor as a Tool for Grasping the Texture and Expanse of Human Reality

We would not be talking about local science if science did not sustain a notion about the universality of order in nature. We would not be talking about a nomothetic version of general science if people had not used imagination and data to grasp the world in the larger population sense. What is the nature of this line of thought, and how can it affect the local circumstances of professional practice?

Imagine sitting in one's home or office: Undoubtedly four walls surround, and there are probably some windows. Our sphere of understanding and direct awareness of the world is very limited to the spaces that we inhabit (e.g., Gibson, 1986). Occasionally, our senses can expand into great distances, as in vision when looking down from a mountain or across an open expanse, but usually they are quite limited. Likewise, our direct sense of humanity, its properties and possibilities, is limited to our ability to meet people and visit the great variety of places that comprise our world. Some do this relatively more frequently than others, as part of their work or recreation, whereas others have very limited exposure. Yet even the most well traveled can scarcely begin to grasp the time-extended actuality of our complex humanity.

A statistical metaphor can help us grasp common and orderly properties of very large collectivities—much larger than we could ever experience directly. In so doing, we achieve ways of looking at the world that transcend immediate circumstances, and levels of explanation that point to influences on lives and thought that would otherwise be completely beyond our recognition. Thus, to find that men and women, as groups, differ in certain spatial or visual search capacities that may be related to evolutionary development (Barkow et al., 1992), or that five major dimensions of personality description seem to account for some of the individual differences we observe in others (Wiggins, 1996), is to gain a way of viewing some of the large-scale influences on the people that surround us, and ourselves. Some of these visions will be incorrect and change with continuing scientific scrutiny. Others will not change and must be incorporated into our world views. Caution is always warranted, but it must be a caution that remains open to the real implications of scientific findings.

When we suggest that the local clinical situation is surrounded by aggregate realities as well as local ones, we suggest that there are phenomena that are general in scope (applicable to each and every member of a set of cases) and phenomena local in scope (present as a special situation in this case) that are operative simultaneously within the frame of our observations. We are to an extent like water molecules riding the ups and downs of population waves as they pass through our region. Professionals must heed these aggregate realities and link them meaningfully to local circumstances, while never assuming that one cannot be plucked from a wave that has risen too high, or from a trough that plunges too deeply below what is level and stable in society. Accepting this and grasping how quantitative tools access and describe these realities, while recognizing their limitations, is key to translating aggregate scientific findings into the local sphere. Foremost is a need to recognize how the averaging that is intrinsic to statistical research necessarily implies that there will be cases that fit well with the general trend of the data, and those that do not. The local clinical scientist needs to be able to assess this issue with respect to findings relevant to his practice.

For example, Loftus's extensive demonstration that memory narratives are fallible, potentially misleading representations of the events they reference suggests the possibility of distortions in memory that might not otherwise be considered. These possibilities must be assessed in the local clinical situation. By the same token, this research does not exhaustively specify the limits of all memory phenomena—and no one ever has suggested that it does. There are limits on the generalizability of any research program. Therefore, it must be recognized that some memories and aspects of memories will be accurate even in the presence of distortion, and, in some cases, distortion may not exist. Reflecting on the variability of results described in such studies (e.g., by looking at the variance of the dependent variables) and the ecological conditions existing in such experiments, as compared with those prevalent in the local clinical situation, is one way of approaching this problem (e.g., Cronbach, 1982; Chapter 9). Another is to look more deeply at the literature where, for example, there may exist other pertinent aggregate evidence, such as evidence suggesting that memory narrative need not always be distorting (e.g., Geiselman, Fisher, MacKinnon, & Holland, 1985).

Reliability and Validity in the Local Sphere

The idea that interpretation and all low-level assumptions based on observation are measurements of sorts suggests that reliability and validity are always at issue. It is the professional's task to determine how they can best be addressed in the local clinical situation. Issues related to the formal quantification of observations and to their concatenation into aggregated measurements are metaphors for the more singular and isolated decisions made by the local clinical scientist in the course of an inquiry. Thus, for example, in reflecting on an observation, one can consider the types of relations being implied by a particular interpretation, be they between observations themselves, in terms of observation–interpretation (or category) relationships, or as a function of category–category relationships being applied to observations. Although it is impractical to question each and every directly given interpretation one makes in an inquiry, there are times when it becomes extremely important to reflect on and to reassess these relationships (Chapters 8 and 9).

Another way the link between aggregate and local realities might be considered is in elaborating the reliability and validity of the various types of local information that the local clinical scientist explores. For example, in identifying instances of general phenomena, such as a link between depression and disrupted interpersonal interactions, the professional might use the standard errors of measurement on key variables (for reliability of a test) and the standard errors of estimate (for validity) to consider the range of possibilities that might be true in particular cases, and use this information to guide assessment of cases at hand. If a patient shows high moderate depression on formally assessed depression, then some range of disruptions in interpersonal interactions are the expectation based on both clinical lore and research evidence (Coyne & Gotlib, 1983; Chapter 8). Descriptions falling outside this range, either too moderate or too severe, might lead the professional to more careful assessment, which would be needed to support the notion that this case has properties not captured in the aggregated findings. Still, even if the expected relationship is noted and fleshed out in the local understanding of the case, care must be taken to remain open to surprises that may have important implications for a case (e.g., a depressed individual gets along very well with everyone except those rare individuals who attempt to get intimate with him).

Reliability and validity of more local sources of information, such as those referencing local cultures, the idiographic elements of the case, and space-time local circumstances in the patient's life and in his interaction with the professional, can also be assessed reflectively using extrapolations from quantitative research methods. For example, local family cultural elements might be assessed by mentally averaging things said by different family members about a problem. In so doing, a normative tendency might become apparent to the clinician that is hidden from direct scrutiny within ongoing family routines and not stated clearly by any single family member. An example of this might be a tendency within a family to limit the range of negative emotions that can be manifested in an interaction via various adjustments in interpretation, even though there may be a considerable range of emotionality expressed across different individuals. This might further manifest itself in sessions that never quite get to the negative emotions surrounding a problem. Of course, such averaging operations may not themselves lead to fruitful analysis of a case, but, insofar as they intensify the local clinical scientist's exploration of available data, they may lead to new discoveries that might not otherwise be considered.

We will examine the reliability and validity of qualitative information in a later chapter; unique and space-time specific settings of local information generally will depend on qualitative approaches to their collection and evaluation. Still, quantitative metaphors can be very useful in establishing that the information given at this level is indeed unique, as opposed to linked to other more aggregate phenomena (e.g., a case history that sounds like the textbook version of a condition such as codependency may lead the clinician to assess carefully the reading of certain books by the patient), and in considering how unique circumstances might themselves relate to, or set a context for, the operation of more general, normative, or quantitatively scalable phenomena.

CONCLUSION

This excursion into the quantitative has barely scratched the surface of an extrapolation from quantitative methodologies and from quantitative research to the local clinical situation. Our main messages here are (1) that such a reflective extrapolation is a possible and informative tool for professional thought and (2) that understanding the basics of the quantification process is critical to any reflective process directed toward using research findings in the local clinical situation (Stricker, 1970). Practitioners must test their world views against scientific findings that are more or less successful in achieving representation of phenomena that are truly universal. Remember that statistics can be calculated on any quantified measure, and any group can have its own statistical characteristics, but not all statistical differences or relationships observed will be theoretically meaningful. Until science, which tends to be slow moving, has opportunity to do so, professionals must translate scientific findings into their own spheres of practice, and act as appropriate interpreters of the under- and overstatement that can be found in scientific and professional writing— indeed they must contribute both to science and to writing. At the same time, they must not act as if their own observation base, in itself, can ever completely represent the general; only with careful theoretical development and generalization across aggregates and individuals can that be achieved (e.g., lithium and psychotherapy have both been shown to work in their respective domains of operation in aggregate studies, and there is a vast history of local clinical evidence that has preceded and coexisted with these studies, mostly unwritten, that supports the larger scientific observation). In the next chapter we flesh this perspective out even more by looking at how quantitative issues are embedded within the larger project of scientific psychology.

6

Linking Theory and Data in the Scientific Study of Constructs and Individual Measurements

> . . . what is chance for the ignorant is no longer chance for the learned.
> Chance is only the measure of our ignorance. Fortuitous phenomena are, by
> definition, those whose laws we are ignorant of.
> —POINCARÉ (1952, p. 65)

This chapter discusses how the quantitative vision is applied in traditional science and its complex implications for the work of the local clinical scientist. Central to this vision is an attitude about the scientific importance of part–whole relationships—as between individual and the collective—methodologically expressed in the belief that aggregation sheds light on general scientific phenomena. Data from collections of cases are analyzed to examine higher-order principles that might underlie the similarities or differences observed, as defined in terms of relationships between variables. The individual case and all other aspects of specificity in science are construed as instances of the combined outcome (main effects and interactions) of general forces in nature. Direct observation of aggregates is required to achieve nomothetic, or truly general, knowledge that is reliable and valid. It is assumed that this knowledge is often difficult to view clearly in the individual case. This may be because of the prominence of error, or because lawful effects are small and only discernible when their incremental and systematic impacts can accumulate with the combining of cases relative to the random and relatively limited impacts of error.

In this chapter we review two classic discussions of this viewpoint, Cronbach and Meehl's (1955) discussion of construct validation of psychological tests and Lamiell's (1981, 1987) critique of traditional scientific approaches to the study of personality. We conclude with Cronbach's (1957, 1975a, 1982) views on the "disciplines" of scientific psychology and the implications of this material for the local clinical scientist.

SCIENCE AS A PROCESS OF VALIDATING CONSTRUCTS

Cronbach and Meehl's (1955) discussion of construct validation in psychological testing is important reading for all psychologists, not only because of its relevance for assessment, but because it is undoubtedly the single best description of the link between psychological theory and empirical data existing in the psychological literature. In light of the importance accorded quantitative data in scientific formulations, Cronbach and Meehl's discussion essentially is a treatise on the relationship between theory and empirical reality. Statistical correlations and group differences identified in the context of experimental manipulations are the primary means by which these linkages are assessed. Many clinicians, including Freud, have been at odds with this aggregated characterization of reality. Meehl (1978, 1994), who in addition to his scientific work, practices from a psychoanalytic perspective, finds no such conflict, but has been very clear about some important differences between aggregated studies and clinical formulations.

A construct is a formal name for a scientific concept. Following the verificationist leanings of logical positivism in its more tolerant received view form, Cronbach and Meehl argued that the problem of construct validation arises whenever a conclusive operational definition for a construct cannot be established. Scientific advance often depends on the acceptance and development of hypothetical constructs that cannot be simply and clearly defined in terms of observation. In a related paper, MacCorquodale and Meehl (1948) had argued that such hypothetical constructs are a necessary part of scientific progress, and that tendencies to avoid their application, which were particularly conspicuous during the 1940s and 1950s, ultimately are misguided. In further extending this line of thought, Cronbach and Meehl developed the idea that any single empirical criterion against which a test—or a theory—might be assessed is itself subject to questions about construct and methodological validity.

Thus, criterion validity, in and of itself, is an inadequate means for establishing conclusively the validity of a test because the construct validity of the criterion measure is no less in question in the validation procedure than is the test being investigated. For example, the demonstration of an inverse correlational relationship between a measure of depression and a measure of success in concentrating on a demanding task would be suggestive, but not conclusive, evidence for the validity of the depression measure and, indeed, for the criterion measure itself. Additionally, it would be one step in enhancing the confidence in the theory that suggested the possibility for such a relationship in the first place. Rather than viewing such criterion-related validity as definitive, Cronbach and Meehl suggested that a singular focus on specific criteria is a temporary means to the end of validating a hypothetical construct. Ultimately, the validity of the construct depends on its usefulness and staying power within a larger network of scientific relationships that Cronbach and Meehl termed a *nomological net*.

Consider a concept like intelligence, defined constitutively as an aptitude and operationally in terms of an IQ test, which in turn is made up of other subtests such as digit span and vocabulary. In the logic of construct validation, the construct of intelligence gets its meaning by virtue of a set of theoretical relationships presumed to exist among these various subskills—such as verbal and performance abilities, which are, themselves, constructs—and a set of empirical linkages with other behaviors, skills, and characteristics. Evidence that vocabulary, digit span, number skills, and so on, intercorrelate in the population would be grounds for imputing an underlying general ability or aptitude in the population. Note that this is not a description of an individual characteristic, but a description of a population characteristic, the observation of which depends on sample information adequately representing the population.

This perspective relies on a belief that individual differences exist in nature as an outcome of underlying, lawful properties common to all in the population. In observing differences, we presumably are accessing these properties. IQ tests have seemed to measure a single construct because actual data collections show that a variety of relevant characteristics intercorrelate, and because such tests can predict other relevant phenomena such as school performance to an acceptable degree. Construct validation continues to be needed even in this highly developed area, however, because these predictions are invariably imperfect. Thus, doubt about exactly what is being measured coincides with evidence supporting the belief that something important is indeed captured by the assessments.

Construct validation proceeds as a process of "elaborating the nomological network ... or of increasing the definiteness of the components" (p. 290). Cronbach and Meehl formally defined a nomological net as an "interlocking system of laws which constitute a theory" (p. 290). These laws relate observable properties or quantities to each other, theoretical constructs to observables, or different theoretical constructs to one another. Constructs or relations that are added to the nomological net must be confirmed by empirical data or by a reduction in the number of theoretical assumptions required to predict empirical observations already established in the network.

Thus, studies supporting what is believed to be the structure of a nomological net, such as an IQ test predicting grades in high school, contribute to the overall picture being constructed at any given point in time. Those that do not, such as an experiment suggesting that attitudes do not predict behavior, raise questions about where in the net modifications are needed. Of course, as suggested in Chapter 3, matters are never as clear as simple views of science would suggest: In addition to the possibility of throwing out the entire theory in a kind of minor Kuhnian scientific revolution, researchers can raise questions about the assumptions involved in the operational definition, about the relationships between variables that were predicted by the theory to exist, about the adequacy of the measurement operations involved in the test of the theory, and so on. Usually, throwing out the theory is not the first choice in a well-established area, and as one considers the complexities and interdependencies of theoretical and operational definitions in a given finding, the difficulty in simply discrediting a theory becomes increasingly evident. For example, despite many years of controversy about mental testing (Cronbach, 1975b), which continues today, the basic structure of testing remains intact and shows no signs that it will be eliminated.

Unfortunately, history suggests that clinging to a theory can be a mistake. For example, the Ptolemaic geocentric theory of cosmology depended on an ad hoc hypothesis about the existence of epicycles (smaller orbits centered on a point that in turn orbits the earth) in planetary orbits (e.g., Bynum et al., 1981). This arbitrary "explanation" of observed planetary behavior, which was not supplanted for 1400 years, shows the extent to which people will go to preserve a flawed theory. The local clinical scientist must guard against the inclination to construct ad hoc hypotheses in an effort to maintain a favored theory. Indeed, the more favored a theory is, the more severely it should be tested (Chapters 8 and 9).

Linking Theory and Aggregated Data

One major contribution of Cronbach and Meehl's work was to establish a place both for theory and for empirical data in achieving valid scientific formulations. Professionals tend to be heavily involved with theory and less so with formal empirical representations of phenomena presumed to generalize to all cases. Alternatively, researchers often are biased in favor of empirical relationships—usually conceived in the statistical sense—over theoretical ones, so we often find very limited theorizing about the limits and implications of findings in empirical studies. Construct validation, although stressing the centrality of empirical studies, allows that scientific meaning occurs within a nexus of understandings, some of which are not empirical.

This vision of the overall process of scientific inquiry offers a realistic view of its complexities, unlike those that simply assume that predictive relationships among variables somehow constitute adequate evidence for the validity of a test or scientific manipulation, without a thoroughly articulated theory. In so doing, simplistic ideas about accepting or abandoning theories based on the success or failure of single studies must be rejected—even though the idea of falsifying a theory through the execution of a critical experiment (Popper, 1959) might continue to provide an ideal goal for experimental work (Chapter 4). Cronbach and Meehl noted that unexpected or negative results may be accounted for by any number of aspects of the inquiry in addition to the possibility that the theory guiding the inquiry is false. Thus, either the measurement devices employed for the predictor or criterion variable may be inadequate, or the design might be a poor or inadequate test of the hypothesis. In any case, positive findings must be viewed in light of the adequacies of the entire network in which they are embedded.

IMPLICATIONS OF THE CONSTRUCT VALIDATION PERSPECTIVE FOR THE LOCAL CLINICAL SCIENTIST

Cronbach and Meehl's work provides an important framework to guide critical thinking in any scientific context, including the local (see also Cronbach, 1982). (We

will discuss some other frameworks for inquiry in Chapter 9.) The construct validation model raises the following issues for our consideration:

A Tool for Critical Analysis of Psychological Research

Construct validation is a framework for considering the integrity of a scientific
report, be it theoretical or empirical. In evaluating a report, the local clinical scientist
should consider how well the nomological net surrounding the study is outlined and
the nature of the assumptions involved in the net. Exactly how does a theoretical
treatise relate to empirical observations one might make? What is the nature of the
supporting observations? How abstract are the inferences one must make to access the
observation base being discussed? It is also important to consider how the findings
described in the report logically link to the empirical realities of practice. Is there a
clear linkage between what is purported to happen in aggregates and that which can be
expected or observed to happen at the individual level? How much do the results
depend on normative assumptions that may not be uniformly distributed across target
populations? Is the theory sophisticated enough to suggest how the lawful relationships identified might operate locally? If theory is lacking, there is reason to doubt that
the researchers have an adequate understanding of what is happening. Similarly, if
straightforward links to the observational level are lacking, then there is reason to
doubt that the authors have thought through the implications of their work. We will
discuss this problem throughout the remainder of the book.

Theoretical presentations and case material can also be evaluated using the
construct validation framework. In cases where empirical phenomena are discussed,
one can examine what sorts of direct and indirect observations are relevant to the
theory (formulation) being presented. For example, a theory of repressed sexuality
may be suggested by a great many observations, including a difficulty in speaking
about sexual matters, a patient's loss of her train of thought when speaking about sex,
complete avoidance of any discussion of such issues, or by all of these observations
and more. On the other hand, some of the same difficulties may be a function of
embarrassment related to one's upbringing, of religious beliefs creating a strain for the
individual in participating fully in the therapy, or of doubts about how the therapist
will handle such a discussion. The local clinical scientist must assess the relevance of
theory and try to generate observations that are consistent with, if not confirming of,
one or more of the most promising perspectives on the material at hand, in effect
filling in a section of the larger nomological net comprising one's case formulation
(see Meehl, 1994, 1995; D. R. Peterson, 1991).

A Tool for Local Theory Development

Construct validation is a framework for considering and analyzing the integrity
of a local theory of a case. If general science operates from nomological assumptions,
then we can think of local clinical science as operating, in part, from "local-logical"
assumptions and a "local-logical" net. In considering the information elements of a

case, we might think of the meaning ascribed to various pieces of information, how they relate to one another, and how they link to empirical-like observations we have made of the case. Part of this may involve recognition of how normative findings from research studies are translated into meaningful relationships among locally generated observations. In this way, clinical judgment might be seen to involve the extrapolation of normative (or theoretical) relationships among data elements to local observations based on judgment of the meaning of the observations collected. "Good judgment" might include extrapolations that are particularly successful in revealing new or confirmatory evidence for one's case formulation. To the extent these data-gathering exercises are not operational in the standard sense (e.g., they are intuitive), they will be difficult to discuss with others, although they still might be a reliable source of information about local circumstances, if treated with proper caution (Chapter 8). For example, a clinician feeling drowsy while working with a patient may or may not be a simple function of how much sleep she has been getting. Considered in light of the ongoing interpersonal interaction and issues being raised in the case, such localized clinician experiences may be fruitful data about the patient's functioning— a theory that can be tested by attending to the contextual details of such events until enough is known to link them to other material in the session, or to reject them because it is determined that the problem originates solely in the therapist and, therefore, is irrelevant to the ongoing work.

Construct Validation Underscores the Critical Link between Theory and Data

Cronbach and Meehl stressed the need for a link to the empirical. Professional science needs to articulate how subtle expert observations and judgments are actually made in the context of the local clinical situation. There is ample reason to doubt that judgment actually operates as a statistical exercise, and any notion that it should do so (Gigerenzer & Murray, 1987; Lamiell, 1981; Lamiell & Trierweiler, 1986; Meehl, 1978). But a commitment to touching base with the space-time matrix, as Harré (1986) has called the empirical endeavor in science, is a commitment to understand, and to be able to discuss, the nature of one's empirical activities in the local clinical situation. These include efforts to identify instances of the operation of general principles; to analyze local cultures; to identify salient, unique qualities of the case, both as idiographic elements and as elements not formally linked to existing theory; and to analyze the space-time local contexts within which observation and judgment occur. The goal is to evaluate the trustworthiness of observations at each level and to assess their broader implications for the case.

The Search for Negative Evidence

Cronbach and Meehl's analysis of scientific psychological testing emphasized the importance of arranging conditions that might reveal negative evidence with respect to one's ongoing theory of the case. The importance of the search for negative evidence is pervasive in discussions of science and scientific thinking (e.g., Popper, 1959). By regularly putting theories to the falsification test—to the point of checking with a patient about one's understanding of what is being said even at a very mundane level—possibilities for enhancing the strength of theory–data linkages are greatly increased. Part of this effort must involve a critical analysis of the adequacy of a particular criterion as a test of a theory (see also Messick, 1980; Tryon, 1979).

Often, attempts to generate empirical data concerning various theoretical issues can be seen to be reasonable but not definitive tests of the theory. Thus, the failure of measures of personality traits to predict measures of behavior, to the extent sought by researchers in the 1960s and 1970s (e.g., Mischel, 1969), was an important realization, but never a definitive negation of trait theory. Important aspects of traits, such as how they represent an aspect of language usage in describing other people, were incompletely specified in the empirical operations associated with the study of consistency in human behavior. Also, new research showed that previous studies were methodologically limited (e.g., Epstein, 1983).

Presently, we are beset with a rhetorical style in scientific and clinical writing that overemphasizes simplistic, straw-man characterizations of previous scientific and clinical beliefs, too often at the expense of scholarly accuracy. Researchers and clinical scholars seek to tout the importance of their own findings, which are invariably presented as evidence for a "new" way of thinking. Perhaps such a style is needed to press home the importance of science in contemporary society. However, we suspect that more careful attention to the caution that Cronbach and Meehl encourage about the integrity of any single scientific finding or theoretical assertion, and reasonable doubt about the adequacy of any single criterion measure or empirical observation in the local clinical situation, might moderate this tendency and put our scientific conversations on a more reasonable footing.

The Analysis of Implicit Theories of Theory–Observation Linkages in the Local Clinical Situation

Cronbach and Meehl suggested that the laws identified in a nomological net may be either probabilistic (i.e., statistical) or deterministic. This is an extremely important issue for the local clinical scientist because of the difficulties involved in interpreting statistical relationships at the local level, as we discuss in detail below. A problem arises to the extent we hold assumptions about the causal nature of such relationships, even though causality may not be supported by theory or data in a nomological net. As discussed in the previous chapter, this problem is particularly prominent in extrapolating from estimates of population correlations between variables to individual cases.

We need to develop new ways of understanding how correlations observed in aggregates may operate at the local level (see below). In the physical sciences we tend to take for granted that physical properties meaningfully go together, quite apart from any association among variables observed in collections of cases. We might, for example, take the height–weight relationship for granted based on our experience of physical objects, and expect the tall person to be heavier. We can even develop a more exacting, albeit still informal, theory where we discuss the skeletal structure needed to support a particular height and show how it is necessarily heavier than one needed to support a lesser height. Because of the transparency of the mechanism involved in this relationship, theories at this level need not draw heavily on formally collected statistical information from populations to establish credibility, even though such information exists in principle. Indeed some of that information would be superfluous to the structural theory being asserted, which, itself, requires exacting measurement that must apply within individuals. In this sense, the reasoning moves from the structural assertion up to the population level rather than the other way around.

Things are not so clear with psychological variables; it is often questionable simply to apply informal theories to individual cases without evidence supporting such application. For example, suppose that family discord predicts depression in the population. We are still faced with how this affects the situation we will observe for the person or family we are working with. If we observe family discord within an individual, how do we understand how that discord relates to the depression we do, or do not, observe within that individual? Are we to assume it is causal, contextual, or simply an independent aspect of life for the individual that has no direct relationship to the clinical problem at hand? Few professionals would accept the latter, weaker interpretations of this linkage. Yet there is nothing in population correlations them- selves to clarify which interpretations are appropriate. Rather, other untested, and usually informal, theory is involved. Another prominent example is in the relationship between psychological trauma and various psychological problems such as poor self- esteem, depressive tendencies, poor interpersonal relationships, and so on. We are in a time where the relationships between trauma and psychological difficulties of various types are seen to be absolute, often without critical evaluation. If one, then so must be the other, as the thinking goes. Yet the existing statistical data are not so absolute as this, even though a relationship does exist between psychological maltreatment and psychological problems (e.g., Finkelhor, 1979), or as often observed, between ob- served psychological problems and later discovered psychological traumas (note these are not the same thing logically). Cronbach and Meehl's analysis is so important because the nomological net surrounding these issues may be more or less strong, yet scientists and clinicians will often assert them with absolute certainty—particularly when the assertions fit existing theoretical and political agendas. Each psychologist must evaluate such assertions on their own merits, and an understanding of construct validation can greatly facilitate this kind of reflection.

In summary, construct validation is a concern for practitioners because it directly addresses the linkage between theoretical formulation and empirical evidence. Con- struct validation is about relationships among constructs, and relationships among constructs and observables. Practitioners draw on constructs and research findings to guide their inquiry into particular problems. We often use constructs to talk about individuals and their lives. Whenever we do so, we, in effect, assign a value on the construct to the individuals that might be compared with other values either actually observed or implicit in our understanding of the construct(s).

Construct validation research is useful to practitioners in specifying the range and typicality of representation of phenomena as they exist in relevant populations. This is useful comparative information. However, practitioners most intensively study individuals and particularistic descriptions of individuals and events, not constructs. There is nothing in the construct validation perspective that clarifies such matters. Cronbach (1975a, 1982) and Meehl (1978) made this problem very clear in later work. To look at this problem we have to get back to the problem of measurement, which brings us to the discussion of Lamiell.

LAMIELL'S CRITIQUE OF PSYCHOLOGY'S USAGE OF QUANTIFICATION

Thus far in our discussion of quantitative approaches we have repeatedly cited Lamiell's (1981, 1987) important work on the limitations of naive applications of scientific aggregation in the study of personality. It is a line of thought that is unrelenting in its doubts about simple generalizations from aggregate studies to the individual. As such, it presents a model for some of the problems professionals face in making the extrapolative leap from the journal article to the clinical situation, and for considering how a useful and logically adequate local clinical science might be framed. It also presents a nice bridge for considering how quantitative approaches link to the qualitative approaches we consider in the next chapter.

Lamiell's (1981, 1987; Lamiell & Trierweiler, 1986) argument began with careful consideration of the stated goals of the science of personality psychology. Personality psychology is a longstanding kindred subject for clinical psychology; not surprisingly, these goals are relevant to the interests of professionals in the local clinical situation. Personality psychology was alleged to focus on the description and understanding of the personalities of individuals (Lamiell, 1987). Yet, popular methodologies for personality research involved the study of individual differences. Therefore, a question arises about the extent to which this methodological perspective serves the stated goal. Lamiell believed there is reason for serious doubt, because—as we outlined above and in the previous chapter—the statistical methods involved in individual differences research address properties of variables, which are only defined in specified groups, not in individual subjects. This creates a logical gap between the variable (data) relationships that are identified in empirical studies, and the substantive interpretive and theoretical statements personologists are fond of making about persons. In Cronbach and Meehl's (1955) terms, Lamiell identified a break in the logical chain running from the empirical/operational level to the theoretical/constitutive level. Short of direct theoretical elaboration of this gap in the nomological nets of personality studies, such elaboration itself being subject to empirical verification, there exists a serious inconsistency in the theory–data linkage that requires attention.

Lamiell viewed this gap as an impediment to the scientific advancement of the field: "whatever other difficulties the psychology of personality might have, [its] unwavering commitment to individual differences research constitutes the discipline's most fundamental problem" (Lamiell, 1987, p. 6).

This perspective may shock some, but it merits careful consideration. To the extent individual cases do not behave exactly like the central tendency of aggregate findings, there is a fundamental nonequivalence between the behavior of aggregates and that observed, or yet to be observed, among the individuals who are the participants in the inquiry. This nonequivalence creates a distance between what we interpret to be scientific generality, as defined statistically, and the specificity of the individual case. Note that the problem is not with the research goal, nor with the methods per se; one could choose to study individuals by other means, such as biographical methods (Rosenwald & Ochberg, 1992; Runyan, 1982), or could be more precise about the theoretical basis for studying individual differences, as we find in evolutionary psychological approaches (e.g., Buss, 1992; Lamiell, 1995). Rather, there are problems with the hidden extramethodological and theoretical assumptions required to support such equivalency when the two are simply taken together (Cronbach, 1975a). These assumptions are rarely considered directly. Indeed, Lamiell's discussion is the only thorough analysis of the problem existing in the psychological literature— although it harkens back to concerns that scientists held long ago about the methodological expedient of aggregating scientific data (see Allport, 1967; Lamiell, 1995; Stigler, 1986). For our purposes, these problems cannot be ignored: It is incumbent on the local clinical scientist to generate evidence for or against the direct generalization of a research finding to a particular circumstance.

Nomothetic versus Idiographic Knowing

Viewed from a somewhat different perspective, the gap identified by Lamiell has to do with the kind of knowledge one considers important for science. Allport (1961) tried to show that aggregate research was not portraying personological science comprehensively by making the distinction between nomothetic and idiographic perspectives. Allport introduced the nomothetic–idiographic distinction based on the work of the German philosopher Windelband (1904). Nomothetic perspectives involve lawful relationships applicable to all individuals. Idiographic perspectives tend to be more historiographic, involving the description and explanation of particular cases. Idiographic approaches, with their emphasis on time-extended historical narratives, are often seen to be clinical approaches, and the problem of bringing nomothetic and idiographic information together is considered a major goal for the professional (e.g., Shakow, 1976).

Lamiell recently has translated Windelband's work from the German (Windelband, 1904). When the philosopher discussed nomothetic principles, he was referring to law and lawlike constructions that identify qualities of phenomena presumed to exist universally. An example would be Newton's laws of motion, which are presumed to apply to all physical bodies in motion, however large or small they might be. Idiographic knowledge, on the other hand, refers to specific cases usually studied and understood over extended periods of time, such as the trajectory of a particular heavenly body, e.g., a comet or an asteroid, and the past and future events surrounding its movement through space and time. Windelband was clear that both perspectives were alive in significant scientific advancements. The key question here, then, is how well do statistically based psychological studies fulfill the promise of the search for nomothetic truth. Allport allowed that statistical research methods were nomothetic: They are presumed to address the common features of the many as opposed to the specifics of a given individual. It is further assumed that the most important, and verifiable, features of human personality are being identified within the aggregate, with specifics being less important (see also Meehl, 1954). This thinking treats most of the specifics of individual cases as "error," or even more loosely, as "sources of error" (see Gigerenzer & Murray, 1987).

Lamiell (1987) suggested that this is where Allport failed to get the idiographic perspective to be taken seriously by the scientific community. He argued that, with respect to the goal of individual personality description, the tools of statistical studies, in and of themselves, are not nomothetic. At best they can be used to study properties of groups, some of which may be nomothetic, but they have no interpretable meaning at the individual level.

It is difficult to accept that time-honored scientific methods might be so out of sync with the needs of professionals. There is little question that population studies can be illuminating, but we must take Lamiell's careful analysis seriously: There is a dearth of theory governing interpretation of aggregate findings at the local level, and for extrapolating from such findings to specific circumstances.

Basic Assumptions of the Individual Differences Approach to Personality and Their Implications for a Local Clinical Science

Lamiell (1981, 1987) outlined the basic assumptions of the individual differences approach to personality as follows. As we go through this material, we will discuss possible extensions and implications for inquiry in the local clinical situation. Many of these points relate to Cronbach's (1957, 1975a) important work on psychology as a scientific discipline, as we discuss later.

1. Human personality is presumed to be structured in terms of a finite number of underlying qualities (attributes, traits, temperaments) that every individual has in some amount or to some degree. A basic scientific goal is to discover these qualities and use them to classify individuals.

Similarly, clinical phenomena or intervention outcomes can be thought to be a function of an unspecified number of influences, some of which are direct or indirect, relevant or ancillary, to the primary work of the professional in the local clinical situation. The important qualities of any such phenomena are, in principle, specifiable in a finite number of such influences. Once discovered, formulations based on this structure are considered to be applicable to all similar situations.

2. It is assumed that components of this general structure can be operationally specified as variables, as dimensions, or as categories of individual differences existing in the population of interest. In strong versions of this thinking (e.g., Nunnally, 1967), aggregate approaches are viewed as the only adequate means for operationalizing an inquiry into this inferred structure.

With respect to local clinical science, components of the structure of the clinical situation can be specified in terms of variables, either as experimental treatments, in which the normative properties of a quality or intervention are emphasized, or as individual differences that serve to influence and occasionally modify how treatments function. Other phenomena observed in the clinical situation, other than treatment outcome—such as a relationship between an individual's intelligence and his or her resilience to difficult life circumstances—are similarly framed.

3. Once the generic personality structure has been identified and operationalized, it can be used to describe the personality of any given individual as coordinates within the larger structure of characteristics. Each person is measured as high on some properties and low on others relative to other individuals.

The generic structure understood to govern clinical situations also is assumed to apply to all such situations and, in principle, one could measure the extent to which certain variables are immediately operative in a specific situation. For example, a therapy can be implemented by a therapist with more or less skill, which in principle can be measured and, if need be, improved with training. Similarly, if verbal skill modifies the efficacy of an approach, that skill can be measured in particular situations as a predictor for how the treatment might unfold.

4. Relationships between variables empirically identified in the generic structure and measures of other overt behaviors (such as personality traits predicting behavior) will reflect general laws governing the relationship between properties of personality and properties of behavior. This is how the structure is presumed to be nomothetic, as opposed, say, simply to being considered a potentially relevant but inconclusive body of findings at a level of analysis different from that of primary interest to the personologist. Aggregate findings are presumed to be the last and most general word on any given topic; they are the most scientific representation of the situation possible and, therefore, they take precedence over all more idiographic representations, which are often portrayed as antiscientific.

In the clinical realm, relationships between variables identified in generic (aggregated) representations of the clinical situation (such as treatment outcome and patient characteristic variables) will reflect general laws of such matters as intervention, pathological process, and healing that influence any similar treatment of the individual cases. These laws may be deterministic or correlational as defined in the aggregate.

Implications for Methodological Practices

Lamiell (1987) provided an example of how this thinking operates at the level of the individual in discussing a central concern for personality psychology, the temporal and cross-situational consistency of personality structure. Failure to demonstrate strong temporal consistency coefficients, which are correlations among personality variables calculated across time and situation, led theorists such as Mischel (1969) to question the viability of trait psychology. Lamiell pointed out that, in this methodology, raw observations are transformed (classified) into data-level variables via a coding operation (see previous chapter). Variables are clustered according to the structure of intercorrelation that exists among them, usually via factor analysis, into higher-level personality trait variables. These correlational relationships define weights for the variables. Assessments for individuals are created by weighting variables according to their contribution to various overarching characteristics and consolidating them (usually by summing) to get overall trait scores. In turn, these scores are converted into measurements, via standardization, according to a measurement model designed to facilitate comparison relative to a chosen reference point, customarily an average calculated across a population domain of interest to the researcher (as in normative measurement models, where a single score is compared to the average of the scores of other individuals, or ipsative measurement models, where a score is compared to the average of other scores for that individual taken across time and situation).

The problem with this approach is that there is no necessary correspondence between the realities of the individual and those of the population the researcher chooses to define (see also Hughes et al., 1993). Population characteristics can change for a variety of reasons, even while individuals stay the same, and there is nothing in the assessments to tell us how to handle this. When scores are to be interpreted relative to the properties of a distribution, then we must accept the uniformity assumptions (Kiesler, 1966) that accompany this action—which professionals will recognize to be increasingly difficult to do as we become more aware of the complexities of individual lives.

Also, although it is possible for traditional work to be longitudinal and, thereby, to avoid some but not all of these pitfalls, research is typically cross-sectional, as if time did not exist in the lives of individuals or in the evolution of populations (Gergen, 1973). Our language has this time deficit built into it as we attempt to frame complex temporal realities in more manageable spatial and object metaphors (Lakoff & Johnson, 1980; Luria, 1981; Vygotsky, 1962). Thus, the dynamic, temporally ordered character of lives is often excluded—as Allport argued but failed to get across as a serious scientific concern. This is akin to a particle physicist saying we are going to stop the world and measure structure as if time, motion, acceleration, and trajectory do not exist. Even if this worked with particles, which are considered to be simple and governed by straightforward mathematical laws, we have no such simplicity or certainty in our thinking about human lives and their trajectories, and how these might be related to the static formulations resulting from our examination of population variables. Moreover, more direct mathematical formulations of laws have not proven possible because there is no theory to support them, although historically, Lewin (1975) and others attempted to produce such theory.

There is little question that differential approaches have made an important contribution to our understanding of human characteristics, many of which directly pertain to our understanding of clinical phenomena. A differential approach can be incisive in some policy and decision contexts where distinctions between and among sets of cases are at issue (e.g., when distributive decisions must be made about who should be hospitalized and who can be sent home). Also, there are uniformities in human populations that merit consideration in their own right. However, Lamiell makes a compelling case that current methodologies do not provide a sound logical basis for a direct move between aggregate and individual levels, and that, consequently, statistical formulations may not be as definitive as they are often portrayed to be.

Aggregates and Individuals

How should observations at the individual level be understood in light of observations made at the aggregate level? Unfortunately, there are no easy answers to this question. Neither correlational nor group difference strategies tell us how two measurements, and most importantly the phenomena with which the measurements correspond, go together in a particular individual. Does height cause weight or vice versa? We can make statements about the nature of physical structure that would deal with this. Only in so doing are we addressing the question of the nature of the link within the single case; statistical observation, without being linked to such descriptive and explanatory levels of theory, cannot address this problem. No wonder clinicians often depend on theories that are not recognized nor understood in more general scientific contexts.

The lack of attention to this problem has cultural implications that extend beyond scientific interpretation. Lamiell (1987) offered a striking example of the results of a political poll in which 90% of the voters say "yes" to a proposal and 10% "no." This would be considered an extremely strong showing on the yes side for the sample as a whole, primarily because it is rare to see this kind of agreement in political polls. But, as Lamiell suggested, it would have no implication at all for how strongly or weakly particular individuals think about the vote. Likewise a 52 versus 48% vote is relatively weak, but this does not mean that particular individuals feel weakly about the issues. Unfortunately, the fallacious confusion of levels of analysis between aggregate and individual is endemic in current public discourse. For example, a recent news story (Borger, 1995) characterizes "most women" as approving of the current president (Clinton), whereas "most men" disapprove. The story gushes about extreme differences between men and women. Yet, we find in the data that 54% of men "disapprove" of the president, whereas 39% approve, and 7%, who responded "don't know," are only reported in a footnote. The data for women reverse this pattern: 37%

"disapprove," 54% "approve," and 9% "don't know." These data show a difference in the statistical sense that is quite large by comparison to many samples, where differences teeter on the brink of virtual randomness (a 50–50 split). Still, the superlative "most" is stretching things with a 54–46 split: Consider how different the presentation becomes when the term "more" replaces "most," or how much better "most" sounds in the 90–10, or even 80–20 split context.

The article quotes a pollster as saying that the president needs women to feel as "intensely" about him as men feel against him. This is a nice metaphor for characterizing the group, but there is nothing in the data about intensity save for a few meaty individual quotes sought out by the article's author. There is no way of knowing if these are representative because sides not conforming to the author's thesis that men and women are in great disagreement are not presented, even though statistically they encompass a large portion of the sample (as in the 46% who do not "disapprove" of the president in the poll). Moreover, we have no way of knowing how many people feel intensely about the position they endorsed in the survey. Only the positing of some form of group mind would admit such a possibility, where the aggregate exactly mirrors properties of the individual. If so, how does this mirroring operate? Where is the theory that would lead us to expect such linkages in the data? Unfortunately, this kind of sloppy use of data can be found as readily in science as in journalism, as Lamiell (1987) elaborated. It illustrates how quantitative data can mislead us when poorly presented and interpreted.

Lamiell does offer an alternative to normative and ipsative measurement models, based on Cattell's (1944) description of interactive measurement. Here comparison is specified in terms of the context of the measurement itself. Lamiell suggests that this is an epistemological approach because it attempts to stay true to the individual's usage of the measurement device, in effect maintaining the scale that the individual uses in making his or her response and allowing that in some circumstances the scale may not be normative—particularly as it might be framed by a research scientist—or even ipsative, in the sense of being an averaging of actual life experiences.

For example, rather than assuming that a response of "four" on a seven-point numerical scale of marital satisfaction should be understood relative to the average response in a given population of say 4.6, it might be considered as an assertion in its own right, relative to what might have been asserted but was not. This can be operationalized by comparing a numerical assertion to the maximum or minimum possible on the given scale—in effect creating a proportion of the total scale that was used to assert one's satisfaction, relative to that which was not used. Lamiell suggested this as one possible means for creating completely individual measurements that hold the promise of general truth without assuming any given researcher knows which comparisons are relevant to the particular circumstance.

This so-called dialectical view of observation and measurement has important implications for local clinical inquiry—for example, how expressive might a child be given a particular family context. To show, via measurement, that the child is very bright and expressive relative to others in his age cohort may be to miss the level of avoided expression in the personal and family context, and the accompanying fear that is often described in psychotherapy. Knowing the normative case may specify something about society and what is possible on average and in the maximum and minimum at any given point in time—for example, children are perhaps as a group more expressive today than they were 50 years ago. But normative information may not reveal what is average or even possible for an individual in a particular context. Of course it might, if the measurement were related to theory relevant to such localized extrapolations, but differential accounts are almost never extended in this way, and such extension would necessarily be theoretical rather than empirical without extensive further inquiry. In this way, Lamiell, through a complicated but compelling set of arguments and empirical demonstrations, captures the sense of measurement having meaning in its own right, locally, that professionals often express in describing their observations.

Relevance for a Local Clinical Science

Lamiell's emphasis on conceptual problems in linking aggregate descriptions to individual ones is highly relevant for the local clinical scientist. The idea of dialectical reasoning associated with interactive measurement is particularly useful. Consider what it means when a patient describes himself as depressed. It is possible that comparisons are being made to others the patient knows (normative measurement; note, however, that such comparison will rarely be normed relative to a representative population description), or to himself at another time (ipsative measurement), but it is also possible that the description entails what is true relative to what might be true but is not (as in an implicit zero point that the patient conceptualizes). The notion that not all possibilities need to be actually available for direct comparison is a hallmark of dialectical thinking. Rather, standards that might not actually exist in the individual's life, nor in the life of any individual, might be applied in self-assessment. Consider, for example, how often intimate relationships and their possibilities are idealized as compared with relationships actually experienced (i.e., actually demonstrable) in a person's life. Or, consider how specific assessments of self and others can be overshadowed by particular life circumstances, such as a recent fight with a spouse that has the patient upset. Still another example might be the common observation in psychotherapeutic work that patients can get visibly better, but continue to describe themselves in old ways for extended periods of time until a more consistent view of what is happening, and of what is possible, develops.

Contrary to assumptions often made about the universal applicability of aggregate models, the key issue here is in determining how the patient construes the measurement situation. In some contexts, the idea that a patient might evaluate himself relative to what he might be feeling but is not, seems more plausible than some general averaging process relative to self or others (see Gigerenzer & Murray, 1987). In other contexts, comparisons of various kinds may be operative, including normative reference points, ipsative reference points, or reference points framed around particular individuals (one's brother) or specific situations one has experienced (that time in the fifth grade).

THE THREE DISCIPLINES
OF SCIENTIFIC PSYCHOLOGY

The issues raised by Cronbach and Meehl (1955) and Lamiell (1981, 1987) are both provocative and perplexing in establishing the relationship between a local clinical science and traditional quantitative science approaches. Therefore, it will be helpful to look at these same issues from a somewhat different angle as framed by Lee J. Cronbach, one of the most prolific and arguably most important figures in scientific methodology in this century. Cronbach has made major contributions to quantitative methodology in the search for a logically adequate means for evaluating systematic effects in light of individual differences (e.g., Cronbach & Gleser, 1953; Cronbach, Gleser, Nanda, & Rajaratnam, 1972). At the same time, he, along with Meehl (1978, 1994), has championed careful consideration of the limits of scientific methods, with a longstanding focus on possibilities for application. A major concern has been the theory–data linkage in psychological research, and Cronbach has long eschewed complacency about what might be accomplished using available methods.

The Experimentalist Perspective

Over the years, Cronbach's work has involved an increasing focus on the relationship between the general and the specific, as in a treatment outcome interacting with patient characteristics. In Cronbach (1957), he argued that applied problems required the combined input from two different disciplines of scientific psychology that had been operating independently of one another. One, which he termed the *experimentalist approach*, follows the tradition of experimental research and relies on observations of group differences, according to the rules of good research design (Chapter 4), to make statements of a general nature about phenomena. In this strategy, direct effects of causal or independent variables are isolated and observed in the group averages that structure factorial research designs. The underlying perspective is similar to that outlined at the beginning of this chapter and to what Darwin (1859/1968) called the *systematist* perspective. In this view, one must accept the belief that there are generalities that apply to all and that in knowing these, one has accessed the important influences on any specific observation. Examples would be the ways the laws of learning govern behavior, or the effects of hormones on motivation and activity. This perspective is most compatible with an overarching metatheoretical position that entails explicit empirical/operational linkages between theory and data, such as behaviorism or cognitivism. It epitomizes an understanding of psychological science as an experimental, laboratory-based discipline.

The Correlationalist Perspective

The second discipline of scientific psychology is comparative in nature, stressing individual differences and concerning matters such as aptitude or personality traits. Because the correlation is the fundamental methodological tool, this is called the *correlational strategy.* This is essentially the perspective discussed by Lamiell (1987). The assumption is that, in addition to any larger homogeneous group effects operative in a situation, there are sources of differences observed across units (persons, stimuli, situations, test items, and so on) that can be meaningfully identified, and that in identifying and labeling reliable differences, one has identified systematic characteristics of human psychology. Given reliable differences, there exists some underlying instigator for these differences that may be discovered by further study. It is further assumed that this instigator exists as a uniform source of variability across the entire distribution of observed differences.

In this approach, the variance and covariance statistics—which are both averaged values—are post hoc means for observing the effects of influential (causal) variables. That is, differences are presumed to result from theoretically given properties of constructs, the effects of which always precede their scientific investigation. This is similar to Darwin's (1859/1968) use of evidence to support natural selection theory: Darwin argued that even tiny variabilities observed in creature characteristics were systematically produced by variabilities and a natural selection process that had preceded the observed effects in prior generations. Similarly, in personality psychology, traits are thought to exist that generate the differences we observe on personality tests. Because of this post hoc quality inherent in the strategy, test construction approaches typically involve a process of rational construction of items and empirical studies to ensure that the items produced actually identify reliable individual differences in specified populations (Allen & Yen, 1979; Nunnally, 1967). Thus, the strategy is strong on comparative classification, but, except for the heritability theory from which these methods originally sprang (e.g., Galton; see Lamiell, 1995) or extensive study of other variables thought to have causal significance for particular measured characteristics, most theories of the differences observed tend to be descriptive-taxonomic rather than explanatory. The strength and meaning of the classification usually depends more on the demonstration of reliability, and concurrent (or predictive) and construct validity, than on explanation of the original differences themselves. This, along with uncertainty about causal directionality in correlation coefficients, gives correlational methods a reputation as being "softer" science than the experimental approach—which holds out the promise of complete, and even causal, explanation of observed effects. Indeed, individual differences, the stuff of the correlational method, are a source of error variance in the experimental method (Chapter 5).

Still, correlational studies are decidedly "harder" than the qualitative approaches most professionals depend on because they are perceived to be objective in the tradition of logical empiricism (Chapters 3 and 7). Successful individual differences measurements, such as the Five-Factor Personality Model (Wiggins, 1996), tend to be those that reliably describe individual differences across a range of situations. Areas depending on the correlational strategy are often characterized by a longstanding debate concerning the preeminence of genetic/constitutional factors or environmental/situational factors in producing observed differences.

A Third Discipline of Scientific Psychology

Cronbach (1957) believed that both the experimental and correlational strategies needed to be combined in applied research, in effect suggesting that interactions between treatments and participant characteristics would be the key to scientific advance in the applied arena. By the mid-1970s, however, Cronbach (1975a) was doubtful that even this merger would be enough. Evidence that higher-order interactions between person characteristics and group treatments (educational) were inconsistent and changed with time and circumstance was of particular concern (see also Bem & Allen, 1974; Gergen, 1973). A major assumption of scientific investigation is violated if the structure of phenomena are not universal and context independent. Cronbach (1975a) suggested that the only solution to this problem is carefully to examine distributions of data for more local effects that may mediate general effects, and to recognize that, within local conditions, all generalizations are "working hypotheses" (p. 125):

> The two scientific disciplines, experimental control and systematic correlation, answer formal questions stated in advance. Intensive local observation goes beyond discipline to an open-eyed, open-minded appreciation of the surprises nature deposits in the investigative net. This kind of interpretation is historical more than scientific. I suspect that if the psychologist were to read more widely in history, ethnology, and the centuries of humanistic writings on man and society, he would be better prepared for this part of his work. (p. 125)

Although Cronbach (1975a) did not propose a third discipline of scientific psychology directly, we believe that, with this remark, a third discipline was born, which we call the local scientific perspective, and which is the subject of this book. This perspective is akin, but not identical, to the historical, idiographic aspect of scientific thought discussed almost a century ago by Windelband, and more recently by Lamiell and others. Later, Cronbach (1982), in discussing a broad strategy for evaluation research, explicitly recognized the need for applied science to be focused on the local, discussed the general issue of extrapolation from formal research findings to local circumstances, and invented a general framework for any inquiry (which we discuss in Chapter 9) to aid this inquiry process. In effect, aggregate analysis is only the beginning of the problem, and more precise links to the individual must follow in the science (Cronbach, 1975a; Meehl, 1978).

Each of the three disciplines of scientific psychology proposes a different kind of information about the structure of reality for the professional to keep in mind. The experimental discipline suggests nomothetic information in a form that emphasizes similarities and commonalities among units. Thus, there are ways in which all psychotherapy sessions, or all school consultations, or all depressed patients, are alike. Similarly, interventions of a certain type, such as a supportive intervention, will yield a predictable outcome much of the time.

Still, even amid this unity of basic structure, there exists diversity. Patient characteristics and properties of the clinical situation inevitably differ from time to time, and in different places. When these differences are recognized to be systematic and influential in determining the outcomes in which we are interested (e.g., who will do well in school? who will be successful as a corporate executive?), we begin to tap into the level of nomothetic information associated with the correlationalist perspective. Consideration of the range and typicality of dimensions of difference is required, as is consideration of the kinds of correlates that might correspond to observed systematic differences. Thus, for example, if we know that individual differences in severity of depression in a community population exist, such as in urban African Americans (Brown, Ahmed, Gary, & Milburn, 1995), we can also consider correlates with this group property as clues to risk for depression among the individuals with whom we work. For example, Brown and colleagues found that changes in residence or stressful events in the past year were conditions associated with diagnosable depression in their study sample.

If systematic differences potentially interact with particular interventions, then Cronbach's (1975a) picture of general properties of interventions and diagnostic conditions operating in relation to individual differences merits consideration. This invites the clinician to consider general properties of the situation in light of specifics of the case cast in terms of relevant individual differences (in effect the individual's value on the individual differences variable). The local clinical scientist can use this sort of information to make comparative judgments about the case in relation to group characterizations of the typical, or average, case. We referred to this nomothetic comparative operation as "instantiation from general to the specific" in Chapter 3 (see also Levine, Sandeen, & Murphy, 1992).

Still, identifying a case as an instance of a general phenomenon is only part of the story, except in those rare textbook cases where the nomothetic formulation accounts for most of the important aspects of the situation. This is true even when such identification involves a complex interaction between normative properties and individual differences. Questions remain about the specific influences of local culture, about the unique life history of the individual, and about space-time local influences on the observational data that are fundamental to the case. The professional's task is to pull together all of the influences of the general and the specific in as coherent and complete an accounting of the case and its specific circumstances as is possible. We believe that the future of methodology for the local clinical scientist lies in the discovery of new and more effective ways of accomplishing these ends.

CONCLUSIONS

The linchpin in the logic of traditional scientific methods in psychology, including what was discussed in Chapters 4 and 5 as well as in this chapter, is the notion that we can create research situations that are controlled and relatively unambiguous from the standpoint of informed public scrutiny. This is the basis for the widespread acceptance, credibility, and legitimation of scientific findings. Our consideration of these issues suggests that the local clinical scientist should keep several things in mind in evaluating scientific findings for purposes of local inquiry.

Reasoned and Balanced Caution

There is no question that the combination of good methods and common sense can lead to convincing research findings, with different areas of inquiry being more or less tractable to the search for clarity and certainty. However, critiques of traditional methodological thought and praxis, including those of statistical inference (e.g., Bakan, 1966; Cohen, 1994; Lykken, 1968) and of the aggregation problem (Lamiell, 1987), doubts about internal validity of even the best research designs (Cronbach, 1982), and questions about local analysis and the problem of localizing scientific interpretation (Cronbach, 1975a; Lamiell, 1981, 1987; Levine et al., 1992; Meehl, 1994; Stricker & Trierweiler, 1995) make clear that it is inappropriate for a local clinical scientist simply to take research findings at face value and to assume that they directly translate into any given local clinical situation. Even when research findings apply precisely, they rarely will account for everything observed, and there remains the problem of how generalities play themselves out in locally unique and space-time specific circumstances. Local clinical scientists must not be distracted from the realities of specific circumstances in order to draw on generalities, nor the converse. Rather, it is always a problem of interpreting specifics in light of what is known, or thought to be known, generally.

This does not mean that the phenomena we observe in the aggregate do not exist in a meaningful way at more local levels, nor that they are somehow unimportant. If the aggregate changed—say there were no correlation between self-esteem and depression—then local observation may well change. But, as Bhaskar (1978) might say, we would then be living in another world, one different from the one we inhabit in its intransitive properties. We can only imagine what such a world would be like. Aggregate phenomena exist, and we glimpse them in our scientific studies. However, careful analysis of our methods suggests that local understanding of an aggregate finding remains a step (or several steps) away until we grasp more precisely the forces, be they from nature or nurture or something else, that link these realities to individuals. The local clinical scientist must see science as incomplete in this way and be very wary of the rhetorical, and, on occasion, polemical forces operating prematurely to make it appear to be complete—particularly those existing in the popular press where sensation will always carry the day over more quiet, reasoned, and complex positions. Certainly, we need to respond based on the best thinking of our science and profession, but there is little justification for acting as if that thinking is singularly definitive.

New Methodological Frameworks Are Needed

The local clinical scientist stands amid the realities of the clinical situation. The most direct observations are local ones. Tools of science and practice, such as psychological testing, may assist the problem of coordinating local observations with aggregate ones not directly available in the clinical situation. Some of the tasks of the local clinical scientist require this link more than others. For example, selection and decision processes, such as initial diagnosis and treatment planning, lend themselves to comparative information (e.g., this patient needs to be hospitalized, that one does not). However, many tasks, including those associated with the implementation of virtually any treatment plan, even the most structured, involve extensive interactions with the particulars, as opposed to the generalities, of a case.

We need to develop ways of understanding how to generalize effectively from the data that are actually obtained in psychological studies, rather than from our wishes, hopes, and fantasies about such data. For example, earlier we suggested that, in looking at how a criterion variable operates at various levels of the predictor variable, it is almost always possible to find cases that do not readily fit the general interpretation of the aggregate information. We need a better understanding of what is possible in single cases, given correlations of various sizes.

Figure 6.1 illustrates the problem with computer-simulated data for two normally distributed variables with a correlation of .55. The top panel shows the bivariate scatterplot for a population of 2000 cases. Note how it takes on the expected upwardly sloping elliptical shape that is characteristic of positively correlated variables. Often, if such correlations are statistically significant (not an issue here because our 2000 cases are, by fiat, the entire population), they are interpreted directly as suggesting that low-valued X cases correspond with low Ys and high Xs with high Ys. Although the scatterplot makes it obvious that this is true in general, it also shows that it may not be true for specific cases. Numerous cases that are high on X, the predictor variable, could not be interpreted as high on Y, the criterion variable. Thus, our most simple and minimal interpretation of correlation becomes questionable at the local level.

This gap between an aggregate property and local exemplars is even more apparent in the lower panel of Figure 6.1, where we have sorted a random sample of 200 cases, taken from the 2000 in the simulated population, on the X variable and plotted their z scores casewise along with their Y z scores. By chance, this sample shows a correlation somewhat higher than that in the population (.62). Note how often low Xs correspond to Ys that are proximal to their own mean (i.e., of average rather than low magnitude), or even on the other side of the Y distribution. The same is true on the high side of both variables. The size of the correlation in this demonstration speaks for itself: What might well be cause for excitement in the more abstract realm of scientific inquiry is sorely wanting in the concrete and specific realm of the professional. We must put aside illusions about the strength of such data and develop realistic approaches to working with their strengths and limitations.

As Meehl (1978) argued, we simply do not have "point" predictions in this type of "soft" science. Indeed, the presence of more than a few noncooperative cases in a given study suggests that locally we have no prediction at all. The example in Figure 6.1 draws on simulated data, so no assumptions of statistical models are violated. In real data, which usually involve smaller sample sizes and less idealized populations,

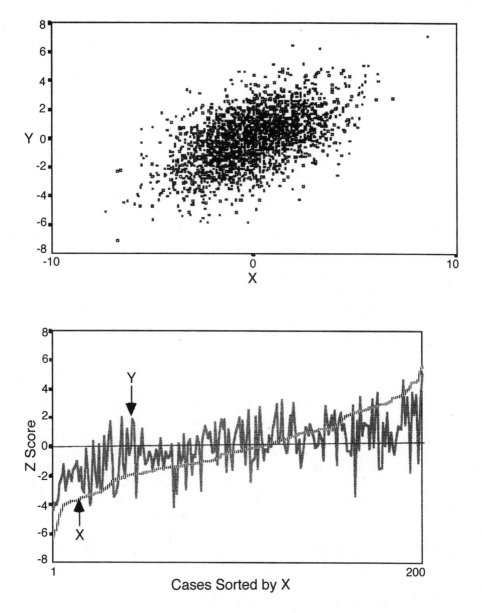

FIGURE 6.1.   (Top) An *XY* scatterplot of 2000 computer-produced cases with a correlation of .55. (Bottom) A line plot of the casewise *z* scores of a randomly selected sample of 200 with a correlation of .62.

such divergence between the specifics of an individual case and the major trend in the aggregate can be even more dramatic. If the correlations shown in Figure 6.1 were higher, then the scatterplot would show a more tightly packed ellipse as it converged on a straight line (a correlation of 1.0), and the Y variable on the line plot would be compact and approaching overlap with the X variable. Lamiell (1981, 1987) suggested that a correlation is truly "general," in the sense of applying equivalently to each and every case, only when its value is 1.0. This leaves a question for general science about what other variables account for the Y variance (error) not described by X. The question for the local clinical scientist is what is happening in this particular case. In principle, both questions have answers; it is simply not clear when and if they are the same answers—which was the basis for Windelband's distinction between nomothetic and idiographic knowing in the first place.

These concerns underscore how general population findings are most useful to the practitioner—usually an administrator, policymaker, or disposition specialist—who is likely to see representatives of the entire scale tested on a predictor and a criterion. In such a broad context, the averaged properties of the predictor–criterion relationship will reasonably—albeit not definitively—reflect the decision-making realities these individuals confront. Other practitioners, who deal with more limited ranges on predictor and criterion variables, will, in fact, work in subpopulations where the more general norms may not exist. There may well be theoretical reason to continue to operate based on the larger population descriptions (usually the default position), but this is an empirical question that is rarely confronted. In some cases, more local norms may be needed to establish the level of evidence an alleged predictor variable might actually offer these practitioners. Restriction of variability on predictor and criterion variables within subpopulations seen by practitioners, which will attenuate the predictive relationship, may limit the usefulness of relationships otherwise quite powerful at the population level. More specifically, this is about the ordered pairs of predictors and criteria that particular practitioners are likely to be dealing with, and a realistic assessment of their predictive and theoretical utility. Traditions of psychological testing have long finessed such problems by supplementing test scores, such as those on an MMPI (e.g., Graham, 1977), with broad qualitative descriptions of expectations for individuals within particular ranges. More attention is needed regarding exactly how these often very useful descriptions are generated and maintained. Recent discussions of criterion-referenced testing are also relevant to these problems (see Allen & Yen, 1979).

Careful Attention to the Theory–Data Linkage

Few of us can readily envision the relationships described by correlation coefficients of various magnitudes in idealized and real aggregates, let alone the complexities of the different forms of ordered pairings of values on the variables possible in specific cases. We are prone simply to accept the general message of a scientific study—if we accept any message at all—trusting that the test of statistical significance makes that message meaningful. The weight of argument, however, is accumulating against this attitude and it is time for professionals to come to grips with the limits of our existing science. This may not require that we throw everything away and start over, as some seem to imply in the science–practice debate. Instead, we need to sharpen our abilities to draw meaningful theoretical linkages across the construct–local reality gap, as discussed by Cronbach and Meehl (1955) so long ago.

For example, even if we cannot produce point predictions in a scientific study, because of limitations of both existing theory and methodology, we can still learn something about the range of possibilities that exists for criterion measures at various levels of a predictor variable. This would at minimum give us a sense of what is possible in a local situation to the extent the situation is comparable to the study sample. What if all reports of clinical science had a discussion of the implications of the residual variance in a regression analysis for interpretation of the results? Quite rapidly, we think, new material would emerge that transcends the simplistic aggregate-versus-error interpretive protocol we now see in the literature. Qualitative profiles of cases having different characteristics, as in being far above or below the regression line in a bivariate relationship, might shed important light on the local facts of such cases, thereby fueling new studies. Rather than treating such facts as error, thus emphasizing the distance between the general statistical formulation and local realities, such analysis combining the aggregate and the individual could facilitate translation of scientific findings and elaboration of the nature of "errors" for future investigations. Both population and individually specific studies are needed, with viewpoints coordinated with what might be the richly connected structure of reality, as opposed to formulations limited to the structure of our methodological disciplines and the systems of rhetoric that surround them. In heeding Cronbach's (1975a, 1982) advice in this way, we might also gain new insights into how relevant relationships operate deterministically, functionally, or simply contiguously. Both local and general science would benefit from such analysis and the dialogue that would ensue.

It is important to emphasize that we are not suggesting that local analysis is somehow more definitive than scientific analysis, nor the converse. Local analysis is neither definitive nor inevitably flawed. As with any science, it is only as good as the care with which it is produced. In addition to being good scholars and scientists in the traditional sense, we are suggesting that local clinical scientists remain open and tentative enough, not to delay action, but to act carefully such that new information can present itself and affect what is happening. We must accept scientific findings that demonstrate their local usefulness. At the same time, we must strive to keep science from extending beyond its reach. George Kelly (1963) made this point about the limits of science some time ago, and it underlies much of the science–practice debate throughout the history of clinical psychology. We need to start heeding this very reasonable caution, rather than simply sloughing it off so that some may argue that they have a better science than others, while others may argue that their clinical theory somehow transcends science.

We began this chapter with a quote from the mathematician-philosopher Poincaré (1952) equating chance with ignorance. He does not leave it at that, but goes on to suggest a more complete view of chance, in which it is composed of both the fortuitous event, which will be forever unpredictable, and the event that we might, but do not yet, understand. More importantly, he suggests that it is the complexity and multiplicity of causes that makes for the unpredictability we call chance or error. Meehl (1978) made similar points suggesting that chance of the fortuitous variety is not really what we should be concerned about. Rather, we need to be more concerned about what it is we do not know, about its complexity, and the limitations on our ability to grasp it using existing methodologies. Clearly, if we are to combine traditional and local approaches, as we are suggesting, we need new ways of talking about the specifics of cases that can handle complexity, that extend beyond current professional theory, and that create the possibility for integration with the stream of scientific discourse.

In Part III we discuss several approaches to scientific thought that are compatible with such an integration and that emphasize the improvement of our ability to describe the specific in ways that might be compatible with scientific formulations.

III

Extrapolations to Local Science from Nontraditional Science and Scholarship

Issues in Qualitative Analysis

> But thought is one thing, the deed is another,
> and the image of the deed still another:
> the wheel of causality does not roll between them.
> —NIETZSCHE (1954, p. 150)

> Words strain,
> Crack and sometimes break, under the burden,
> Under the tension, slip, slide, perish,
> Decay with imprecision, will not stay in place,
> Will not stay still.
> —T. S. ELIOT (1943, p. 19)

Qualitative research has become legitimate practice in the past 15 years. Qualitative methodologies are steeped in the rhetoric of innovation and in the rejection of what is thought to be the rigid and biased past of positivism. They carry all of the philosophical debate we have discussed in earlier chapters, and hold out the promise for overcoming the sins of omission, such as attention to matters of gender, ethnicity, and culture, that have received too little attention in quantitative studies.

Is this the long-awaited means for the scientific redemption of the professional, the means to attack the problem of specificity in phenomena that seems so lacking in quantitative science? Is it the greening of methods that will put practitioner ways of knowing back in the center of psychological science?

To answer questions such as these we must consider the history of debate about quantitative and qualitative methods as it relates to the philosophical, pedagogical, and political issues we have discussed throughout the book. It is a story of philosophical and methodological preferences, and the rather arbitrary raising of certain phenomena to methodological and scientific ascendance over others.

In this chapter we discuss the design and execution of qualitative research and how these methods can be extrapolated to a local clinical science. We will discuss how the qualitative–quantitative research distinction revolves around decisions about how to represent phenomena. In quantitative research, the emphasis is on the material properties of objects and events such as they are represented through assignments of numerical measurements (Lamiell, 1987). Quantitative analysis involves the application of the language, symbols, logic, and properties of mathematics and the number system to represent psychological phenomena in a reliable and valid fashion as defined within the logic of the system (Chapters 5 and 6). In contrast, qualitative analysis emphasizes properties of phenomena as represented in a linguistic system, usually natural language. Unlike numbers, which have a few useful properties that can be applied to many different situations, words are complex and seemingly without limits in their ability to label, codify, and interlink properties of phenomena. As used in everyday conversation, they are laden with subtlety and nuance that can defy any direct characterization. Because the rules governing linguistic systems and their coordination with phenomena occurring in the world are seldom clearly delineated and consensual, the operations involved in analyzing qualitative data are not as systematic and uniform as in quantitative analysis. Nonetheless, as numerous authors have recently shown (e.g., Miles & Huberman, 1994; Patton, 1990), it is possible to reduce equivocality in qualitative representations, and thereby achieve reliability and validity, by treating qualitative information in more systematic ways. We will discuss some of these strategies. We also will discuss how the scientist's direct confrontation with phenomena in the world is often more clearly discussed in the qualitative methodology literature than in the quantitative.

The local clinical scientist is like an anthropologist, entering a vaguely defined, but endlessly complex, open system of language and symbols where even simple descriptions can be difficult. An awareness of the "cultural clash" implicit in all entries into our patients' lives is useful in managing many of the pitfalls of clinical work recently being discussed, such as cultural diversity issues. Beyond that, however, the tools of qualitative analysis offer explicit ways of conceptualizing and handling such thorny issues.

BACKGROUND

Qualitative methods have been around for as long or longer than have quantitative approaches in the psychological and social sciences. Professional psychology is arguably more grounded in qualitative information, such as case studies, than it is in quantitative research. Quantitative methods only came into their own in the 1950s and 1960s, with the rise of methodological behaviorism. Still, the exclusivity and critical nature of quantitative approaches to the alleged achievement of certainty have deeply influenced our thinking about observation and research in the human sciences. Paralleling the debate between scientists and practitioners about how psychological practice should be legitimized, the psychological scientists looked on the qualitative science of Freud and other professionally oriented innovators with suspicion. Self-report data, the bread and butter of professional inquiry, were seen as laden with bias and nonspecific sources of unreliability (e.g., Runkel & McGrath, 1972). Only operationalizations directed toward precise assignment of numerical codes in order, systematically and exhaustively, to represent variation in observable phenomena of interest were considered adequate representations for an empirical science. Quantification itself seemed to carry a magical power instantly to legitimize a project.

Countering this attitude of exclusivity in science were pleas for more qualitative perspectives. These were tied to theoretical debates about the importance of studying human experience, as opposed to human behavior, as a means to the end of understanding social processes (e.g., Berger & Luckman, 1966; Geertz, 1973; Phillipson, 1972). Mostly they were directed against the strong behavioristic position in vogue through the 1920s and reaching a peak sometime in the 1960s. Recall that quantitative research, as framed more or less tightly around the goal of studying human behavior, was strong on specifying the limits of certainty in an inquiry and the means by which certainty could be enhanced. This, for example, was what Campbell and Stanley's (1963) work was designed to accomplish (Chapter 4). In its strongest form, only physically defined behavior observed reliably, in the statistical sense (Chapter 5), was the admissible observation base in a research program. In turn, the range of non-behavioral methods—many of which are central to the operations of the practitioner (e.g., interviewing)—and nonbehavioral orientations toward the substance of the human sciences (e.g., the study of subjective experience) were viewed with suspicion. At best, they were considered as preliminary to the real science that would follow when the appropriate experimental work could be accomplished.

Critics of this rigidity in science argued that matters of subjectivity were of the essence and that such matters required interpretive methods (e.g., Harré & Secord, 1973; Schutz, 1962, 1963). Thus, qualitative approaches like depth interviewing (often considered as the clinical method) or participant observation necessarily were the heart of the scientific inquiry. Methodologically speaking, this perspective shifted attention from rigid rules of certainty to the problem of directly examining phenomena of interest, however fallible such work might need to be. For example, Glaser and Strauss's (1967) grounded theory approach, which is, in a sense, an instruction guide for ethnographic inductive science (see below), proposed stretching the inquiry out as one way of staying true to phenomena while managing the questions about certainty raised by behavioral researchers (see also discussion of replication by Barlow et al., 1984).

Today, several other agendas have been added to the discussion and, in an extraordinary move in a historical sense, a good deal more of the discussion has focused on purely methodological questions than on substantive matters (e.g., see Denzin & Lincoln, 1994). Guba and Lincoln (1994), in discussing the rationale for qualitative methodologies, described four different perspectives as the conceptual underpinnings of scientific inquiry: (1) *positivism* (see Chapter 3); (2) what they term *postpositivism*, which is a kind of fallibilist realism we discussed in Chapter 3 and which we favor; (3) *critical theory*, which emphasizes the sociopolitical context within which inquiry takes place and which uses the insights of analyses of political and economic self-interests as a basis for critiquing scientific work; and finally, (4) *social constructionism*, which in some recent versions is completely relativistic as to the nature and substance of scientific inquiry. There is a great deal of confusion surrounding these various agendas, their alleged implications for scientific inquiry, and the often spotty scholarship on which many allegations are based [e.g., Kuhn's

(1970) position is often used rhetorically without careful attention to its substantive implications]. There does seem to be a common ground in concern about what is not being done in the traditional framework.

In keeping with our characterization of critical pedagogy, we will tend to downplay the critique here, just as we have downplayed the claims of certainty in regarding more traditional approaches. Instead, we will focus on issues raised by the qualitative methods literature as they might aid the local clinical scientist in managing the link between general knowledge and specific local realities.

CONSIDERATIONS OF A QUALITATIVE SCIENCE IN CONTRAST TO A QUANTITATIVE ONE

Guba and Lincoln (1994, p. 106) discussed some of the concerns about received view science that support the need for the development of qualitative approaches to inquiry. They listed several critiques that they described as internal to the "paradigm" of scientific inquiry: (1) loss of context, as when numerical codes are assigned to an observation and the informational context of the observation is lost; (2) exclusion of meaning and purpose as the physical properties of human behavior take priority in the inquiry; (3) divergences between general theories and the common understandings existing among individuals residing in local contexts; (4) inapplicability of statistical generalizations to individuals, as we have discussed in previous chapters; and (5) emphasis on verification rather than discovery—sometimes, they feel, a scientist just needs to explore what is going on.

Guba and Lincoln (1994) also listed several questions about the assumptions often associated with the basic notion of conducting a scientific inquiry: (1) facts are theory laden, so verificationist thinking is theory bound; (2) different theories might account for the same so-called facts (i.e., the problem of induction); (3) facts are value laden, making science not value free, as indirectly contended in some presentations of the scientific position (e.g., Ayer, 1952); and (4) the inquirer and inquiree are in a human transaction in the human sciences, thus affecting the objectivity of any inquiry. Each of these is viewed as an argument for introducing qualitative approaches. Even more, the latter are seen as providing a basis for modifying the entire project of science as regards human studies.

For our purposes, the argument favoring qualitative research approaches reduces to a need to examine relevant phenomena, within all of the complexity of their natural occurrence, based on theories of the nature of subjectivity and sociality, as we describe below. Such theories must recognize points of human similarity between the observer and the observed, and knowledge and self-interest, as they manifest and reverse roles and perspectives in the course of a clinical relationship. Our perspective toward qualitative methods and their justification is scientifically oriented and, therefore, our presentation fits with Guba and Lincoln's representations for *post-positivism*. We presume there to be a reality transcending the simple constructions of any set of individuals, but also that, with increasing care, theory, and fruitful inquiry—some of which might be qualitative—the distance between conceptualization and the structure of phenomena can be reduced (Manicas & Secord, 1983). Accordingly, we emphasize the possibilities for qualitative methodologies to enhance discovery and problem solving in the local clinical situation.

Next we look at several issues in the debate about qualitative research that offer useful perspectives for local inquiry. Following this, we will consider innovative methods and reconsider old methods that will contribute to these ends.

Precision in Science

The history of the debate between quantitative and qualitative methodologies revolves in part around the issue of precision in an inquiry. It is a bit like the bandwidth–fidelity issue in psychological assessment (Cronbach, 1984). If a construct or a narrative can capture a great range of phenomena, in all of their subtlety and uniqueness, then it has wide bandwidth, but one might question its fidelity in representing the essence of the situation. Also, all aspects of the representation may seem equally important, with no focus or commitment to the central issues involved. Alternatively, great precision might be mustered to represent a single property that is thought to be the essence of the situation as simply and accurately as possible. If so, there is high fidelity, but limited bandwidth, and important qualities of the situation may be lost. Psychological scientists have tended to place fidelity above bandwidth in attempts to represent a few properties in as reliable and consensual a manner as possible. Clinicians have tended to look for more complex and thorough representations of a case, and are willing to allow a little (or a lot of) slack in portraying any single element of the inquiry. Qualitative characterizations are clearly tending toward the clinicians' side of this spectrum.

Subjectivity versus Objectivity

A major issue in the debate about the qualitative–quantitative distinction hinges on notions of subjectivity versus objectivity, and the roles each play in science. Once again, the positivist perspective is often seen to occupy one end of the continuum (the objective end) and constructionism the other (the subjective end).

The notion of objectivity carries several connotations relevant to local clinical inquiry. It references phenomena that are perceived, or imputed, to be out there, consensual, public, positivistic, and precise (i.e., implying no surplus meanings). Another interesting connotation is captured in the phrase "objected to." The referent of an objective characterization is placed in opposition to something else. *Webster's* defines the term *objective* as "existing as an object or fact, independent of the mind, real." It is "concerned with the realities of the thing rather than the thoughts of the artist or writer … without bias or prejudice." Note how this definition directly contradicts any notion that facts are simply the products of mind. The concept is old, coming from the Latin *ob*, toward, or against; and *iacere*, to throw. It is "to throw against the senses" (Skeat, 1989). We may indeed have doubts about uninterpreted givens in science (Gergen, 1985; Manicas & Secord, 1983), but it is difficult to argue that certain phenomena seem to be thrown against our senses, in opposition to any mental machinations, more so than others.

The idea of subjectivity has similar roots: It comes from the Latin prefix *sub* for under and *iacere*, to throw. Literally, it means to throw under. It connotes the inside, the hidden, the nonconsensual or private, the nonpositivistic, and the imprecise. *Webster's* defines it in opposition to objectivity—the persistent theme in the discourse of science with its detractors—as "of or resulting from the feelings of the person thinking; not objective; personal." Even if history does not always clearly conform to battles between traditionalists and innovators, as these stories are often told, there has indeed been a developing preference for the subjective in recent years in contrast to a longstanding striving for the objective.

Forms of Subjectivity

Once we have decided to study subjectivity, there remains a question of what aspect of subjectivity we will study. There is significant ambiguity in this decision. To illustrate the problem, we consider four different ways we might look at subjectivity.

Everyday Subjectivity

First, consider subjectivity as commonly understood. At its simplest, this is taking the subjective to be whatever an individual says about him- or herself. If we understand what the person says, then we understand something about subjectivity. We get along quite well with this simple assumption day to day. Our world does not require great precision for our words to be good enough communications about our subjectivity. If a person tells his friend he is hungry as they walk past a restaurant, that is generally enough to decide to enter or not; the friend does not need to know exactly what is required to satisfy the hunger, nor to verify that the hunger actually exists in some more objective physiological sense, in order to produce an adequate response to the remark. At least this is true most of the time. If it turns out that the hungry individual has just committed a crime and is looking for an excuse to get off the street, the remark about hunger may turn out to have a different meaning to the friend at a later time. Even the simplest communications can carry deception, and a great variety of other ambiguous and deeply human meanings (Goffman, 1974). Such is the richness of human communication and the stuff of human drama.

Accepting communications as common understandings is generally a fine approach to inquiry into subjectivity, even in a variety of research contexts and local clinical situations. If a patient says she received a phone call from her mother, it is usually sound to take it as given, following the conversation to other important material about what happened during the call. But then there are times when the whole simple picture can change, as when it turns out that the phone call follows a day after the patient called her mother to relate a disturbing piece of information about events in her life. If the clinician is unaware of this prior event, and if the patient is not ready to talk about it, then the entire phone conversation can cast a misleading subjective light, even though certain aspects of the patient's account of the call may be very directly presented and apprehended by the professional.

Accepting subjectivity in the everyday sense is something we must do, but it is a policy fraught with pitfalls from a scientific perspective. The problem is not unlike the fundamental ambiguities surrounding the simplest notions of positivism, as in our page number example in Chapter 3. Simple subjectivity is only simple and accurate if we have no particular reason to seek increasingly greater precision, as we often must in science and in local practice.

Actual Subjectivity

Questions about everyday subjectivity originate in another possibility, which is almost paradoxical when considered in light of the scientific controversy about whether psychological science should stress the objective or the subjective. What about the actual subjectivity of the individual? In the phone call example, this might involve the patient's experiencing both what she described in the session—for example, something disturbing about the way her mother spoke to her—and that thing she might have experienced but failed to muster the courage to talk about—for example, the conversation she initiated with her mother the day before. Therapists often treat such material as unconscious, but there is little evidence to tell us one way or the other whether it is unconscious or not, and there remains considerable ambiguity about exactly what a notion of unconsciousness—as opposed to something preconscious or simply unspoken—might mean in a specific clinical situation. Whatever the case, it certainly means something more than ideas not mentioned in the course of therapy sessions, even though that is the primary source of evidence for any notion that an idea, later revealed directly, was unconscious.

The idea that we can consider actual subjectivity is intriguing from both a scientific and a practical perspective. Such a notion does not necessarily require that we get wrapped up in the language problems that worry many qualitative methodologists, and that were outlined by Wittgenstein (1958) and Vygotsky (1962). These revolve around the observation that the meaning of an attribution of some continuing subjective state, like loneliness, becomes increasingly difficult to grasp as we look to locate it in increasingly specific contexts. Rather, the notion of actual subjectivity merely entails an interest in identifying, to whatever extent possible, the experience of an individual as it is experienced in some space-time context.

A concept like *loneliness* may well capture aspects of this time-bound experience. But it is also true that the individual being examined might well have produced a think-aloud commentary of exactly what was being experienced moment to moment. If such material were produced, it would obviously be limited by the ability of the speaker and the ability of language, as it exists in our culture, to capture the phenomena experienced. Nonetheless, this does not mean one cannot pursue a trajectory of tying language with increasing specificity to the experience, and thereby finding a level of detail that is adequate to a particular inquiry (Chapter 3).

We might, for example, find out that the reference to loneliness by a male patient is actually coordinated with a period of feeling sad and alone, and quiet crying to himself during a weekend when no one calls. This might be a time during which this person reflects on the lack of an important, longed-for relationship in his life. At the same time, even greater detail about the context of the loneliness may reveal that this weekend followed several days of unusually intense and intimate contact with friends who, for some reason, are not included in the loneliness narrative. It still may be accurate to describe this time period, and indeed much larger portions of the person's life, as "lonely." Yet, the pursuit of material approaching actual subjectivity, as specified in space and time, may add considerably greater insight into the explicit meaning of the loneliness concept to the individual.

Objective Subjectivity

Moving to a somewhat higher level of theoretical abstraction, we might ask a paradoxical question about the objective aspects of subjectivity. What aspects of it are effectively flung in front of the senses of the client, and in turn given to the professional as immutable aspects of the story being told? What is it that contributes to this narrative? To what extent is the narrative actually based in sensorial material, as opposed to interpretations that are more or less subject to unfolding and development however immutable they seem at a particular time—as constructionist theory suggests?

For example, a psychotherapy patient may say that a parent drinks heavily, and might construe this as evidence of being hated. This may be an important part of the patient's self-narrative, and may indeed capture a longstanding, and frequently considered, interpretation the patient has of events in his life. Yet, the drinking aspects of the story may be more concretely given than the "heavily" interpretation, which may be considerably more sensorial than the "hating." In effect, the interpretation is objective in itself, but subjective in its coordination to events in the patient's life. The local clinical scientist can identify objectively, in the course of the therapeutic relationship, the subjective and objective aspects of the narrative as a means to helping the patient see possibilities for change. The ability to see old events in new ways is an alteration of subjectivity known as reframing (e.g., Safran & Segal, 1990).

Inaccessible Subjectivity

As with our earlier discussion of the perception of simple objects like the page number, some aspects of the subjectivity of another, and indeed of one's self, will be accessible and reasonably describable in a given language community, and other aspects will not. A notion of pursuing objective subjectivity via qualitative methodologies is a process of moving oneself toward the accessible to whatever extent one can, and of finding ways to render the inaccessible as perceivable as it can possibly become. Still, there remains an element of inaccessible subjectivity, some of which might involve stories untold—as is often realized later as the thing that should have been said in a situation—and some of which involve things not conceivable because there is no language to describe them. It seems likely, for example, that women experienced themselves as being treated in ways that caused them concern and annoyance, and many other feelings, long before the women's movement came to its recent level of fruition. Yet, insofar as they did not have the language of social oppression or political action, they were unlikely to have seen and presented this phenomenon as an issue subject to change, or, in many cases, as a gender issue at all. Language provides a means of analyzing experience (Vygotsky, 1962), and because language itself evolves in society quite out of our individual control (although we are free to make up new words and combinations of words if we wish to do so), there are limits to the ways we can see and describe our experience at any given time. This is not an excuse to stop looking, or to assume that no accuracy is possible in the linguistic codification of experience. It only means that a lack of precision is endemic to the process, and there must be a level of openness and flexibility if the range of possibilities that actually might exist within a given local context can find their way to the surface. The idea of "getting in touch with one's feelings" is itself a relatively recent cultural conception, springing from the use of language to access inner life and to explore once deeply private realms for purposes of helping. We are a long way from having developed a language system (formal or informal) that can handle the complexity of professionals' experience in the course of their everyday inquiries into human problems.

We have to admit to a bit of intellectual sleight of hand here in suggesting unusual notions like *objective subjectivity*. The point is not to burden our thinking with too many distinctions, but rather to underscore how local clinical scientists are very often engaged in a process of inquiry into the subjectivity of another without giving much thought to assumptions being made about how that subjectivity is accessed. There are undoubtedly forms of knowing, perhaps of a holistic variety, that are engaged when persons interact with one another and that allow them to access important aspects of subjectivity. For example, an unconscious process, or even a narrative schema (Bonanno, 1990; Safran & Segal, 1990), may reveal itself in multiple observations of what is and is not brought into the conversation over an extended period of time. Professionals must become more aware of how these subtle expert forms of observation and inference operate and must practice their effective usage (see Chapter 9). Nonetheless, professionals must also remain cognizant of the pitfalls in any pursuit of subjective understanding. Subjectivity is not, and can never be, simply and completely objective—as would support the displays of certainty often seen in professional conversations (e.g., Meehl, 1973). This is true however much qualities of one's professional experience of a patient may seem to be thrown against one's broadly defined senses. The most reasonable position to take with respect to the complications of subjectivity in the local clinical situation is one of moving back and forth within a balanced dialectic between doubt and certainty (Chapter 8). Qualitative methodologies offer useful models that are designed to assist one in thinking through such problems.

The Biases of the Scientist

Qualitative information and a whole body of material that can be described as self-report data have often been questioned on the grounds that they represent various forms of bias not relevant to research questions. Research on interviewing has shown that interview outcomes can be greatly affected by characteristics of the interviewer (Mishler, 1986). There can be no assurance that information pertaining to subjectivity of a particular individual is not equally as reflective of biases of the researcher. Certainly the range of answers possible depends on the question(s) asked. Because human interaction is extremely complex, even very subtle influences, such as non-verbal phenomena, are possible. In response to this criticism, proponents of qualitative methods have emphasized the richness and relevance of qualitative information, downplaying possibilities for bias. Recently, there is even recognition that interviewer effects must be part of the understanding of the data (e.g., Mishler, 1986; Weiss, 1994).

Sociality in Science

It is important for psychologists to understand that a good deal of the debate about the use of qualitative methodologies and the methodological proposals actually being made are primarily focused on social issues. Apart from the interviewing found in psychotherapeutic traditions, qualitative methods are the principal domain of the nonpsychological social sciences, such as anthropology and sociology. This can be difficult for the psychologist to grasp; there are huge areas of overlap between the psychological and the other social sciences. At the same time, there are some fundamental differences that must be considered in evaluating qualitative methodologies for a local clinical science. There are many ways in which the credible usage of these methods depends heavily on social conceptions that psychologists are often unaware of, or unwilling to adopt (e.g., Mills, 1959; Rappaport, 1977).

What do we mean by social? Social conceptualizations are directed at the description and explanation of social entities. Social entities always involve more than one individual, and the focus is on understanding the structure and dynamics within and beyond the social entity. In contrast, psychology often focuses directly on the individual, making no claims for the applicability of its concepts for social phenomena. Inquiry here is directed at the understanding of the structure and dynamics of phenomena within an individual. When considered at the individual level, subjectivity can seem so deeply personal that the idea of experience shared with others can seem to have no meaning. Thus, from this idiographic perspective, we tend to concentrate on the richness, complexity, and uniqueness of the individual. Qualitative methods, such as depth interviewing, are designed to illuminate the unique biography of the individual (e.g., Runyan, 1982). Any generalities drawn from such material address how individuals with particular biographical characteristics or perspectives manage in their worlds. As in our discussion of quantitative studies, the distinction between what is true in a collection of humans and what is true for the general individual—that is, for each and every individual in his or her own way (see Lamiell, 1987)—is blurred in this thinking.

A social perspective looks directly at the collection rather than at the individual. It might also involve biography, but, in so doing, there is relatively greater attention to the social aspects of that biography. The perspective of the individual is viewed in light of his or her membership in a collection of perspectives existing because of a particular structural location or status within a social milieu. Mills (1959) has called this social viewpoint, and the insights that accompany it, the *sociological imagination*. Thus, sharedness and the operation of larger societal structures are emphasized more than uniqueness, in a way that is not dissimilar to the quantitative step of combining observations assumed to be similar enough that meaningful generalizations can be made based on their common, or average, qualities. This sharedness need not be quantitatively derived, however, for it is also possible to observe shared properties within social groupings that are qualitative in nature and that seem to reveal something important about shared experience and the nature of social process. This observation often is most apparent if one is an outsider, as in the anthropological situation where a researcher enters a cultural milieu different enough from the one from which she comes to make any insight seemingly profound (e.g., Donner, 1982). Adopting the outsider perspective more locally requires comparison with some standard, such as an emphasis on evidence of difference between the observed grouping and some presumed-to-be commonly held notion of "everyperson."

The social perspective is at its best when it illuminates aspects of a phenomenon that are invisible without it, as in Sampson's (1985) and Cushman's (1990) recent call for a more social view of the self (see also Markus, 1983; Markus & Nurius, 1986). The concept of the self, although starting from a distinctly social perspective in the work of Cooley (1930) and Mead (1934), has evolved into an extremely individualized characteristic—as if the self is carried solely within the individual and is unrelated to the social context in which it is embedded.

The attention to sociality implicit in recent discussions of the need for qualitative research methods can easily be misunderstood or forgotten by psychologists. Or, it can easily be transformed into a kind of informal social theorizing without appropriate awareness of the accuracy and applicability of the social assumptions and observations one is making. We cannot all be sociologists or anthropologists, however much such ideas have currency in popular thought. This becomes a potential problem when a practitioner adopts a political position or an intracultural perspective that might exclude or render problematic certain local observations that might be important to a particular case. By the same token, careful awareness of social context can greatly assist one's ability to grasp particular phenomena. For example, a woman may well experience power issues in relationship to her spouse even though she may never interpret them in the same way as certain feminist political positions might dictate. Understanding of the larger social issues, when combined with openness to whatever form it takes within the individual, can open up fruitful conversations about such matters.

Interpretation from the social perspective is different from the presumed exercise of empathy toward an individual (Trierweiler & Donovan, 1994); it assumes as much attention to the observer, the social context of the observation, and one's knowledge of that context as to the observed (Schutz, 1962, 1963). Moreover, in viewing subjectivity through a social lens, certain empirical qualities that are of great interest become apparent. For example, we can see that, to the extent language is used to access subjective phenomena, experience is tied to linguistic symbols existing within a larger sociocultural context. These symbols may affect experience and constrain— or facilitate—how that experience is understood, by an observer (e.g., Whorf, 1956). They exist independent of any particular user, societies work hard to make them refer to a limited range of phenomena and situations, and their usage is heavily dependent on particular sociohistorical contexts. Perhaps most compelling of all, they allow for even very complex meanings to be shared among individuals, and this sharedness itself is a social condition that can have enormous impact.

Consider for example how shared views about the value of public education increased throughout the nineteenth and twentieth centuries until a vast public education complex was created in this country. Sometime in the 1970s serious doubts about the value and success of this project, particularly in large urban high schools, began to be voiced amid changing economic and social conditions. Such views had not been given much credence prior to that time. Although, overall, the shared commitment to public education remains strong, there are signs of doubt in the debate that were far more limited at an earlier time. In this way, public debate can be thought to create more or less sizable pockets of sharedness of viewpoint around a particular issue at any given point in time.

In like fashion, but on a smaller time scale, psychotherapy styles have come in and out of fashion; psychoanalysis, for example, which had once been considered a liberating force, came to be viewed as an oppressive tradition and, more recently, as "too expensive" an endeavor for the health care system. Yet, even as this is happening, the seeds for its revival are being sewn (Jacoby, 1986). To the extent viewpoints like these are shared, or at least accepted, in societies, they can have great impact on historical conditions. But shared meaning, even in very local circumstances, as between therapist and client or within an intimate couple, can have considerable impact on events and experiences of events within the local domain.

Attention to the inherent sociality in a qualitative inquiry, thus, makes otherwise impalpable subjectivity more concrete as meaning, language, and social relationships are interpreted at a higher level of analysis. Much of the current discourse around disempowerment of different groups in society involves the application of social forms of inquiry, analysis, and interpretation to psychological phenomena and traditions. Most importantly, looking at matters from a social perspective calls for an examination of the subjective as well as the objective, and subjectivity can be interpreted in terms of comparisons among larger social units. Differences in subjectivity can be compelling and obvious when cast in intercultural terms (e.g., Triandis, 1972), as in an anthropological study of strikingly different cultures (e.g., Donner, 1982) or in terms of hidden differences that exist within our own culture, such as the social systems of youth on the urban streets (Whyte, 1981). Social subjectivity, as manifested in language and in forms of interaction, is more empirically accessible in the social sphere than within the individual, and concerns about the impact of investigator bias are less prominent when the inquiry is understood as a social inquiry. The problem of bias remains, however, and must be given due heed when attempting to apply the larger social thinking locally. Additionally, the collective frame of reference allows quantitative approaches to be used as well as, or in combination with, qualitative ones (e.g., Triandis, 1972).

The Intriguing Exploration of Otherness

Another way of thinking about the underlying social premise of qualitative approaches to inquiry is to recognize that such methods spring from the often extraordinary excitement we experience in observing something different from ourselves—that is, as long as the difference is not threatening. If quantitative methods require emphasis on our similarities and differences as physical human objects, then qualitative methods require emphasis on our similarities and differences as experiencing human subjects. The study of otherness is inherently interesting and, perhaps, most vividly revealed when an aspect of cultural reality that we take for granted is viewed in contrast to a dramatically different conception of that reality when viewed from another culture. If the differences are large enough, the importance of such examination speaks for itself. Thus, anthropological studies have been justified using qualitative methods, despite how heavily "scientific" (meaning quantitative in this context) social sciences have sought to become. Experiments are not needed for us to be intrigued by Whorf's (1956) famous contention that certain Arctic cultures have many more words for differentiating snow than do most mainland U.S. cultures, although experiments might well be used to examine and verify such a finding. Yet, the prospect of one's neighbor down the street describing a given snowfall differently from oneself would generate little scientific interest. Partially this is because of implications for general versus local understanding. It also is related, in no small part, to an idea that some subjectivities are more well formed, more useful to one's understanding of the world, and more worth pursuing in their own right, than are others, and that some of this pursuit should be scientific. We can dismiss our neighbor's view of the snowfall with little thought; however, Whorf's idea that language actually leads some cultures to perceive the world differently than we (who are presumably in Whorf's culture) is another matter. One can immediately envision a polite conversation with someone from another culture about the snow, seeking to understand the distinctions that are being made; the neighbor may or may not receive such consideration. Why is this so?

Although there is not sufficient space here to answer such a complex question, we can say that it has something to do with the sacred and the profane of scientific and professional life, and with what we value and what we consider mundane. As such, the argument for the qualitative study of subjectivity usually requires extensive justification of why a particular subjectivity might be important for one's understanding. This is obvious to the professional in the local clinical situation, who has been justifying the pursuit of subjectivity in his formulations for generations. But it is not obvious at that point where science and practice bridge, and, as a result, it should be understood that qualitative methods carry with them the need to show carefully how a subjective examination fits into more general scientific questions. In this sense, qualitative studies provide good training for professional life. Note that this has also been true of traditional quantitative studies, but the sense that the methods carry weight of justification, more so than the theory addressed in a particular study, has obscured this need to justify one's work. It is doubtful that qualitative methods, however sophisticated they become, will ever be given the blind credence that the quantitative approaches have enjoyed—which may explain some of the intensity of the philosophy and political rhetoric brought to bear in discussion of qualitative social and psychological sciences (see Denzin & Lincoln, 1994). Nonetheless, the press to strengthen the link between theory and inquiry is a benefit to all (Chapters 6, 8, and 9). To study otherness, one needs to explain why the results are important and interesting, and how we will learn something we do not already know. In turn, the best studies will be those that reveal something about actual subjectivity of an identified other that was previously unseen or unseeable.

The work on *Women's Ways of Knowing* by Belenky et al. (1986) is a particularly interesting example in revealing how individuals who are not necessarily dedicated to a traditional academic way of knowing understand their world. Viewed within the context of this interview-based research, the concept of knowing is, itself, transformed forever. This type of empirically grounded innovation has long been an objective for empirical science, be it quantitative or qualitative (e.g., Cronbach & Meehl, 1955), and shows how framing the interest in otherness can set a context for fruitful qualitative explorations.

Emic and Etic Aspects of Qualitative Studies

The discussion of qualitative research is in large part about what has been termed the *insider–outsider* debate in cross-cultural studies (Headland, Pike, & Harris, 1990). Pike (1967) identified the emic aspects of a study as those having to do with the view held within a cultural community. Anthropologists are often interested in accessing this view and, therefore, they hold back on bringing general concepts from their science to bear in a particular situation. Instead they concentrate on describing what is observed within the natural setting of the community. This within-community focus is an attempt to grasp the emic aspects of otherness, and it is obviously a goal shared by many professional psychologists with respect to the experience of their patients.

Supplementary to emic ways of knowing within a culture are etic ways, which involve the application of general constructs, presumed to apply to all cultures, to particular cases. To operate from an etic perspective, a researcher might seek to identify how an etic construct operates within a cultural community. For example, the research may be interested in how social distance is maintained within different cultural contexts (e.g., Triandis, 1977), assuming it is a universal of certain types of societies. The task then becomes one of measuring that construct within a given culture. Similarly, when a professional applies professional constructs to local cultures, such as the psychiatric classification system, he is operating from an etic perspective. Obviously, if emic and etic observations are compatible, there is no problem in doing so. However, if they are in conflict, where, for example, an individual's intracultural view of normalcy is in conflict with a professional's view of psychopathology, or where the etic construct seems to miss the boat entirely, then a debate will ensue. A fascinating example of combining emic and etic information so as to grasp a social problem in a productive way is Sarason's (1971) examination of change within the education system.

Relevance

It seems obvious that subjectivity and any communication about it will involve the selection of material that is relevant to the current interests of the individual (e.g., Miller, Galanter, & Pribram, 1960). Understanding relevance is a major goal of qualitative inquiry into subjectivity. Yet, there is surprisingly little literature directly addressing this problem. The social phenomenological theory of Schutz (e.g., 1970) offers a particularly illuminating examination of subjective relevance that merits study by psychologists. We cannot provide a thorough presentation of this theory here, but we can offer some concepts as a brief introduction to Schutz's perspective.

Schutz focused attention on the individual's immediate sense of reality, which is phenomenologically bigger than any particular situation. The person experiences being surrounded by an expansive subjective reality much of which is taken for granted (typified). He called this subjective sphere the *life-world*. The life-world is composed of the commonly recognized or typical, which Schutz referred to as *typifications*.

One aspect of the life-world is a *theme*, which reflects the interests, actions, and intentions of the individual, and a horizon, which provides context for the unfolding of the theme. Themes are constituted of various topics for interest and attention, and there exists—and the individual assumes there to be—a surrounding array of identifiable matters (e.g., objects, persons, events, interpretations) that are intrinsically related (relevant) to a given theme. Note that this thinking is very similar to recent beliefs about concept formation where object features are thought to be relevant to particular concepts (Neisser, 1976; Rosch & Mervis, 1975). All of this occurs within the context of a *stock of knowledge at hand*, which is the knowledge base available to the individual to interpret a situation and all aspects of life that come into attention.

When local circumstances (typifications) pertain to the existing interests and understanding of an individual, Schutz referred to them as *relevances*. Experience entails various forms of relevances, which are the stuff of the life narratives an individual might tell. These concepts raise interesting possibilities for exploration of individual subjectivity in any circumstance (e.g., they provide a useful framework— see Chapter 9).

More recently, Sperber and Wilson (1986) drew on contemporary cognitive theory to discuss the problem of relevance directly as a problem of human communication. This recent work is exciting both because of the thread it adjoins to the work of Schutz and others—even though these modern authors did not mention the earlier work—and in providing additional useful perspectives on the problem of grasping subjectivity of a specific other. They suggested that the problem of relevance is actually one of understanding the context and specifics of interpretation itself, an important issue for qualitative research as many authors have argued (e.g., Lincoln & Guba, 1985). In focusing on verbal communication, they presented a picture of relevance as linking old and new information. Present information is deemed relevant in light of an ongoing interpretation of the world that exists before and extends through the present. In so doing, new recognition, insights, and possibilities are realized that might not arise if events were actually pulled from their continuous temporal link with the past. Sperber and Wilson discussed how communication has an inherent relevance-generating process that, at root, seems to be interpersonal. They elucidated the concept of *ostension* in communication, which refers to the two levels of information often seen in communication pragmatics (see also Watzlawick, Beavin, & Jackson, 1967): the information that is the subject of the communication, and the ostensive information, which is the communication of the intent to communicate something about the information being discussed, that comes automatically with the conversation. This aspect of communication ensures that certain relevances will collect around the conversation even though many specifics of the actual communication refer to experiences unique to participants, which may be difficult to actually describe in unique detail, and which may go unnoticed if the content of the material directly discussed is the only object of attention.

This formulation is clearly related to multiple levels of information to which clinicians must attend in executing their role. For example, a patient mentioning a dream in psychotherapy suggests something about the patient's intent that is important for the clinician to understand. At the most obvious level, the dream may be an important experience for the patient that she feels should be discussed in the therapy. Alternatively, the intent to communicate about dreams may be more about what the patient perceives to be the actions of a good patient, in which case the ostensive communication is not as clear as it may appear. There are numerous other possibilities. Sperber and Wilson's analysis offers many useful ideas that could assist clinicians in generating strategies for handling such ambiguities in communication with their patients.

As an aside here we should note that much work in cognitive psychology and, more generally, cognitive science pertains to the problems of analyzing subjectivity and qualitative analysis (e.g., Ericsson & Simon, 1993). We believe that more clinicians need to become involved in translating this material into useful frameworks for analysis of the local clinical situation (e.g., Bonanno, 1990; Turk & Salovey, 1988; Chapter 9).

Summary

The issues surrounding qualitative methodologies and their place in psychological research are complex and intriguing. Miles and Huberman (1994) summarized three ways qualitative methodologies have been approached. These show how essential sociality and the interest in otherness are in justifying qualitative methodologies. They are:

- *Interpretivism*, which is based in notions that human action must be interpreted. Interpretivism is essentially subjectivist and explores a domain that natural science presumably cannot grasp.
- *Social anthropology*, which involves ethnography, extended direct contact with a community, naturalistic observation, and often a participant-observer stance. Social anthropology tends to be descriptive, focusing on culture, life history, grounded theory (see below), ecological psychology, and narrative studies.
- *Collaborative social research*, in which social activists seek out researchers to accompany and describe their work, following from the notion that research can have practical consequences (same goal as local clinical scientist). The emphasis here tends toward field experiments, policy analysis and recommendation, and the "action science" of Argyris, Putnam, and Smith (1985).

We can supplement this summary with three major substantive uses for qualitative research approaches in the context of scientific examination of phenomena of interest to professionals. These have great bearing for the local clinical scientist. Qualitative approaches are useful in:

- *Exploring subjective phenomena not previously examined*, or about which there is a lack of knowledge (e.g., the study of views of the idea of "mental health" in a community setting)
- *Allowing for and analyzing opened textual, free response, or narrative information* provided by clients or research participants (e.g., a description of a person's sexual development during an anamnestic interview)

- *Exploring how particular relationships between variables identified at the population level might actually operate in the lives and experiences of individuals.* For example, class and race have been shown to be related to a variety of healthy issues in the United States (Williams & Collins, 1995). Although aggregate data may have no direct implication for how things work for particular individuals, qualitative methods might be used to understand how an individual assigned a value on a social class variable might actually experience the world in such a way as to participate in the kinds of health outcomes identified at the aggregate level. For example, particular individuals from the higher social classes may experience more confidence and less stress in their social milieu because their social position is discernible both materially and implicitly in their overall countenance. Therefore, even if the stress of social situations, such as employment, is related to health outcomes, such as hypertension, then we might find that narratives of such higher-class individuals do not often contain stories of higher job-related social stress. Or, when they do, other compensatory elements may be available, such as frequent dramatically resuscitating vacations, only possible because of the resources available to such individuals. Elements of these stories might also be unique, such as a higher-class individual who experiences stress in employment no matter what resources are available. Others might be shared enough that researchers can use the qualitative information to identify new questions for examination of the population relationships. Qualitative data allow for this examination of the relationship between aggregate conceptualizations and individual realities.

SOME QUALITATIVE METHODS

In quantitative research, the rules for moving from measurement to data analysis and data display are well worked out. Much of the technical details are handled using existing statistical programs. There are questions of exactly how results should be presented and interpreted that draw on the creative and theoretical skills of the scientist. But the format for the presentation and the range of arguments allowable are generally clear. Not so in qualitative studies. The operations in qualitative research are designed to put the researcher in the presence of phenomena, rather than to act as operational definitions for phenomena. Moreover, the methods by which one moves from direct observation to data presentation and conclusions lack the precision in definition possible when using numbers. Of course, this need not be a disadvantage in that the operations involved in moving from a research plan to research conclusion(s) can be tailored to the research question; often such steps are obscured by the routine nature of statistical analysis. Nonetheless, there is considerable work involved in these steps and no assurance of success for any particular approach.

Miles and Huberman (1994) offered a useful summary of approaches to qualitative data analysis that have kinship with familiar quantitative approaches. There are three overarching operations involved in qualitative analysis: data reduction, data display, and conclusion drawing and verification.

Data Reduction

Data reduction involves the always formidable operation of reducing large amounts of qualitative, usually linguistic, information to a lesser amount that captures important structure in the data. It is a process of focusing, simplifying, abstracting, and transforming the raw data. The researcher is required to make choices about what to keep and what to select out in answering a question logically linked to the data. In this sense, the researcher is an active processor of the information and an instrument of analysis. Professionals necessarily engage in similar information reductive operations to deal with the often unorganized and chaotic data of practice. The process is not dissimilar to the quantitative operation of averaging, which is a major reductive operation, but as we have suggested, it is neither as systematic nor as definitive a summarization as in quantitative procedures. However, when properly executed, qualitative data reduction may be more closely linked to the operative theory of the researcher than in a typical quantitative study.

Data Display

Data display involves the systematic ordering of qualitative information for presentation so as to reveal and underscore relationships, processes, and structures existing among elements in the data. This might be accomplished with a summary textual table similar in purpose to the statistical summary tables found in quantitative studies.

Miles and Huberman (1994) discussed a variety of displays that can be used as examples for asking creative questions. For example, a matrix crossing a series of events with different categories of information can be useful in illuminating how particular situations go together. Such displays can be ordered around time, roles, or concepts. Multiple cases or sessions can be ordered temporally or on the basis of some organizing construct or theory. Even implied causal maps can be drawn to show how events come to be, either in one's theory and observation or in the ways research participants construe causal relationships. Readers are encouraged to consult Miles and Huberman (1994) or Tufte (1983, 1990) to explore some of the virtually endless array of possibilities that might be developed to address particular issues.

For example, an association could be demonstrated between a patient's relationship with a sibling and his sexual concerns via a table showing that his discussions of his sexual difficulties are proximal in time and theme to seemingly unrelated issues about his sister over the course of the treatment. Such tables can also reveal content links in the material discussed that are not apparent to the patient or the therapist as they unfold across an extended time period. In effect, qualitative displays order verbal and, particularly, narrative information so as to reveal the important and useful elements while pushing the confusing or the distracting into the background. They are a means to raise the practical signal value of the material above the noise existing in its complexity.

Conclusions and Verification

Conclusion drawing and the ultimate verification of a research finding are subject to the same issues in qualitative studies as they are in traditional quantitative research, although the problems associated with this domain of research operations are perhaps more apparent than in traditional quantitative research, where methodologies are widely accepted as handling problems for the researcher. Once the researcher has made a commitment to certain aspects of the data, then whatever empirical results follow from that commitment must be brought into the conclusion, whether compatible with the researcher's views or not. In this sense, qualitative data are no less empirical than any other form. Thus, questions about generalizability, replicability, and validity of the information–in the sense that it addresses the substantive questions it presumes to address—are as important here as in the traditional quantitative experimental frame of reference.

The information available for data display will set limits, albeit often broad ones, on what can be said in one's conclusions. This is true both in exploratory and in confirmatory qualitative studies. Some believe that qualitative data can be manipulated to say anything, and certainly this is true if one is willing to leave out, or not look at, important aspects of the data. This also can be done in quantitative studies. But assuming the research is conducted in an honest and thorough manner, qualitative data, judiciously considered, will reduce the range of possible answers to most research questions. Thus, our psychotherapy patient's sexual problems may seem to revolve around his masculine identity. Yet, the discovery of a proximity of complaints about his sister with times when the sexual issues were prominent in the therapeutic conversation may suggest that problems with women are also part of this concern. Further pursuit of this hypothesis, however, may reveal that feminine qualities noticed in the sister, which the patient rejects in himself, are more relevant to his sexual problems, leading to a revision, in whole or in part, of the operating formulation. If links can be discerned between those qualities of the sister and the patient's view of women in his life and his sense of his own failing as a man, then this line of thinking may lead to important new insights about the patient's sexual issues. Alternatively, further exploration of the historical information in the psychotherapy may show that the temporal proximity of sister conversations and sexual complaints is not as clear as originally thought. If so, other lines of inquiry might better be pursued. In this frame, notions of confirmation, reliability, and validity refer to useful and defensible leads to be pursued and the evidence that suggests that a particular focus is paying off or not (see Stiles, 1993).

The Conceptual Framework

An important step in any research endeavor comes in the framing of the research question. In mainstream scientific work, this usually involves a careful analysis of the published literature in an area as a means to raising questions logically related to what has been done previously, and that represent an advancement in knowledge about the area. It can also involve a theory about how phenomena operate that is linked to an operational plan for executing the research. The same is true in qualitative studies, except that the literature is relatively more sparse and, because basic data collection and analytic procedures cannot be taken for granted, the theoretical framework is relatively more important. Even in very inductive, observational studies, a framework of some kind is implicated even if only to guide when and how the observations are collected. Frameworks need not be strong theories of phenomena, as they need only guide attention to certain aspects of the phenomena in question to be useful (see Chapter 9).

Webster's defines a framework as a "frame of reference, a set or system (as of facts or ideas) serving to orient or give a particular meaning." In this sense, a framework, even a very rudimentary one, can serve an important heuristic function of guiding attention to potential relevant observations, of raising questions, and of keeping an inquiry going when we might easily fall into complacency. Miles and Huberman (1994) discussed frameworks as involving the things of the research, such as concepts, entities being studied (e.g., people, communities), and the relationships that exist among them, as in order, attachment, implication, covariation, flow, and influence. A good framework provides a first step in identifying the who, what, when, and where, or structural aspects, of phenomena, and the how aspects in the ways relationships among structural entities are constituted. Frameworks can involve virtually any means of communication, including visual diagrams, lists of conceptual propositions, mathematical formulas, or even a poetic statement that carries meaning beyond its direct linguistic connotation.

Miles and Huberman provided several compelling and instructive examples of theoretical frameworks that, although requiring careful study, can be useful in accessing important qualities of the phenomena being investigated and in illuminating the central trajectory of the researcher's thought. Frameworks often are useful organizing tools for pulling together what one thinks is going on in a phenomenon and for clarifying how the conceptual tools one has available might function. They also are useful for critical analysis.

Figure 7.1 provides an example of a framework used by one of us (Trierweiler) in conceptualizing a hospital inpatient consultation performed some years ago. The lines reflect direction of influence and flow of information leading ultimately to the report sought by hospital staff about a patient. Such a framework may not be definitive even in its own terms, as in accurately reflecting information flow—the consultant, after all, also affects systems as well as patients. However, it was extremely useful in providing a context for reflection on observations the consultant made throughout his

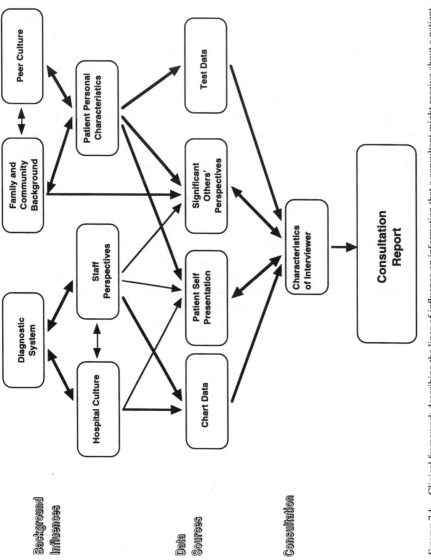

FIGURE 7.1. Clinical framework describing the lines of influence on information that a consultant might receive about a patient (thick lines indicate direct or strong influence probable; thin lines, indirect or mild influence probable).

contacts with the patient and the site, and was helpful in interpreting the meaning of various forms of information given in the consultation and in raising questions about information still needed. Note that this framework could be a preliminary model for a qualitative study where various bits of information could be classified according to the framework (see below) and evaluated for their ultimate impact on the report (e.g., the strictures of the diagnostic system may have inordinate influence in some cases). Also, note that frameworks may serve to suggest what is not being considered as well as what is. For example, economic issues were not prominent in the framework in Figure 7.1 although they might well be made more explicit today. More about frameworks is provided in Chapter 9, where we look at the contribution such devices can make to clear and critical thinking.

Note that both frameworks and the data displays one hopes to produce serve the important function of linking one's ideas with information presumed to exist independent of one's viewpoint. This may even be information about oneself. Thus, for example, one may use a framework or a time-ordered display to explore one's own notes about a clinical case, thereby reducing an overwhelming task to a maximally focused and efficient exploration. Considering the relationships a client has as they are mentioned in the course of sessions and how they correspond to major issues or themes identified in the therapy can provide extremely useful information about the ebb and flow of sessions across time, as in the case of the client's sister mentioned earlier. Qualitative methods, to the extent they involve familiar tools like interviewing, and the analytical tools discussed by Miles and Huberman, serve this important role of bringing ideas and data together, and they are of great value to the critical thinking of the local clinical scientist.

Codes and Coding

One major way theory is linked to qualitative information is via a formal coding operation. Chunks of information are identified and codes, or categories that have a descriptive or interpretive function, are assigned to these chunks. The operation of generating codes is similar to the quantitative data generation process described in Chapter 5: Observations are assigned numbers that link to theoretical properties or constructs of interest to the researcher. This is also true in qualitative studies except that the assignments are typically not numbers, but rather categories or lower-level concepts that summarize the raw qualitative material.

Codes can follow from theory. For example, Stern's (1985) theory of infant development might suggest codes applicable to mothers' descriptions of their interactions with their infants, or they can be generated via a more inductive process from qualitative material already collected and summarized in a useful fashion, such as verbatim transcripts of free response interviews (see below).

There is a sense in which coding, like measurement in the quantitative frame, entails the basic operation of assignment of meaning to the raw material of scientific observation. In this sense it is very similar to the inquiry task regularly facing professionals. Diagnosis, for example, involves the coding of information gained in diagnostic interviews into a nosological framework, such as DSM-IV (American Psychiatric Association, 1994). Similarly the symptoms, which make up the syndromes identified in a diagnostic structure, are themselves codes for more specific information that arises in the course of a clinician's interactions with a patient and with other clinical information existing about the patient. Such codes always involve both a descriptive and an interpretive function in the sense that some aspect of the information is isolated from the other information in an implicit chunking operation (e.g., a report of depressed feeling might receive more focused attention in the diagnostic frame than a comment that "life is not as meaningful as it once was"), and then it is categorized (coded) to reflect the existence of some phenomenon described within the classification system. A comment about not being able to sleep through the night becomes the symptom of "early morning awakening," and so on. In the logic of traditional science, the code is a sign for the observation, which in turn maps into the higher-order descriptive and interpretive structure (Creighton & Smart, 1932; Sullivan, 1954). Formal diagnosis aside, all clinical and professional interpretation involves the coding of information at some level, even if implicitly, and inclusion in a larger structure of meaning for the professional. As we argue in greater detail in the next chapter, this is why the categorical logic of traditional Western philosophy and science remains important to local clinical scientists, regardless of whether they operate within a quantitative or qualitative framework.

The aspect of scientific qualitative coding that is perhaps most useful for the local clinical scientist is the invitation it carries to look more planfully and precisely at the qualitative information existing in the clinical situation. Scientific constructs, subconstructs, and observations, and the codes each entails at its own level of analysis, should not be held at a distance from the clinical situation. Rather, they can be vivid and alive to the extent the professional can bring them into the actual operations of professional inquiry. Sometimes they will simply provide a means for considering what is going on (the descriptive function of codes), often they will provide a level of order and explanation (the interpretive function), and occasionally they will yield new insights and directions for inquiry and action that otherwise would not exist (the heuristic function). For example, in family therapy, vivid examples of enmeshment in real interactions among family members might provide a basis for concrete discussion of how assumptions and emotions of different family members impact family interactions (e.g., Trierweiler, Nagata, & Banks, 1995).

More broadly considered, codes can raise possibilities for understanding that are fundamentally local and that greatly extend the researcher's empirical grasp of phenomena to which there may be no direct access (such as conditions that are time extended or that involve higher levels of analysis, such as family, organizational, or cultural groupings). Miles and Huberman (1994) described *pattern codes*, which are higher-level inferential or explanatory codes, that might be assigned to observations once linkages between events are understood. For example, topics discussed at different times in psychotherapy may be recognized as related to common underlying themes. Separate mentions of the joys of traveling, of the wonderful city in which the patient grew up, of the difficulties in leaving home as a young adult, and of issues in striving for success on the job may suggest an underlying pattern or theme related to difficulties in identity development and in the achievement of independence in the context of "the wonderful situation created for the patient by her hardworking parents." Such hypothesized linkages can be "tested" by a clinician by coding conversations about these matters in her notes and then by looking for other information proximal to the discussion that might suggest that the identified theme is operative. Although no one else may ever read these notes, the possibilities for a concrete and specific understanding of how the clinical case formulation is generated and tested can be worth the effort. Coded sections that do not support the attributed theme can also be identified and explored for material perhaps not immediately apparent to the clinician. Such exploration might lead to fruitful modification of the clinician's working hypotheses.

This example brings up one other important function of codes and coding, the indexical function (Patton, 1990). Records are useful for professionals, but they can quickly become too massive and difficult to digest, as is true with all qualitative data. However, if codes are assigned to reflect a clinician's understanding of situations as they develop, then new access to sets of information that might assist inquiry becomes available. This is particularly true if notes are computerized and the search function of a word processing or database program can be used. For example, mentions of the patient's family, collected within and across several sessions, can be readily examined together if properly indexed. Computers can accomplish this with key words embedded in text in ways that can be useful in a professional's reflections. In this way codes enhance the merging of the professional's interpretations of phenomena with the ongoing material of professional inquiry and action. The more carefully and systematically this is accomplished, the higher is the probability that new or confirmatory observation can be made across time and circumstance in the professional interaction, and complex matters can be more efficiently scrutinized.

The Grounded Theory Perspective

Many who advocate qualitative approaches to research believe that theory-driven inquiry is inherently distorting (e.g., Morse, 1994). They tend to advocate inductive approaches where the substance of the inquiry arises out of direct contacts in the field. One of the most influential works on this process was Glaser and Strauss's (1967) *The Discovery of Grounded Theory: Strategies for Qualitative Research* (see also Strauss & Corbin, 1994). As the title of this work implies, the focus was on how theory can be generated via interaction with empirical situations in the world. In this view, theory generation is the primary purpose of research, and it needs to be graspable to those studied, as well as to the researchers (also an agenda for Schutz, 1962). Thus, in the grounded-theory approach, which was written for sociologists, an understanding of subjectivity as it exists in the world is an important part of the theory to be produced, as is sociality.

The emphasis on theory generation includes a strategy for collecting information that will ensure that the researcher is exposed to phenomena of interest, in ways where categories and properties relevant to understanding those phenomena can emerge in the process of the research. Obviously, this sounds like the open-ended approach to inquiry favored by many psychological practitioners. Glaser and Strauss (1967) described a process of careful sampling and comparisons between groups that might produce meaningful insights. This type of research is less product and more process oriented: Hypotheses are generated based on field experience, theory is elaborated, and then brought back into the field for assessment of its fit. The goal is to generate theory that is coherent at the highest and lowest levels of abstraction and formality, and that links behavior and experience in the world to scientific formulations.

Glaser and Strauss (1967) proposed the *constant comparative method* as a means to achieve this goal. This involves (1) coding and constantly making comparisons between incidents sharing codes in common, explicitly noting similarities and differences; (2) working the material resulting from these comparisons into a theory in which different categories are integrated and in which theory-linked empirical events can be elaborated (e.g., they give an example of how nurses working with dying patients "recalculate" patients' loss as nurses come to know them better and how these changes in their observations relate to the "loss" story ultimately told by the nurses, and to how the nurses, themselves, cope with death in their work); (3) delimiting the theory as it becomes increasingly focused on certain aspects of events, and consolidating categories as this becomes possible and meaningful; and, finally, (4) writing the theory based on the material generated, which will include both description of observations and notes about how categories have been generated, used in the research, and integrated into larger themes and conclusions.

The grounded-theory approach captures the intuition of many in the social sciences—which is also highly valued by many professional psychologists—that discovery is still possible and is needed in localized inquiry, that it is as important as anything currently existing in the literature, and that science must include a naturalistic observational component if it is to advance. Many local clinical scientists follow an approach similar to this in professional inquiry. The difference is that, in writing within the scientific frame of reference, Glaser and Strauss and numerous qualitative methodologists more strongly emphasize that the approach must be systematic, carefully documented, and oriented toward the generation of relevant and meaningful theory. Local clinical scientists can greatly benefit from adapting this thinking to clinical situations where both local and general descriptions of a case may benefit a treatment.

Reliability and Validity in Drawing Conclusions from Qualitative Data

In traditional research designs, questions of reliability and validity of the measurements and the findings are central. Both are defined in terms of applied statistics.

Qualitative studies also raise questions of reliability and validity, although we can no longer depend on the orderly structure of statistics to tell us how successful we have been in achieving these goals. The logical argument that underlies a scientific conclusion, which is typically hidden in the rigid logic of statistics and research design, is looser, more clearly verbal as opposed to mathematical, and is bound to the particular audience to which it is addressed (e.g., participants in the study, the professional community, a dissertation committee) (Stiles, 1993).

Drawing on the thinking of numerous authors (e.g., Lincoln & Guba, 1985; Manicas & Secord, 1983; Miles & Huberman, 1994; Stiles, 1993), reliability and validity in qualitative research design reduce to three classes of questions. In reading through these, consider how directly they capture some fruitful questions for local clinical scientific inquiry.

Reliability/Dependability

Can we trust that the data collected and summarized accurately reflect that which we, or any of a class of like researchers, would have collected under similar circumstances, were it actually possible to repeat those circumstances? Is this true both for the breadth (range) and depth (detail) of the information given (e.g., did the respondent tell the whole story to the extent it could reasonably be expected)? Furthermore, to what extent are these data bound to the particular circumstances of their collections (e.g., time, researcher, location)? Would other researchers, given the same data, have performed data reduction operations the same way?

Validity/Credibility

Given dependable data, is there reason to believe that the data bear on the phenomena being investigated in the way the researcher claims they do? For example, a respondent in a study of work life may report "feeling overworked." This might lead the researcher to a discussion of the workload demanded by an organization. However, this seemingly logical linkage may lack credibility to the extent there does not also exist direct evidence that this worker's statement communicates a perception that the organization's workload is too great. Other meanings for the statement might be relevant, such as "there is no reward for the work accomplished," "I wish someone would take this burden off my shoulders," "I am having problems balancing the demands of my personal life with the real requirements of a particular type of work," or any of a number of comparable connotations of the original statement. The point here is that there is considerable equivocality as to the meaning of particular statements respondents might make. Therefore, credibility is increased to the extent each piece of evidence is explicitly placed within the larger context of the respondent's relationship with his or her work. The threads of logic and relevance that lead to credible discussion of a particular datum are best revealed when the description of the phenomenon—in this example, the respondent's perception of work—is as complete and comprehensive as possible. The anthropologist Clifford Geertz (1973) described this as "thick description."

Warranted Assertability

Drawing on a notion discussed by Manicas and Secord (1983), we can push this thinking beyond the data themselves into the conclusions we presume to derive from the data. Remember that, even in quantitative studies, conclusions are, for the most part, interpretive. Can we say that the conclusions drawn from the data are warranted, both because the researcher has given us reason to believe that the data are both trust-worthy and credible, and because the chain of reasoning linking the results to the larger discussion of conclusions and implication of the work is clear and plausible? Does the work adequately deal with plausible rival perspectives? Although that is inevitably a judgment call, the researcher can facilitate the warranted assertability of a conclusion by writing research reports wherein the logic leading to a conclusion is absolutely clear, and wherein the range of alternative conclusions have been consid-ered and ruled out. In turn, the reader of a research report can test the warranted assertability of a conclusion by making sure the chain of logic leading to the conclusion is clear and plausible, and by consciously attempting to frame alternative conclusions not addressed in the report. Unfortunately, by these standards, warranted conclusions are rare in a wide range of scientific studies, whether qualitative or quantitative. This, however, should not discourage us from trying to strengthen this aspect of our work.

Some Activities or Techniques for Enhancing Reliability and Validity in Qualitative Studies

Now let us consider a sampling of some of the numerous activities and tech-niques that exist in the literature to address these goals (Lincoln & Guba, 1985; Miles & Huberman, 1994). Most are self-explanatory and have direct implication for a local clinical science. Think about how they relate to reliability, validity, and the generation of warranted conclusions in the professional context. We will offer some possibilities as we move through the material.

Prolonged Engagement

More contact, with proper effort, should yield more data, and it should be increasingly likely that evidence can be mustered in support of one's conclusions. Of course, in the real world there are economic, ethical, and practical conditions that might inhibit this aspect of professional inquiry. Still, it is useful to consider what one might have if contact were prolonged or intensified, and how this might render current conclusions more humble than they might otherwise be.

Persistent Observation

Seek salience in an inquiry, that is, those elements and characteristics of the case that are of greatest relevance to the intent of the inquiry, and focus on those. Avoid being distracted by other matters unless they force themselves into the inquiry because they are found to be highly relevant. A good framework, even one generated and updated regularly for a particular case, can help one from being distracted by the complexity of lives and the social world. Still, complexity sometimes will be the relevant reality, and the scientist must respond to it accordingly.

Triangulation

This involves multiple measures or measurements, and essentially is a process of observing the same phenomenon via several different methods or perspectives. The differing approaches should be independent of one another to the extent possible so as to rule out contamination. For example, if a person reports being religious, he is independently confirmed to attend religious services regularly, and religious material can be observed on his bookshelf, these various observations are beginning to render the report itself plausible in a certain sense. Of course, how it applies to the individual, and indeed whether these distinct observations are ultimately linked in the individual's character, requires additional assessment. In professional work, multiple investigators and multiple sources of evidence may not be possible or practical. Still, one can construct deeper assessments by recognizing the kinds of information such sources might yield were they available. In addition, the internal consistency of a patient's report, such that details corroborate each other and converge on a common understanding, is an example of local triangulation.

Peer Debriefing

Exposing oneself to a disinterested peer to review an investigation and look at one's interpretations of data can be extremely useful. Like supervision in professional work, it is an opportunity to clarify both one's thinking and what is affecting the work.

Member Checks

The data analytical approaches, interpretations, and conclusions are checked by members of the respondent sample. The notion here is that a good qualitative analysis should be credible to participants (Stiles, 1993). Regular check-ins with participants will avoid certain personal and institutional biases that may affect the inquiry. At the same time, they may also endorse a parochial vision of the problem to which participants cling. Ultimately the researcher must take responsibility for the analysis. We believe the same is true for the professional. Professionals will gain trustworthiness and credibility in their formulations to the extent they are able to present them comprehensibly to their clients and incorporate in reasonable fashion the clients' response to such presentations. Still, it is incumbent on the professional to take responsibility for the overall quality of the inquiry.

Weighting the Evidence

Some evidence is more concrete and convincing than other evidence. Thus, it might reasonably receive greater weight in some circumstances, though care must be taken to evaluate the context within which such evidence seems stronger and to avoid getting carried away with the strength of an interpretation simply because it is supported by concrete evidence. Many a great mystery tale has been told about how the seemingly concrete in evidence can lead an investigator astray because the interpretive context within which it is embedded is not given due heed (e.g., Doyle, 1891–1892). When hard and soft evidence lead to differing conclusions, a new perspective may be required to understand the data.

Making Contrasts and Comparisons

Contrasts and comparisons are essential to any inquiry, and even to the possibility of knowing itself (e.g., Bateson, 1972, 1979). Virtually any statement identifying a quality of an object or event, or even labeling the object, distinguishes it in some way from what it is not. We have seen that the search for similarities and differences is central to traditional quantitative science, and so it goes with qualitative inquiry. The trick is in determining which elements or qualities of elements to compare. Often theory will guide one's choices. At other times, careful observation and playing one's hunches will be required. In multicase studies, one can look for subgroupings of respondents, or situations within respondents—for example, things said, or the ways things are said—that seem to go together. In the local clinical situation, points of similarity or difference within a case, or across cases having some common background, can provide hints about matters otherwise unseen.

Ruling Out Spurious Relations

Caution about accepting an apparent but, perhaps, spurious relationship in making one's interpretations of events should be a basic rule of social life. Qualitative researchers must carefully assess relationships that become apparent during the course of a study. The more obvious the relationship observed, the greater scrutiny it requires in that it becomes increasingly difficult to rule out. It is particularly difficult to modify or replace a belief in a relationship between variables and events that readily fits one's conceptualization, or worse, one's general beliefs about the nature of things. This problem is especially noticeable for therapists doing marital and family work. Often, their existing beliefs about what is possible in intimate relationships can affect their beliefs about the constraints operating in the relationships of their clients. Only careful attention to one's beliefs, with open recognition of how much they are supported by clear evidence as opposed to mere assumptions about what is true, can free one of these imprecise implicit theories.

Documentation and Auditing

Documentation, organized so that it might actually be understood by an outsider, is always an expensive proposition. Nonetheless, preparation for an audit of the data collection, reduction, and analysis is a solid way to enhance the credibility of a project. This means that all matters are documented, and the documents are actively used in drawing conclusions for the inquiry. This calls for patience, tenacity, and a good deal of self-awareness so that one can actually reconstruct the inquiry process. Even more, it requires a tolerance for ambiguity, as conclusions are kept in abeyance or in preliminary status until all of the data are in and the entire operation can be reviewed. A powerful source of credibility for an inquiry lies in having the project so clearly designed and executed that an outsider could (and would) arrive at the same conclusions as the researcher.

It is clear from this list of strategies, and any reading in the qualitative research literature, that much depends on the honesty and integrity of the researcher. This involves more than just telling the truth—people believe they are honest—to include efforts to avoid cutting corners; becoming overly secure in one's own perspective; or failing to look in the inconvenient, uncomfortable, or messy shadows of an inquiry. The goal is to incorporate a sense of responsibility, availability, and openness to the public into one's inquiry in the service of credibility, even if one's work is never actually scrutinized. It involves being able to explain one's formulation to a knowledgeable outsider and to evaluate its fit with the central realities of the situation.

The notion that psychotherapy, for example, is so private that it cannot be understood by another would not be consistent with the scientific ethic. The relevant knowledge need not be simple and superficial; it may require some understanding of details not readily available to nonprofessionals, and even some specific knowledge of how a particular professional conducts herself. Nonetheless, scientific credibility depends on the professional's ability to generate a straightforward (if not simple) account of all of the material from the case. Being available to public scrutiny is, in the last analysis, merely an expression of an aspiration to clarity in one's thinking, of the wish to approximate truth, as opposed to simply conforming with convention, and of the habits of mind that spring from these values.

SUMMARY AND EXTRAPOLATION

Qualitative research procedures are so close to the typical ways practitioners operate that their extrapolation to the local clinical situation is obvious in most of what we have discussed. However, we do want to underscore certain issues associated with this research tradition that the local clinical scientist would do well to keep in mind.

Sociality and Its Relevance to Practice

Many ideas that professionals depend on take on specialized meanings within the context of their common experiences and interests that will not readily be apparent to nonprofessionals. Nonetheless, it must be kept in mind that ideas do not simply exist for the cognoscenti within a particular discipline. Sooner or later, all important ideas pertaining to health and well-being will find their way into the common language of society. Professionals must recognize that this will happen, with or without their input and blessing, and ready themselves to manage both the positive and deleterious consequences of this evolution. Moreover, as professions compete in the health care marketplace to sell their perspectives on psychological dysfunction (witness, for example, how definitive the biochemical perspective on depression seems in any psychopharmaceutical advertisement), the coordination between commonly used ideas, their actual professional usage, and the phenomena that they reference in a particular context may become all the more strained. In the face of the popular media's deliberate manipulation of experience and its labels, professionals must redouble their efforts to gauge how words are actually being used in particular circumstances.

When all patients are talking of dreams and the unconscious, of abuse and codependence, or of the impact of social oppression, it is no longer clear that language is opening the same window to human suffering that it once did. This social context for an inquiry may have important implications for one's conceptualization of specific cases. We would, for example, not be pleased to learn that our understanding of a case depends as much on a patient's conceptions and misconceptions of professional theory, as represented say in the popular press, as on that individual's actual experience of a problem. Without careful assessment it can be difficult to determine exactly what is true (e.g., consider the false memory debate). The social analyses that underpin qualitative methodologies can make us more aware of this aspect of our profession's mutually influential interaction with society.

Language is a basic tool for both public and professional discourse and from a scientific perspective it involves more than simply structures in the brain and psychological development: It also is a social symbol system that exists apart from any given individual or group (e.g., Luria, 1981; Vygotsky, 1962). The call for sensitivity to the subjectivity of our patients encourages the development of perspectives on human problems that are less distant and socially demeaning than are some of the esoteric constructs of certain practice traditions—which often imply blame, weakness, or pathology and which often require practitioners to simply rely on authority to define the meaning of clinical observations. Working directly with the substance of a conceptualization as reflected in the actual interpersonal and social conditions that exist for a patient can serve to confirm or raise questions about one's ongoing case formulation. If traditional practice constructs are indeed valid, then there should be cogent ways of understanding their social implications, and there should be social evidence in the form of comprehensible linkages between the construct and what is actually observed in the local clinical situation. Thus, for example, repression should be representable at interpersonal levels as well as in a clinician's inference about the intrapsychic, and enmeshment in a family should have some identifiable interactive consequences that can be represented to the family in a comprehensible fashion.

In short, professionals need to take special care to ensure that the language they use to represent a particular local clinical situation—including a whole case and events within a case—is as precise and carefully linked to solid evidence as possible. If the operative constructs are abstract, then links to more clear and straightforward data, such as specific events or client interpretations of events, are needed. Although it is likely that some professional constructs will be more amenable to this endeavor than others, and there will continue to be an element of uncertainty as the professional hypotheses develop into increasingly well-supported formulations, the effort will reduce the possibility that the formulation has strayed away from important facts in the case. Because there are no guarantees in local analysis, measures that improve the probability of accuracy are all the more important (Chapter 8).

The Fact of Otherness

When dealing with human beings we are always dealing with an individual who, like ourselves, has views, more or less strong, about the nature of things. This is particularly true in psychological inquiry, where the subjectivity of the other is a major access route to phenomena of interest. Otherness and dealing with otherness can be either a strength for our science, to the extent we do not get overinvolved in human problems and lose sight of alternative possibilities that might usefully fit a client, or a weakness, if we become too distant from the actual experiences that drive communications about problems in the client's life. No matter how much we get to know someone we work with, we are ultimately always outsiders in that person's life, and we must take care not to confuse our own experiences and ways of evaluating matters with theirs. This does not mean that empathy cannot be a powerful professional tool, just that it should be regularly evaluated for its accuracy and completeness. (It is not, for example, a good situation when we skillfully pick on some aspect of a patient's experience only to have the cooperative and appreciative patient remain silent about some other aspect of that experience that we failed to recognize.) Like anthropologists entering another culture, we must remain cognizant of our skills and limitations, our ability to communicate, and our reasons for being there. It is a pervasive fact that our expertise is marketed in society by a number of means, including our science, and that, as psychologists, there is an expectation that we will manage the focus on the other in the service of that individual's health and human possibilities. The work of qualitative scientists, as in anthropological studies, can be of use in developing a professional understanding of this emic–etic contrast implicit in all professional work.

Clinical Science as Qualitative Science

There is a sense in which many clinicians already act as qualitative scientists who are indeed vindicated by the recent trend for greater appreciation of this form of work. Beyond that, however, the rise of qualitative methods in the science also raises unavoidable questions about the quality and relevance of the information produced by our inquiry. This should encourage professionals, once again, to look at how we obtain information, at how we examine its reliability and validity, and at how linkages between operative theory and actual data are drawn. We suspect that all can benefit by tightening this inquiry process, by putting our biases and predilections aside for a time—perhaps to be rediscovered if they actually work well—and engaging in a process of reflection and empirical and logical evaluation of the quality of information we operate on. If nothing more, the fact of constructionism and uncertainty in qualitative inquiry is reason for maintaining an appropriate level of humility in our work.

The development of new ways of evaluating our work and the quality of our inquiry that move beyond aggregate outcome studies will undoubtedly benefit every aspect of the profession. In the next chapters we take up matters of critical thinking that assist the development of the scientific attitude in the local clinical situation and provide models for moving an inquiry forward.

Logic, Critical Thinking, and the Local Clinical Scientist

Scientific work . . . demands the utmost candor and openness of mind. . . .
One must be willing to abandon any theory as soon as it is found to disagree
with the facts. And this is by no means an easy thing to do. When one has a
theory which suffices for nearly all the facts, there is always the temptation
to cling to it, and to neglect or explain away any troublesome or
contradictory facts.
—CREIGHTON AND SMART (1932, p. 332)

There is no royal road to logic, and really valuable ideas can only be had at
the price of close attention.
—PEIRCE (1878/1955, p. 40)

True science teaches, above all, to doubt and to be ignorant.
—MIGUEL DE UNAMUNO Y JUGO

PRELUDE: SHERLOCK HOLMES, A CASE OF IDENTITY AS THE LOCAL CLINICAL SCIENTIST

Sherlock Holmes would have a bewildering time were he to pursue training in
scientific professional psychology. He might wish to apply his celebrated method to
the investigation of mind, but he would find our scientific ways frustrating. In his
training, he would learn a great deal about psychopathology, psychotherapy, developmental and social issues across the life span, and perhaps a bit about himself. He
would learn about research methods and statistics. He would find that there are more
journal articles than any one investigator could ever read, and theory abounds. But in
the end, he would find that methods he perfected for his criminal investigations are
largely absent in our training.

Holmes's approach was based on knowledge, observation, and logical inference.
To be sure, there is a fair amount of knowledge to be had in modern professional
psychology, but much of it comes to us via authority, both professional and scientific.
Thus, there is distance in that knowledge even in its application. We suspect Holmes
would be surprised by our inattention to the details of local habit and lifestyle he often
used in his detective work.

And what of observation and logic? Holmes would find little explicit attention to the former and virtually none to the latter. These are skills more appreciated in another era, when a youthful science promised to reveal the secrets of human nature. They also are the skills of more concrete realms of inquiry like criminal investigation, where Holmes could spin trifles into elegantly logical webs of inference about human events. Practicing psychologists use science to legitimate the knowledge base of the profession, but we have never been completely satisfied with scientific methods. Besides, science has changed in the past century; the lonely struggle to interpret nature has been supplanted by big money institutional science, and the scientist is as often a master entrepreneur as a master of logic and evidence. Among professionals, Holmes would find more than a few eyebrows raised to his unbridled scientific enthusiasm.

There are good reasons for this professional ambivalence. Science has developed enormous prestige since Holmes's day; it offers unsurpassed mastery of the material world. In scientific psychology our knowledge of genetics, neurochemistry, cognition, behavior, interpersonal systems, and the larger impacts of culture, gender, and ethnicity is greater than at any other time in history; our prejudices about psychological problems are fewer and our choices for treatment ever expanding. Why wouldn't practitioners want to be affiliated with such productive enterprise?

Yet science is also a place where space shuttles explode and rain forests are ravaged. There are inevitable costs and compromises in accepting science as our way to knowledge. The clinician is acutely aware of this: Science, with its complexity, aggregation, and conservative values, tends to obscure the fundamental insight that knowing a man or woman is knowing how he or she thinks and feels and makes life meaningful, across circumstance and a lifetime. Because science is the public face of our profession, the clinician has been left with the lonely, often secret, task of making psychology relevant to people, somewhere on the interface between the conceptual world of science and that of everyday common sense. It is a daunting task fraught with ambiguity about what is real; clinicians go to colleagues or significant others for help with this problem, not to science.

Holmes, having read Chapter 3 of this book, might be dismayed to hear that his romantic notion of a direct scientific confrontation with reality is not possible, even in principle. He would find us still debating the assumptions that undergird psychological practice, practicing and thinking about practice through a virtual Babel of theories and perspectives, and unable to agree about which phenomena are fundamental to our discipline. He might wish that these matters were settled, that clinical training consisted of sleuthing a client's forgotten thought or hidden intention, but ultimately, like the rest of us, Holmes would have to join the intellectual culture of psychology as we close out the twentieth century.

Holmes is a quintessential local scientist. He would undoubtedly devote himself to convincing us of the merit of his method. For example, he might argue that we avoid presupposition with our clients—not to throw theory away, but to hold it in abeyance in a posture of openness and receptivity. But this is only the beginning; he would also want us to notice details, especially seeming trifles, and absences as well as presences.

He would want us to put our thinking to the test of public scrutiny, with client and colleague (we should all have a Watson!). He would suggest that we be skeptical about appearances, that we "stay close to the data," and that our understanding of the situation be well grounded in the particulars of a case before theory is even mentioned. We would be warned to treat impressions with caution, especially those favoring our pet theory, but avidly to seek the evidence that supports them, and that which does not. He would teach us to evaluate the certainty of our evidence, and caution us to separate observation from theoretical rhetoric.

The image of the brilliant Holmes at work reminds us that truly spectacular insights emerge in toying with evidence, not in simply applying facts or theories learned from some far-off authority. It also reminds us that science resides in the "deep structure" of our professional work; we are ultimately scientific investigators of the local conditions of psychological suffering. Science is more than a course in statistics, a laboratory, or a source of "miracles" for colorful portrayal on public television. It is a way of thinking critically and concretely about a problem, of inviting others to participate in the inquiry, and of developing new ways of looking at our world. The quality of this work depends on our assumptions about what is real and what is important. Holmes would have much to teach us about using evidence, even intuitive evidence, to develop compelling, localized accounts of human events. In the end, he might even convince us that his version of science is what we clinicians have been trying to achieve all along.

LOGIC AND CRITICAL THINKING
IN PROFESSIONAL PRACTICE

We have suggested that local clinical scientists be "critical investigators of local (as opposed to universal) realities who are knowledgeable of research, scholarship, personal experience, and scientific methodology; and who are able to develop plausible, communicable formulations for understanding essentially local phenomena using theory, general world knowledge including scientific research, and, most importantly, their own abilities as skeptical scientific observers" (Trierweiler & Stricker, 1992, p. 104).

Toward this end, we have focused on how standard methodological thought in science can contribute to localized inquiry. This chapter goes a step further by exploring tools of logic and critical thinking that focus on alternative possibilities for understanding local phenomena when definitive science is lacking or when the application of scientific thought is ambiguous. In effect, we take up the questions raised by a Sherlock Holmes in pursuing scientific ideals in the context of specific cases.

This chapter combines some old and new material in examining the classic relationship that has existed between science and logic (e.g., Cohen & Nagel, 1934). As the study of logic has become more specialized and abstract, the basics, which are still quite useful to clinicians, have been deemphasized in training. Meehl (1954, 1960, 1973, 1978), Meehl and Rosen (1955), Cronbach and Meehl (1955), and Cronbach (1957, 1975a) have thoroughly examined logical issues related to aggregated judgments. Here our focus is more on thinking strategies for improving single judgments.

In the recent literature, an expanded, more functional version of logic has been discussed within the contemporary frame of critical thinking (e.g., Baron & Sternberg, 1987; Dauer, 1989; Levi, 1991). Gambrill (1990) focused on the errors of thinking that pervade professional practice. We will discuss some of this material below.

Some Definitions

Logic

Logic is a complex topic. Its definition and subject matter resides somewhere between the nature of general thought and the nature of good, or correct, thought. It has roots in the rhetoric of Socrates and the syllogism of Aristotle, in the natural science of nineteenth century Europe and the United States, and in the ever-expanding web of scientific inquiry that has characterized the twentieth century (e.g., Bynum et al., 1981; Cohen & Nagel, 1934; Creighton & Smart, 1932; Dauer, 1989). There are both mathematical and philosophical versions of basic logical concepts (Burke & Foxley, 1996). In the first part of the twentieth century it was virtually equated with science, in keeping with the logical positivist perspective. "Logic may be defined as the science of thought, or as the science which investigates the process of thinking" (Creighton & Smart, 1932, p. 3). In line with the interests in the properties of successful science, it also has been concerned with the nature of evidence.

> Logic may be said to be concerned with the question of the adequacy or probative value of different kinds of evidence. Traditionally, however, it has devoted itself in the main to the study of what constitutes proof, that is, complete or conclusive evidence . . . the latter is necessarily involved in determining the weight of partial evidence and in arriving at conclusions that are said to be more or less probable. (Cohen & Nagel, 1934, p. 5)

This last point is extremely important for our concerns. Logic is a tool for determining what would be needed in principle to answer a question definitively. In so doing, it also provides a standard against which to evaluate the incomplete evidence that we will inevitably have in the clinical situation. We have argued that the traditional tools of our modern science, such as research design and measurement theory, give us idealizations against which to compare available data in thought experiments and the like. The study of logic was a foundation for the creation of these methods.

> Logic . . . is involved in all reasoned knowledge (which is the original meaning of 'science') but is not the whole of it . . . all science [is] applied logic, which was expressed by the Greeks in calling the science of any subject, for example, man or the earth, the logic of it—anthropo*logy*, or geo*logy*. (Cohen & Nagel, 1934, p. 191)

Critical Thinking

In a sense, critical thinking is about self-supervision, about expanding one's view of situations such that choices can be made to enhance the fit between observation, inference, and professional interventions. To get to critical thinking, we must first understand thinking itself. Traditionally, to think is to exercise the mind, judge, consider, or suppose (Skeat, 1989; *Webster's*). The idea of exercising the mind is important: Valuable thought may require effort to see things in new ways—and this will not always be easy.

Baron (1994) offered a useful, updated, cognitive information processing view of thinking as a tool in decision making. Thinking is defined as a process of search and inference (pp. 4–5). "Thinking is, in its most general sense, a method of choosing among potential possibilities, that is, possible actions, beliefs, and personal goals" (p. 6). This definition emphasizes an instrumental quality. The generation of possibilities, goals, and evidence that expand and deepen one's understanding of the local clinical situation is a major goal of clinical inquiry. Baron noted that *possibilities* are possible answers to a question, *goals* are criteria for evaluating possibilities, and *evidence* is any belief that helps evaluate the fit between goals and possibilities (see also Ennis, 1987).

The term *critical* is rooted in a Greek term referring to "a judge" and "able to discern." The term *critique* comes from the same Greek root as *criterion*, which is "a test" (Skeat, 1989). The term *critical* has become an oddly negative word in recent times. An older *Webster's Collegiate Dictionary* (Gove et al., 1971) stresses finding fault, the actions of critics, and a point of crisis, or crucial. A newer *Oxford American* stresses the same three, but only the "moment of crisis" without the additional connotation of "crucial" (Ehrlich, Flexner, Carruth, & Hawkins, 1979). Somehow the notion of quiet discernment has been lost to us in this culture when judgment is an issue. Discernment, which is to perceive clearly with the mind or the senses, is the central issue for the local clinical scientist. Also, we emphasize a notion of critical that seeks the crucial (the very important or necessary) evidence and interpretations and their implications. Critical evidence and interpretations may or may not be negative. The local clinical scientist must put herself in a position to see clearly, and to act based on that vision. To this end, critical thinking is discerning judgment dedicated to exploring the crucial and distinguishing the crucial from the not crucial.

Skepticism also is an interesting term. In newer thinking the skeptic is one who doubts, who is inclined to disbelieve truth claims (Ehrlich, et al., 1979). Again, the older usage may be more cogent: Skepticism was doubting, hesitating, from the French *sceptique*—"one who is ever asking and never finds." It is also related to the Greek term meaning thoughtful and inquiring (Skeat, 1989). Critical thinking may certainly be affirmative as well as questioning and doubtful. Indeed, the task is to find and affirm those perspectives that are most supported in the local situation. Skepticism should be considered a means to the end of critical thought, not the end in itself. A skeptical attitude complements the scientific perspective, it does not define it.

Objects, Categories, and Classes

In our discussion of logic we use the term *object* to refer broadly to any person, object (including words), or event.

There are two issues involved in assigning a category to an object: (1) we are associating that object with the meaning of the category in the culture in which we reside (the various levels of local information setting are relevant here) and (2) we are assigning that object to a class of similarly described objects. It is a matter of historical debate whether the meaning of a category is equivalent to the class of objects associated with it, but we need not have a solution to this concern for the logic of categories and classes to be useful to us. Rather, we can use the logic of categories and classes to help us consider alternative possibilities raised by empirical observations made in the local clinical situation. In considering the *categorical* aspect of linguistic extensions to a particular circumstance, we are concerned with the empirical and conceptual adequacy (truth) of the category assigned in a particular instance. In considering the *class assignment* aspects of an assertion, we are raising questions about the appropriateness of the collection of objects associated with the category. These are two aspects of the same essential problem of assigning appropriate and instructive terminology to clinically relevant objects.

Overview: Logic and Critical Thinking in Basic Problem Solving

How does one think critically? The answer to this question depends on the domain of information one is observing and one's skills in recognizing properties of events within the domain. At length, it is about recognizing and evaluating alternative formulations.

Consider the observational perspectives outlined by Shakow (1976) (naturalistic, subjective, participant, and self) that we discussed in Chapter 2. A patient may be presenting material related to a theme that the world is against him and a constant source of pain. The *naturalistic* observer may see an individual who has many skills that are not being implemented for reasons that have not yet emerged (and which may be suspected by the therapist). Yet, the *subjective* observer may recognize a sincerity in the perspective being displayed and real pain in the client's experience. The *participant* observer might feel a "pull" to provide sympathy and understanding, and the *self* observer may be aware of a slight impatience with the patient. Now, one could follow a standard therapeutic protocol in the face of such information complexity (e.g., remain silent, explore problematic cognitions, interpret the therapeutic relationship). But better, the critically thinking therapist will recognize equally the legitimacy and importance of all observations, and indeed to some extent all possible responses, and determine a way to bring the qualities of each into the therapy.

For example, if it is early in the treatment, the therapist may recognize the difficulties the person is having with others, but at the same time, wonder aloud how this goes along with being one who obviously has considerable skills in other areas.

The goal might be to expand the information coming from the patient and create an interpersonal dialogue. Later on, as the patient slips back into his habitual mode of responding, the therapist may simply wait silently for the patient to recognize this pattern himself, aided by the earlier conversation that brought this style to the attention of both.

In preceding chapters, we have established that the major tools of science—aggregation, randomization, replication, or consensus—are not available to regulate local observation and decision making. Methods can be specified in practice traditions and to an extent they can even be verified by science. However, even the most perfectly designed clinical method offers no assurance of perfection in its application to specific instances. Mechanical, manualized approaches to treatment may work within the specific domains for which they are designed, but inasmuch as psychological interventions extend beyond these rarefied instances—for example, beyond symptom relief into an individual's style of relating to self and others—it is unlikely that simple rules can ever be specified comprehensively enough to cover all situations. This may be one reason why so many questions are being raised about clinical utility as well as efficacy in considering the psychotherapy effectiveness problem (e.g., Goldfried & Wolfe, 1996; Hollon, 1996; Stricker & Trierweiler, 1995; Strupp, 1986). Ultimately, clarity of thought itself is the front-line tool by which observations and decisions are evaluated in specific local circumstances.

Categories and Propositions as the Tools of Inquiry in Open Systems

The clinical situation will be both familiar and novel. Inquiry involves gathering information that supports what is known, clarifying what may be ambiguous, and evaluating the existing understanding (assessment) of the case against new evidence as it emerges. The clinical situation is analogous to the laboratory, but it is decidedly not the closed system the laboratory strives to become (Manicas & Secord, 1983; Stricker & Trierweiler, 1995). Only conceptual closure is possible in an open system. Thus, much of the data gathering is not purely empirical but rather is, itself, guided by theories of psychological difficulties in the relevant domain, and by standard forms of practice (e.g., face-to-face contact in a time span of 45 to 50 minutes, multiple interviews with members of an organization, observation of a child in a free-play context). It also is guided by the operational and conceptual tools related to the professional's working model of the case.

For example, a behaviorist working with a child who is exhibiting problematic behavior in a classroom will observe the child's behavior and relate it to antecedent and consequent conditions observable in the environment. Conditions thought to increase the probability of the behavior will be eliminated or modified to mitigate the antecedent–behavior–consequent pattern supporting the behavior. In turn, appropriate behavior incompatible with the problem behavior (e.g., sitting quietly as opposed to getting out of seat and talking) may be reinforced in the child. To accomplish these ends, the clinician may become directly involved with the child, or work indirectly through guidance of the actions of others. The intervention may involve the modification of the behavior of the teacher, other children, or the child's parents.

The above example illustrates an intervention strategy for applying behavioral learning theory to classroom behavior (e.g., O'Leary & O'Leary, 1972). The theory involves recognition of certain categorical qualities in the clinical situation (behaviors, antecedent and consequent conditions, and so on). These in turn are related to one another in the context of the unique properties of the case (e.g., the behavior occurs in a particular classroom, observable at a particular time). Propositions are generated about how the various categories of information intermingle and interact, and actions are developed to ameliorate the conditions so identified that are considered problematic.

The same operations are relevant to any theory of a case. Psychodynamic theories may focus on derivatives of unconscious conflict identified in session material as it is understood by the therapist. To this end, certain evidence, such as dreams, may be accorded greater attention than other material. In interpersonal approaches (e.g., Benjamin, 1996; Kiesler, 1982), the emphasis may be more on properties of interpersonal relationships; in feminist approaches (Hare-Mustin & Maracek, 1986), evidence thought to reveal gender-influenced power relationships will receive relatively greater emphasis. Even cultural theories (e.g., Nagata, 1991; Sue & Zane, 1987) involve assumptions about evidence and the meaning of that evidence. Theories only gain their meaning in the efforts of the professional to apply them in actual clinical situations. One could say that it is the ability of new theories to offer plausible rival hypotheses about phenomena not previously recognized, or to reframe phenomena, that is their ultimate contribution to our knowledge base.

Ultimately all information comes from observing and listening to the patient, from an understanding of the meaning and circumstances surrounding the information, and from a theory or model for organizing the information that is developed by the therapist—based in science or a practice tradition (e.g., Kanfer, 1990). Usually, there is a favored set of interpretations associated with theories that are brought into the clinical situation by the professional. The local clinical scientist model suggests that these favored interpretations should be a point of departure for inquiry rather than inevitable ends impervious to the influence of local evidence.

Reasons for Clinicians to Be Concerned with the Study of Logic and Critical Thought

Why should a clinician be interested in logic and critical thinking if she already knows where to look for familiar answers to her questions? Why change a view that is accepted implicitly, that may be grounded in good training with an esteemed authority? Why exert extra care when one already knows what is true, when one has a favored perspective for viewing matters such as this one, when one is, after all, an expert?

There are no easy answers to such questions and therein lies the problem. Science and practice traditions are presented as so definitive that the need for additional analytic tools, and nonspecific ones at that, can be difficult to engage. Logic is not the most popular academic topic, in any case, which may explain its post-World War II dismissal from the center of the curriculum of an educated person. Particularly in the social sciences there is an aversion to anything so abstract and seemingly disconnected from matters of substantive interest to the scientist. Yet, in deemphasizing the study of logic, apart from research and statistical logic, we have missed an opportunity to raise important questions about the nature of argument in our scientific, scholarly, and practice pursuits.

Consider now several reasons that an understanding of good logic can be helpful to the local clinical scientist. Not only are these arguments reasons for pursuing the study of logic and critical thinking, but they also illustrate an open but critical skepticism; we do not have to accept a particular critique but we do need to consider it fairly. This list adds to the reasons cited in the literature for heeding science and bringing it into the operations of everyday practice (e.g., Barlow, 1996; Goldfried & Wolfe, 1996; Hollon, 1996).

Intuition and Authority Need to Be Assessed Carefully

Beliefs based in a priori thinking, tenacity, intuition, or authority (see Chapter 4) need to be treated with caution. These sources of belief are too powerful not to be scrutinized. Professionals get beliefs from a number of sources including formal and informal training, influential supervisors, the psychological literature, personal experience, professional experience, institutional and economic priorities, moral belief systems, the public media, and so on. Unfortunately, given the level of commitment and effort involved in learning about practice traditions, the range of alternatives to one's favored locally operative beliefs is often not carefully considered.

Consider beliefs based in authority, as in the ideas of a favored supervisor. Authorities gain their authority via their position as clinicians and scientists, and the cogency of their arguments. What they offer, however, is not truth, but rather possibilities for consideration. All such offerings merit consideration, but few justify blind acceptance. Authority-based beliefs are not inevitably flawed, but they can be strengthened and improved by putting them to constant test. Testing allows effective beliefs to prove their accuracy and utility relative to alternative possibilities.

The operations of intuition need special scrutiny. Intuition implies something known immediately without reasoning (see below). Observations about subjectivity of self and other in the clinical situation often come to us as intuitions (e.g., a sense of hidden pain in a presentation of a relationship with a loved one). Intuitions might be thought of as a set of implicit assumptions, interpretive preferences, or tacit recognitions that may operate outside awareness (cf. Reber, 1989) (e.g., an assumption that a patient's description of problems with her parents accurately reflects actual parent motivations, that a patient's financial stability is the result of his own labor, that a child who is the misunderstood object of larger systemic issues operating in a family cannot be held culpable for aspects of his behavior, that in a well-functioning therapeutic relationship everything that might be of interest to the clinician has been talked about, or that an elderly Chinese man will be cared for by his family). Intuition can be accurate and powerful, or inaccurate and misleading. Although intuitions may not arise from reason, reason (logic) can be used to test their veracity. It is the ability of intuition to lead to accurate, penetrating representations of real situations that makes it so powerful and influential. To leave intuitions untested and unchallenged is to miss some of this power.

Not All Evidence Is Equal

This is a major complaint of Meehl (1973) in his self-described polemic against weak thinking in case conferences. It is also a basic tenet of modern conceptions of applied logic (Dauer, 1989). The problem is that evidence does not always tell us how to think about it, yet, inevitably, some evidence will serve certain ends better than other evidence. As Meehl suggested, more experienced and broadly informed perspectives on the meaning of evidence must be given due respect, as representing the positive aspects of authority. At the same time, an open attitude suggests that any grounded perspective might be beneficial in illuminating the local clinical situation. Thus, in case conferences and elsewhere, the local clinical scientist must balance the I-already-know-the-answer position of the experienced professional against the all-evidence-is-equal position of the novice. Even a weakly framed observation made by an inexperienced colleague, when properly understood and contextualized, could yield important insights. We need tools for evaluating evidence of all kinds and for allowing the most central evidence to emerge as an understanding of the case deepens. We need free and open conversation, but freedom of expression should not be allowed to compromise the strength and cogency of a conceptualization.

Language and the Observation of Psychological Phenomena

Attaching language (constructs) to human psychological events is the essential task of the local clinical scientist. Nonetheless, it is an imprecise endeavor that needs continuous updating and careful evaluation. There often are hidden assumptions involved in particular attachments that would be of great interest to us were they considered directly. Conscious effort will be required to reveal these assumptions.

To illustrate, consider the situation where a clinician asserts some quality of a patient, say, that the patient is socially avoidant and self-deprecating. A whole array of other observations that are consistent with this picture may also be available; for example, the patient may hold a job that requires little direct contact with people. However, even assertions richly supported by observation and direct experience may distract from disconfirming evidence even as they inform. For example, once the socially avoidant aspects of the patient's presentation have been categorized, the clinician may begin to perceive other aspects of the person as reflective of the category without any directly supportive observation (as in new, intuitively consistent observations or in reflective inferences). This aspect of categorization has long been known (Bruner, 1973) and recently has been called *confirmatory bias*, *representativeness heuristic*, and *illusory correlation* (Kahneman et al., 1982; Turk & Salovey, 1988). Consistent with the previously recognized data, the clinician may assume that the socially avoidant individual has no positive interactions or relationships. In actuality, the person may have an array of successful interactions that are simply not part of the presentation of self that is generated between clinician and patient (e.g., he may go to church and do things in the community that would surprise, or there may be satisfying relationships among members of the extended family of the patient). Logical analysis suggests that such possibilities may exist however a person presents and that there may be great benefit from exploring information not represented directly in the primary presentation.

There Are No Locally Simple Relationships between Actions and Outcomes, Observations and Inferences

Some things we know as clinicians are given directly in our experience of a patient, some by inference. Some of our interventions work, some do not. Behavior, thoughts, and experiences are not independent, nor do they operate in simple unidirectional fashion. Intuition often will connect with something substantial but there are not guarantees that it reflects accurate interpretation.

It is easy for professionals to fall into habits of making simplistic if–then statements between actions and outcomes, observations and inferences in their work. For example, Bakan (1956), in discussing the importance of logic in clinical inquiry, cited Rogers's (1955) comments on the clinical attitude as a means of accessing the experience of the other. This involves an open stance and suspension of judgment. It is a very good description of one aspect of clinical method and experienced clinicians will have a basic idea of what such an open stance is like. Yet questions arise: How does one open up and what is the nature of opening? Can one assume that any particular style is always actually opening? Does active interest actually lead the patient also to open up? Alternatively, does looking and acting neutral do so? Enacting openness and a patient-centered approach with an obsessive individual may be reason for the patient to doubt that he can actually be open with his experience. On the other hand, being assertive, which may seem to run counter to openness, may in some cases actually facilitate a sense of safety and clarity. Asking direct questions and even sharing an opinion may facilitate freedom of expression in the patient. These ideas can be raised and explored fruitfully in the local clinical situation.

The Logic of Thought and Emotion May or May Not Be Different

Clinicians tend to associate logic with thought and intuition with emotion. Yet there is no particular reason that this needs to be the case. For the patient, the logic of thought and that of emotion may or may not differ in a particular situation. Likewise for the practitioner, accurate thoughts and accurate intuitions will both be valuable. Logical analysis can help to describe the similarities and differences between what is thought and what is experienced and enacted emotionally in a case. For example, in marital work, a man who argues vehemently for his view of problems in the marriage may or may not actually be attempting to dominate the situation, although he might well be perceived that way by his spouse and perhaps even by the therapist. Often, he may have a sense he is merely defending himself against his powerful spouse. A woman, on the other hand, in perceiving dominance in his manner, might become angry and frustrated as she attempts to express her own position. This is all quite apart from the issues being discussed and the *reality* of the couple's circumstances. This emotional dance can be analyzed for what is and is not revealed in the same way as the issues being discussed might be. To notice and describe such phenomena is to use language to analyze an otherwise ambiguous situation (Vygotsky, 1962). The language of emotion demands no less accuracy than does the language of objects and events.

In any case, the clinician faces an inevitable problem in tying thought to what might be fundamentally emotion. Clinicians often assume that their intuitions about emotional events are definitive. There is little reason for such confidence. The relationship between thought and emotion is controversial (James, 1890/1950; Lazarus, 1984; Zajonc, 1984). There is reason to believe that both always exist (Schacter & Singer, 1962) and this fact needs to be represented in our thinking regardless of which one has priority in one's clinical theorizing.

There Are No Hard Boundaries in Soft Science

The objects we observe are selected from a larger information field with fuzzy as opposed to clear boundaries. Diagnostic categories, for example, are often thought of in categorical terms, as if there are clear boundaries around a classification. There may be good reasons for doing so with some diagnostic categories such as schizophrenia (e.g., Meehl, 1995; Meehl & Golden, 1982). However, there also are reasons to believe that more dimensional representations might do a better job in some diagnostic situations in handling heterogeneities within diagnosis such as comorbidity of disorder (Clark, Watson, & Reynolds, 1995). To the extent there exists unclarity and doubt about the integrity of any classification, either formal, as in diagnosis, or informal, as in simply attributing a characteristic to a person or event, there is a need for the local clinical scientist carefully to explore alternative formulations of a case.

Fashions Change, Old Problems May Not Be Solved

One has to be disturbed that the concepts used in the soft sciences change with fashion in increasingly rapid cycles (see Meehl, 1978). Our society has developed a virtual cult of newness. New ideas are valued simply because they are new, however flimsy are the arguments for their superiority over more established viewpoints.

Unfortunately, new thinking may not be as good as it appears to be. For example, in the past 25 years, eating disorders have gone from being very rare to being everywhere; trauma theory, once a secondary viewpoint, has become a favored interpretation that is promulgated with moralistic zeal. Do we really believe that these changes are simply the discovery of something previously hidden from view? The problem is that even as we discover human problems that need attention, we cannot be sure our efforts quickly to identify and treat them are not also distorting need, as new service markets are generated and as the media attempt to represent mental illness to the public. Recent times have demonstrated beyond a doubt that when matters of the consulting room become part of the public discourse, much activity is mobilized (e.g., Loftus, 1993). However, there is no clear evidence that people are better off than they used to be, or that the problems that used to occupy the attention of patients and therapists in an earlier time are any less relevant today.

This influence of the times is apparent in all areas of science. Logical analysis will not diminish such influences. However, it does encourage critical evaluation of the primary messages of the times, acceptance of the useful, and due caution toward potential distortions.

Distinction between Aggregate and Individual

As discussed in Chapters 5 and 6, the distinction between an understanding of aggregates and of individuals must be inspected in each local clinical situation. If evidence exists that an aggregate formulation is applicable (e.g., that this individual's apparent aptitude, educational background, and achievement conform to what population studies suggest is true of people in general), then proceeding with the general scientific characterization is justified. Alternatively, evidence contrary to the general formulation (e.g., evidence of inconsistency between aptitude, background, and current achievement) suggests that population evidence for an applicable subgroup may be needed. In any case, local information also will be needed for a complete description of how a population characterization does or does not apply to the particular case. Errors of logical typing involve the confusion of the individual with the group and vice versa (Watzlawick, Weakland, & Fisch, 1974). They are widespread in areas of the public discourse where propositions thought to fit a general category (e.g., *men* or *women*, *blacks* or *whites*, *Republicans* or *Democrats*) are ascribed to particular individuals. The impact of such confusion is pernicious in two ways: (1) It may hide local variation such that individuality and uniqueness is obscured, and at the same time, (2) it may hide instructive similiarity and consistency that actually exists between group and individual levels. One outcome of this confusion of the objects of our language (group versus individual) is the tendency to make sweepingly uninformed attributions about local realities that are transported into the clinical situation in the guise of scientific expertise (e.g., any woman who is supportive of a troubled man is codependent; any man is out of his element in emotional conversation).

In the next section we discuss some ideas of logic that can help avoid these problematic situations in local clinical inquiry.

A PRIMER OF LOGIC AND CRITICAL THOUGHT
FOR THE LOCAL CLINICAL SCIENTIST

For those with some background in logic, the usual disclaimer applies: As in our discussion of philosophy of science in Chapter 3, we are not attempting to solve the problems of logic, but merely to ask how selected insights from logical inquiry contribute to the real tasks of the local clinical scientist. There is no single approach to critical thinking. There are many ideas about how thought can go awry. Here we begin the process of linking logic and critical thinking more explicitly to the training of professional psychologists.

As a point of departure for this discussion, let us revisit the clinical situation where a professional first encounters a new client. The initial encounter can be considered an open information field. The face-to-face element has a clear temporal boundary. There is also a reflective component that extends into the future for both client and clinician. In principle, if information during the initial encounter does not get into the professional's memory, then it is not available for reflection. The information heeded [we are using this terminology in the same sense as Ericsson and Simon (1993)] is subject to a virtually endless array of interpretations, and new questions to be addressed at a future encounter can be considered. Clinicians often attempt to operate from a position of suspended belief—indeed, it can seem as though there is competition between different perspectives with regard to which approach and assumptions access this position best. An open stance allows the client to offer information about his or her own perspective on the situation. However, even here, the extent to which this information is actually registered and integrated into a larger clinical formulation is subject to the ability and judgment of the clinician.

Clinically important information may involve a particular event in space-time, or a whole range of encounters across an extended time period. The clinician's task is always to observe, apprehend meaningful information, and interpret it in a way that facilitates healing for the patient. The extent to which this process is patient or clinician driven will vary with circumstances, including the theoretical perspective of the clinician and of the patient, and the particulars of the therapy (e.g., a short-term setting).

The task of logic and critical thought is to isolate circumstances where examination of alternative possibilities in specifying an observation or in framing an interpretation might prove useful. An understanding of the formal properties of logical thought can help in raising critical questions to extend and focus an inquiry—much like those identified around research logic in Chapter 4.

Consideration of the Source of an Observation and a Proposition

Several authors have discussed how aspects of logical analysis can be applied to critical thinking in everyday life (e.g., Dauer, 1989; Levi, 1991). The possibility of merging logical and empirical analysis is particularly relevant to the examination of interpersonal and social experience insofar as much of this experience is time extended and referencing phenomena that are not directly available for scrutiny. Some characterizations of the world are easier to accept than others. Dauer (1989) called these *unproblematic propositions*. Because we will not be able to analyze carefully every proposition about the local clinical situation, establishing what we can take for granted will reduce the amount of material we must scrutinize carefully. Unproblematic propositions are those that give us little reason to doubt them and that might be considered a reasonable foundation for higher-level inferences.

Dauer's Candidates for the Unproblematic

Dauer (1989) described five categories of information that promise to be unproblematic.

Observational Statements.   Observational statements involve the traditional empirical stuff of science. In the local clinical situation, they might include direct observations of self or other or, more often, descriptions of observations made by the patient or other significant participant in the treatment. They might also include test data or relevant archival data (e.g., a school record). Statements describing subjective states might also be considered observational (e.g., a patient reports feeling depressed).

In this context, observational refers to the understanding that the producer of the proposition has directly apprehended the situation described. Of course, just because a statement is observational and, therefore, tending toward the unproblematic does not mean we must take it as given—although often we will. It is important to remember that because the observation is framed in language, there is an interpretive step involved that may require assessment (cf. the relationship between observation and data in Chapter 5). Aspects of a statement that are not in doubt, and their meaning for the client, can be explored by the clinician.

Keep in mind that observations are not equivalent to the inferences derived from them. For example, we must distinguish the clinician's inference of depression from her observations of the way the patient acted and spoke on which the inference was based. A more general example of this distinction can often be found in newspapers. For example, a news headline stating "Candidate A Ahead in the Polls; Candidate B Needs to Revive Campaign," suggests an observational statement that is unproblematic and verifiable with regard to the polls, but an inference with regard to the need to revive the campaign. Dauer (1989) distinguished the directly heeded from that which was directly heeded, but now is only available in memory (see also Ericsson & Simon, 1993). This distinction has important implications for understanding the referents of verbal material generated in local clinical interactions as we discuss in the next chapter.

Facts Based on the Claims of Experts. The claims of experts are often treated as factual based on observations that might have been made in principle if conditions were right, as in a claim about an event that actually would have been observable in the past; they are based on numerous observations that have been summarized (as in accepting the experience-based assertions of a teacher and supervisor); or they are based on noncontroversial inferences drawn from observations. Scientists and other experts regularly make public claims that are more or less taken as true. Thus, we take it as unproblematic that scientific claims that depression and anxiety are separate disorders are accurate claims and that there exist data to this effect that have actually been collected. [There are also data to the contrary (e.g., Taylor, Koch, Woody, & McLean, 1996).] Here we must attend to a difference between data actually collected, and collective or widespread consensus that operates in professional cultures (paradigms). There certainly are conditions taken as fact that may not have any actual data other than professional sensibility associated with them. Also, there are inferences and assumptions made within research and clinical paradigms that are not necessarily intrinsic to the data enlisted to support them. For example, the fact that maintaining a certain attentive distance, and even silence, may work to assist freedom in patients' presentation in many psychotherapy cases (e.g., Paul, 1978) does not ensure it will work for all cases. Nor is the common interpretation of this position—as a means to the end, say, of free association—necessarily accurate in all circumstances. The empirical/factual quickly shades into judgment and authority in our field. Local clinical scientists who are aware of this, and who retain an open awareness of how facts and assumptions come to them, will be able to adjust when factual beliefs begin to distract from local realities.

Intuitive Knowledge. Dauer (1989) set rather severe restrictions with respect to intuitive claims that might be considered unproblematic. Such claims must not depend on particular observations or past learning, but rather only on a limited amount of reflection (e.g., $2 + 2 = 4$). This is an instructive definitional baseline for contemplating how intuitively given thought might actually be unproblematic. However, as commonly described in professional psychology, intuitive knowing involves more overlap between observation, prior learning, reflection, and intuition such that a rather complex awareness may arise at a particular point in time with little reflection (e.g., a well-dressed child is being cared for by someone, structure is needed to maintain order in a classroom, individuals usually act on behalf of their own needs and interests). Obviously, this expanded definition widens the doorway to sources of doubt about the intuition.

More broadly considered, intuitive claims are a subset of the a priori knowledge (see Chapter 4) that is accessible with fairly brief reflection. Intuitive knowledge is interesting in that it seems to come to us directly based on what we already know. An example might be the recognition of pain in a patient's description of a family reunion, or the insight that phrases repeated in different contexts may mean that something important is being withheld in the presentation. In a sense, intuition is the linkage of several seemingly unrelated events in a way that may lead to additional insights.

To be sure, intuition can be both useful and dangerous in the local clinical situation. Much of the intuitively given information in professional interactions will be unproblematic much of the time, and therein lies the trap. Intuitions can seem so unproblematic that motivation to explore their veracity may be lacking. Yet, conscious efforts to do so can yield powerful results. For example, intuitive awareness of the pain a patient experiences can have a powerful therapeutic impact. However, singular attention to pain, or overweighing its importance, may diminish needed attention to sources of strength and coping not intuitively given in a particular circumstance. Because intuitive knowledge may not be accurate or shared with others, the wise practitioner will regularly assess the accuracy and relevance of basic intuitions about a case.

Some believe that claims of intuitive inspiration are lazy answers to unexplored mental processes. Others find the romance and drama of intuition inspiring in their own right. The local clinical scientist should be able to enjoy the power of sudden understanding while still laboring to uncover relevant cues, to assess their veracity, and to evaluate the validity of the intuitive, soon to become logical, links drawn between them. Neither the romance nor the logic is the problem with intuition; the problem lies in our strange notion that the two cannot coexist in a scientific analysis.

General Claims of Science. The general claims of science are about the implications of scientific laws and principles for our general understanding of the world. For example, few today would consider the structure and function of bodily organs to be unrelated to health, because there exists an enormous amount of science that suggests otherwise. The discovery of laws is a major aspiration of received view science, as outlined by Cronbach and Meehl (1955) (Chapter 6). Laws of behavior, psychopathology, interaction, and relationship, once known and identifiable in the local clinical situation, could have profound implication for professional action.

If, for example, we can assume that the big five personality characteristics (Wiggins, 1996) actually constitute a structural law of individual differences in personality in the human population that is applicable to each and every individual, then each individual should be meaningfully locatable on such dimensions (see Chapter 6). Another example might be when treatment X is thought to yield positive outcomes with problem A and is empirically demonstrated to do so. The local questions involve the extent to which the treatment is being applied correctly—according to the law—in this particular case, and whether it is producing the same kind of outcome alleged by supportive scientific claims.

Although there is little logical or scientific justification for doing so, psychologists often can be heard asserting lawlike scientific claims based on the findings of single studies. Similarly, lawlike assertions arise from often questionable commonsense extrapolations from scientific findings, as we discuss below. Some laws are also paradigm specific, which means fruitful alternatives outside the paradigm may not receive sufficient attention.

A major gap between science and practice arises out of the differences in operation and emphasis between the activities of psychological scientists in presumably establishing lawful relationship (as in the examination of statistical correlations), and the activities of practitioners in the observation and assessment of individual cases in real practice situations. We have tended to confuse the search for general scientific laws with all science, without recognizing the pervasive need for active development of the implications of more general lawful thought to all sorts of applications. Some of these developments must be considered to have purely local implications, which is a major reason we need to develop our grasp of thought, observation, and inquiry at the local level. We need to promote a tradition of working out these implications as scientific findings and theories come to light. This work would both reveal controversial issues and assumptions, and provide practitioners with a set of midlevel conceptual tools for locating evidence in the local clinical situation. We discuss how general and local science might be bridged with explicit conceptual frameworks in the next chapter.

As suggested in Chapters 5 and 6, problems may arise in assuming that correlational relationships, framed as lawful relationships between variables, can be directly extrapolated to the local level without examining supportive local details. We will discuss this further below in looking at specifics of correlation in the context of logical analysis. Undoubtedly, direct extrapolation of the interpretive gist of the correlation is most reasonable when the relationship is understood in the context of a strong nomological net (Cronbach & Meehl, 1955).

When the search for instances of lawlike relationships works well, it can be very helpful to inquiry. For example, suspicion of bipolar illness may lead to questions about how money is handled or about periods of heightened activity that could enhance certainty about one's suspicions. There are informal, non-definitively established laws that operate in clinical lore and procedure, for example, that a patient's open self-expression has a healing property. Such phenomena may be widely observed, but they will not necessarily achieve the status of a scientific law because of our inability to establish definitively their truth. Actually, there are surprisingly few laws that are simply applicable in our field or in psychology in general. Instead, there are informal notions that are treated as laws in professional communities.

General Claims of Common Sense.   Commonsense claims involve information that is supported by many confirming instances that are easily accessible to all, that is widely acceptable to adequately informed individuals, and that is so accepted as to be resilient to discomfirming instances, which are quickly explained away (Dauer, 1989).

Aristotle described common sense as involving possibilities common to all sensation (Bynum et al., 1981). Today it is the common sensibility, that which is understood by all and available to normal good sense that is based in life experience. For example, people cannot see through walls, things do not just disappear, if a patient is wealthy the money must have a source somewhere and this may have implications for the treatment, or if a marriage is described, there was a ceremony at some time.

Both everyday common sense and professional common sense are relevant to the local clinical scientist. Inasmuch as problems can develop when professional common sense runs counter to local everyday common sense, everyday common sense may receive too little attention in professional formulations. For example, taken-for-granted professional views of childrearing practices—particularly those of a quasi-moral nature that may be grounded in suggestive but nondefinitive scientific data, such as a preemptive bias against the use of physical punishment—may conflict with those accepted as common sense in a local community. This is a matter of local culture that requires careful assessment by the practitioner to determine if working with local common sense may not actually be a superior strategy to asserting the authority of the professional perspective. Because common sense can seem so broadly acceptable to the professional, it can lead to an arrogant presumption of superior knowledge when there may be little actual ground for such presumption. The integrity of perspectives that are grounded in science or in professional experience is of the essence in matters of nonshared common sense; premature application, acting as if basic questions were answered definitively when they were not, poorly serves clients, clinicians, and the profession.

Ideas rooted in the common sense of the professional are undoubtedly more prevalent than formal laws in professional work. In acculturating to a profession, one develops a shared sense of what is true, of what works and what does not, and of the ground rules for professional operation and decision making. For example, it is professional common sense to the psychotherapist that 45 to 60 minutes is an adequate period of contact for most clinical interventions. Depending on one's goals and theoretical perspective, anywhere from one to five visits per week is a commonsense amount of therapy needed to progress.

Other commonsense ideas have to do with understanding the patient's life. In order to communicate, we must have some basic understanding of what a patient is telling us, and time constraints will ensure that we will be unable to explore carefully each bit of information (in some forms of treatment there may be little or no exploration). Thus, care is needed in managing the commonsense assumptions intrinsic to human conversation. Many insights given in common sense will be true; common life issues often will be understandable at a commonsense level. However, common sense, of both lay and professional varieties, offers no guarantees of accuracy. Training oneself to pick up important spots in a dialogue where understanding may diverge from the patient's reality will undoubtedly be beneficial.

Unexamined professional common sense can go seriously awry in grasping locally unique and space-time specific phenomena. For example, most clinicians would accept that a patient who is a successful law school student must be working hard enough to get good grades. A clinician who has been through years of schooling will have a basic understanding of the required effort based in his own experience. Of course, this commonsense perspective, which is also personal for the particular practitioner, can also be very misleading to the extent that the patient has different skills and work capacities than the clinician. For example, if the patient reports working very little to be successful, considerable ambiguity surrounds the meaning of "very little," such ambiguity usually being poorly served by commonsense assumptions of the clinician. In the end, although a pragmatic professional common sense must be considered a major source for the "laws" governing our practice, only continuous assessment will ensure a sensibility that is well connected with local circumstances.

Problems with the Unproblematic

Ambiguity pervades the territory of the local clinical scientist. In discussing candidates for unproblematic evidence, we have repeatedly pointed to problems. In effect, there are no unproblematic data in the local clinical situation, just varying degrees of ease and clarity with which phenomena might be identified. There is strong and weak evidence, but the boundary that exists between problematic but obvious data, and potentially even more problematic categorization and inference, is subject to interpretation. The local clinical scientist must use the tools of logic, science, and substantive practice theory to narrow the range of alternative possibilities.

Fundamental Logical Connections between Elements and Descriptive Classes

Basic features of logic provide us with an overview of what is possible in the propositions we might generate to describe and analyze phenomena in the local clinical situation. Each time we name or describe a person, object, or event, we are creating a proposition that is subject to logical rules.

Negation (Not)

Negation may be the most important logical operation. Some things are defined in terms of assertions (affirmations), others as negations—as in what is missing that might be there. Negation picks up the idea of the complement: An assertion negates the complement and vice versa. Whether we realize it or not, we are tacitly comparing the individuals we observe with a model of what normal should be like for them if there were no pathology. This model may or may not be the same as the average of an individual differences distribution, but it is locally normative given the particular patient and particular clinician, nonetheless. Judgment of what is absent depends heavily on the clinician's model of the local reality. Some of the most pathological conditions are specifiable as much in terms of what is lacking as in terms of what actually exists. For example, positive symptoms of schizophrenia, such as hallucinations and delusions, have a better prognosis than so-called negative symptoms (e.g., alogia or flat affect) that are defined by observed absences (e.g., Andreasen, Arndt, Alliger, Miller, & Flaum, 1995).

In addition to unethical actions, antisocial personality disorder is a pathological absence. The antisocial individual has no close personal relationships, and treats people as objects to be exploited. It would be surprising to find such a person deeply involved with someone. Negation raises a question about how one assesses absence. How, for example, does one assess absence of depth in relationships? DSM-IV refers to behaviors like lying or infidelity (American Psychiatric Association, 1994). The point here is that the assertion of a category such as antisocial personality involves boundaries that need to be assessed (e.g., How accurate is the attribution of the disorder? How pervasive is the behavior identified?) and complementary negations that may also need to be assessed (e.g., Are things absent that should be absent if the attribution of the disorder is accurate?). In so doing, hidden points of strength and/or vulnerability might emerge that would otherwise remain in the shadows.

Reflection on the negations associated with an assertion can help to reveal circumstantial limits that may exist for a case. For example, severe substance abuse can make it difficult for intimacy to develop within a couple, however much they might wish for intimacy in their sober moments. If that substance abuse is strongly linked to the local culture of family and friends, then the problem is even more intractable. Understanding limits in this way may lead to useful predictions about the course necessary for a successful treatment. The assessment of a negation also has relevance for evaluating emotional presentations, as when presenting the pain shrouds the pursuit of the pleasure that may actually drive particular acts. Because emotions are often strong when an individual seeks professional help, it can be easy to ignore the complements of those emotions, even though, save for the most severe and chronic disturbances, such complements must exist for the person at some level.

It is important to remember that if something can be asserted, then it can also be negated. To suggest that a patient looks depressed is also to assert that he does not look not-depressed. Often this fact is overlooked, even though it can have dramatic implication in overextending interpretations of patient data. For example, to note that a patient tends to be impulsive is to note a quality that, in some cases, can have major impacts on the patient's well-being and possibilities for a stable life (if such is desirable). In so noting this characteristic of the patient, however, we may miss carefully planned aspects of the patient's life that are not at all impulsive. A patient impulsive in love relationships may be very careful and organized on a job, or with respect to a creative activity, that may not be brought to the therapy as readily as the painful relationship issues. Impulsiveness reflective of the patient's impatience with another, which might have an opportunity to come out if the contrast with other life areas is revealed, is different from that driven by other issues. Some clinicians will say that what is not brought into the treatment is not relevant to the clinical process, others will say that it is more relevant. Whatever the belief, the clinician's grasp of the local clinical situation is influenced by judgment of what is and is not revealed in the patient's presentation. It is good policy to reflect regularly on the implications of negating the major descriptive propositions in one's inquiry as an exercise in evaluating the supporting evidence.

Conjunction (and)

We regularly combine characteristics as we come to know the individuals we work with. At least two characteristics are needed for a conjunctive statement. As we combine descriptors, we become increasingly specific about the case in question. Indeed, specificity is largely the result of the increasing uniqueness that attends the combination of more and more characteristics within a particular individual. Whether these characteristics blend, interact, or simply coexist within the individual is food for further inquiry. For example, an individual may be wealthy, abusive, and lonely. Reflection on how the abusiveness relates to the wealth may lead to a somewhat different picture than reflection on how it relates to the loneliness. Only additional inquiry might reveal how particular combinations of characteristics are manifest in a unique life. For example, the abusiveness may originate, in part, in a way of life intrinsic to the development of personal wealth. At the same time, this outcome of wealth seeking may be intrinsic to the patterns of loneliness observed.

Unpacking the meaning of even simple conjunctive propositions can have major implications for inquiry into a case. It is important to take care in one's assessment as increasingly specific material is examined: Conjunctive statements are only true when both properties are actually present. Unreliable or inaccurate identification of one or both can be very misleading as one reflects on their combination and calls into question the validity of any inferences based on the false premise.

Disjunction (or)

Sometimes it is unclear which characteristics (predicates) apply but we have a sense of the possibilities based in our experience or in an applicable theory. Thus, a school phobia may be a function of fears of something in the school (e.g., problematic interactions with peers), of something in the home (e.g., fear that in leaving home something dreadful will happen there), of something between school and home, or of some combination of these (multiple determinism making everything more complicated). In this way, disjunctions imply different pathways in an inquiry that often will be incompatible.

Another way of thinking about disjunctions is as alternative rival hypotheses for understanding particular local circumstances. Usually, disjunction implies a need for additional inquiry to clarify which pathway is most fruitful. If an inquiry and subsequent treatment go awry, it can usually be traced back to some point where a disjunctive choice was possible and either was not heeded or a choice was made that in retrospect may not have been justified. For example, the decision to treat an individual rather than a couple can be a difficult disjunctive choice when couples issues are clearly related to individual problems. Opinions vary broadly about the best policy in such situations. Local clinical science seeks justification that extends beyond our preferences for particular modes of practice. Therefore, disjunctive choices available in such situations should be considered on their own merits. Awareness of the choice is the first step, careful evaluation the next. In this way pathways with maximal justification can be recognized and choices can be made and then comprehended retrospectively if matters do not go as planned. For example, some cases of depression that are related to couples issues may not be completely resolvable in the context of couples treatment, even though substantial progress can be made. Understanding this from the very beginning can facilitate a clinician's recognition of what is and is not successful in the couples treatment and facilitate referral or implementation of additional treatment for problems not handled in the couples work.

Each setting of local information (see Chapters 2 and 3) implies a set of alternative possibilities, many of which will be disjunctive. Some will be inclusive, meaning a or b or both. Some will be exclusive, meaning a or b, but not both. For example, in making a diagnosis (identifying an instance of a general theoretical category) a patient may be showing signs of an obsessional condition or outright thought disorder, or both, or neither, depending on the evidence available to the clinician. The same patient may present a local culture in which the obsessional material is supported, as in religious obsessions, or not. At the space-time local level the clinician has to evaluate whether the interview evidence supporting the attribution of obsessionality was actually obsessional material, or a reflection of efforts to avoid even more anxiety-arousing topics during the interview, or both.

Implication (if–then)

Science and practice are replete with if–then (conditional) statements, many of which are implicit: If the patient has early morning awakening, then the diagnosis is depression; if the individual had a frightening experience, then it was trauma and the person has posttraumatic stress disorder; if a child says abuse is happening, then it must be true; if there are symptoms, then there must be unconscious conflict; and on and on. An important task for the professional is unpacking the meaning of general if–then propositions in science and in the local clinical situation. Another is to become aware of the set of important if–then propositions that the patient and clinician carry about what is happening in the patient's life and in the course of the treatment.

We often associate if–then propositions with causality. The *if* part is the antecedent, implying temporal precedence as described in Chapter 4; the *then* part is the consequent in such statements. It is important to note that, from a logical standpoint, the truth value of implicational statements depends on the circumstances of both antecedent and consequent. In most formulations, the implication statement is only false when both the antecedent (a) is present and the consequent (c) is absent, in effect "falsifying the statement." The statement remains true for the three other possibilities because it cannot be ruled out: *a* present and *c* present, *a* absent and *c* present, and *a* absent and *c* absent. We can decide how viable the statement really is only when *a* is present, in which case *c* must be present for the statement to be true or absent for the statement to be false. When *a* is absent, then the presence or absence of *c* does not tell us whether or not the statement is true, so the statement remains true by default. If a particular patient experiences anxiety when family members argue, then this proposition remains true if there are no arguments and there is no anxiety, or if there are no arguments and there is anxiety (anxiety may be caused by other things as well). The anxiety observed today, in the absence of evidence of an argument, does not rule out the proposition that arguments cause anxiety in the patient. Of course, there is also a problem that arises when the antecedent is mistakenly identified as present (as when a prior experience is deemed frightening when it actually was not), so that the entire test of the proposition is no longer valid.

Traditional logical conventions aside, there is some arbitrariness to this choice of leaving a proposition true under the indeterminate condition of the antecedent being absent. We could argue that there should be no such acceptance of truth under indeterminate conditions, which is a more conservative position that may be more appropriate to empirical and scientific determinations. (This is the reason for saying a theory must be refutable given the data for it to be an acceptable test.) We could allow other possibilities to exist than the simple judgment of true or false for indeterminate cases. We could say that a statement should be considered false rather than true when conditions do not permit a determination—although this would not solve the indeterminacy problems. Clearly, unlike logical analysis in the abstract, the local clinical situation demands that we allow for uncertainty. But this shows a commonly observed flaw in clinical thinking: When a consequent is observed without a given antecedent, such as low self-esteem without the identification of a traumatic condition in the past, a proposition that trauma caused the observed low self-esteem is indeterminate. The important thing here is the indeterminacy; speculations about antecedent conditions should be accordingly humble.

Equivalence

Two or more elements are treated as equivalent to one another. This is often assumed without careful analysis (e.g., certain events and trauma—even though evidence for traumatic nature may be questionable, pleasure seeking and moral looseness, success or goal attainment, and satisfaction or happiness). Sometimes what are actually conjunctive hypotheses about one or more characteristics are treated as though they are equivalent. For example, an individual's failure on a job is equated with being treated poorly by the boss, when aspects of the patient's motivation may also be at issue; or particular arguments within a couple are equated with poor communication, when some arguments may be based on actual conflicts where aspects of communications are accurate reflections of the participants' intent. Equivalence can be meaningful in pointing out common features of characteristics that may be inappropriately separated. For example, conflicting couples may stress the differences between them and ignore, or take for granted, areas of profound similarity and equivalence of purpose (this is also an example of negation). Conversely, it can be misleading to assume equivalence without supportive evidence. For example, normative population studies assume within-population homogeneity. As discussed in Chapters 5 and 6, this works well for population summaries and interpopulation comparisons. However, it does not follow that any two or more cases from the population should automatically be treated as equivalent without supportive evidence to this effect. For example, differences between ethnicities that are very real at the population level may be inappropriately transported into conversation about individuals and small groups at the local level. Recall that population correlations rarely approach 1.0, so generalizations from population findings are always probabilistic (see below). If these constructions hide important points of intragroup dissimilarity and intergroup similarity, then instantiation of the general finding distorts local realities.

Basic Properties of Propositions

If we accept that any time we link a construct to an object we have, in effect, assigned that object to a class of similarly assigned objects, then there are several properties of the assigning propositions that are useful for reflection. Cohen and Nagel (1934, pp. 35–39) described several distinctions that are notable in generally descriptive propositions. First, they may reference quantity. Traditionally, this has been accomplished by the presence of quantifiers such as *all*, *some*, or *none* (e.g., all ravens are black). For our purposes, we would add a specific instance identifier (*this* or *that*) which may imply uniqueness in a specific case even as we assign it to a general category and its associated class (e.g., this raven is mottled gray). Second, the proposition contains a reference to a quality, such as the color of the birds in the above example. The array of qualities is as endless as our language—which, of course, means it is not endless, but rather simply very large and complex. Third, propositions can be exclusive or exceptive. An *exclusive* proposition is one where the meaning of one idea is predicated on another exclusively, such as "only the depressed are suicidal." An *exceptive* proposition is one where something is denied the group identified by the subject of the sentence (e.g., no individual with bipolar illness exhibits delusions of thought insertion). Fourth, propositions reflect some distribution of the meaning of the propositions to the identified objects. So-called *distributed* propositions imply all objects in the class—in effect a population in the statistical sense (e.g., all individuals with schizophrenia exhibit poor social skills). *Undistributed* propositions refer to an indefinite part of the class—in effect of subpopulation (e.g., some cases of PTSD are exacerbated by poor levels of functioning prior to the traumatic event). The terminology is not so important here as is the awareness of the basic properties of thought captured in this analysis of propositions. In particular, it underscores how our descriptions of phenomena link local circumstances to general properties that preexist in our language community, and, thereby, these circumstances are assigned to classes of objects presumed to have actual existence in the world.

There are four basic forms of propositions that describe the classifications that are thought to come into being as soon as a distinction is drawn by an observer. These are: all As are B, no As are B, some As are B, and some As are not B.

These assertions are fundamental to any classifying statement. They can be readily illustrated using diagrams first described by the Swiss mathematician Euler in the eighteenth century (Figure 8.1). Each row of Figure 8.1 is described next.

All As are B. Note that the subset and superset can be either A or B. If A were the superset, then the descriptive sentence would become "Some As are B," as described below. Logically, the structure of subset and superset relations should not be reversed, but this is common confusion in professional thought. Subset and superset relations involved in various specific assertions made in clinical work often are imprecisely identified and may be unknown. For example, consider a belief held by a clinician that a particular depressed patient has thoughts about suicide whether he admits it or not, which is based in another belief that all depressed individuals have suicidal thoughts at some point in their depression. If this latter assertion is pictured as above, then depressed individuals with suicidal thoughts are a subclass of individuals with suicidal thoughts. Alternatively, if the belief were that all individuals with suicidal thoughts are also depressed, then the subset–superset structure of the assertion would be reversed. We are likely to hear both types of assertions in clinical discourse without any clarity about which assumptions are operative. Although this may not have serious implications for identifications in cooperative cases, it can make cases not conforming to our implicit, incorrect theories difficult to identify.

Note also that the all-As-are-B assertion includes the situation where A and B are identical, in which case the subset–superset issue is not a concern.

Some As are B. The conjunction of characteristics can involve various degrees of overlap among the classes described by the proposition. Note that if the overlap is partial, as on the left side of Figure 8.1, then the conjunction actually describes three subgroups: As that are not B, As and B, and Bs that are not A. Reflection on how these subgroups might actually exist in a relevant population can be helpful in assessing the viability and usefulness of the asserted conjunction. This parsing of the overall class when an undistributed relationship is specified has major implications for local interpretation of correlational relationships, as we discuss below.

Some As are not B. These diagrams are the same because in negating a conjunction we are implicitly asserting its possibility and vice versa.

No As are B. We are unlikely to assert this type of exceptive relationship locally because we are more inclined to describe what we see rather than what we do not see. However, it is often a useful strategy for testing one's assumptions to seek evidence refuting a negative hypothesis. For example, if one assumes a child cannot understand a complicated adult interaction ("No children understand adult interactions"), it nevertheless is useful on occasion to assess just what the child might know. Occasionally, responses of surprising depth can be obtained, which, of course, refutes the quantifier of the larger proposition (assumption).

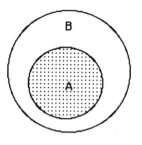

or

Some As Are B

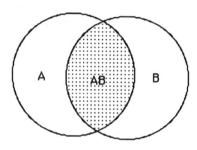

or

Some As are not B

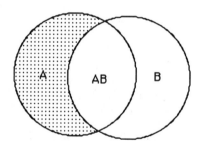

or

No As are B

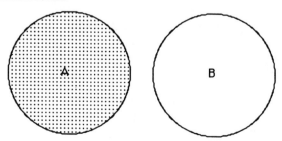

FIGURE 8.1. Euler diagrams depicting forms of proposition associated with classification. Shaded areas are referenced by the proposition.

Gambrill (1990) discussed Euler diagrams in the context of inappropriate stereotyping, that is, inappropriately confusing the individual with group in both misattributing individual characteristics to all group members and the reverse. Stereotyping seems inherent to labeling and it is unlikely that we can avoid it. However, if one remembers that there is always an implicit implication that a larger set of objects might also contain the relationship unless otherwise stated, and one learns to assess realistically the uniformity and diversity likely to exist in such a group, then stereotyping can play a less pernicious role in local inquiry. The worst stereotypes are based on extremely naive and uninformed characterizations of groups and it is surprising that some of them would continue to play any role in professional discourse. Such a lack of information about the basic characteristics of our society and local cultures is unacceptable in scientific professional practice. For example, once-common stereotypes about men and women, and their attitudes toward one another, are becoming of increasingly limited descriptive value and of virtually no scientific value. Yet there is little doubt that in continuing to describe a class of men separate from a class of women, new stereotypes and assumptions are being born, some of which will be retained as productive descriptions, and some undoubtedly to become the misattributions of the future. As we suggested in Chapter 5, we need to learn how to develop reasonable understanding of the defining properties of populations we work with, and, in this context we should add, of the populations from which our descriptive constructs are drawn. Such awareness will afford the possibility of modifying our views if evidence runs against deductively or inductively based characterizations in the clinical situation.

The Laws of Thought

Most discussions of logic deal with the so-called laws of thought, which originate in the writings of Aristotle (Cohen & Nagel, 1934; Dauer, 1989). Although as laws governing thinking they are highly questionable, they are useful in considering assumptions about boundaries as we assign categories and classes to our observations. In particular they specify the nature of crisply bounded categorical information, as opposed to fuzzy or continuous boundaries. It is instructive to look at the fundamental nature of crisp boundaries in an effort to better understand the nature and limits on the fuzziness we actually experience in the world of practice.

The laws are stated as three intuitively obvious principles:

The Principle of Identity

An object designated as A, is A. In effect, the object designation is consistent with the meaning of the category. Alternatively stated with an emphasis on the truth value of a proposition: If a principle is true, it is true, there is no alternative in actuality.

The Principle of Contradiction

No object can be both A and not-A. If the object is described by the category, it cannot be described by the negation of the category. A proposition cannot be both true and not-true.

The Principle of the Excluded Middle

Any object must be either A or not-A; it cannot be in between. A proposition is either true or false.

Obviously, these "laws" set up a stronger categorical boundary than many clinicians would feel comfortable with in the clinical situation. Indeed, few designations in human psychology would support such distinct boundaries. However, if one looks at the way natural language is used, particularly in designations of physical objects, then one can see how Aristotle and others might have come up with lawlike principles such as these (see Rosch & Mervis, 1975). They all can be contradicted by particular circumstances. Nonetheless, they illustrate clearly what we implicitly strive for in framing strong truth statements about the nature of matters in the clinical realm. To the extent we are arguing for any description we would develop in the clinical situation, we are effectively setting up boundaries of this potentially misleading variety. Of course, if we choose not to make strong arguments (if these can be avoided— see next chapter) our thinking may seem too fuzzy and noncommittal, albeit, perhaps, more attuned to realistic complexities (a fuzzy logic exists for conceptualizing this complexity; e.g., Zimmermann, 1996). The laws of thought and their deficiencies for our purposes raise questions about how we should present our beliefs about clinical cases.

Boundaries are always a problem in any analysis. This has led some to assert that there are no nonconstructed boundaries (Chapter 3). However, practically speaking, we can say there are reasonable boundaries and consistencies across categories and their usage, and this is why certain positions, like psychoanalysis, do not disappear despite critiques. Indeed, the basic idea of reliability of measurement is rooted in the laws of thought. As discussed in Chapter 5, reliability is a process of classifying phenomena in a consistent fashion across some relevant domain of generalizability (e.g., raters, time, items, situations). It seems likely that we came to this idea of generalizability because we already had some notion of how classification was logically supposed to behave when working correctly.

One critique of science in relation to professional work is that we come in with concepts striving toward boundaries as characterized in classical laws of thought, but work with phenomena that do not necessarily lend themselves to this kind of thinking.[1] However, if we use the laws of thought more as tools than as prescriptions, then they have important implications for a local clinical science. In a practical

---

[1]Contemporary work on fuzzy logic (e.g., Zimmermann, 1996) may prove a useful alternative to the crisp boundaries assumed in the laws of thought.

diagnostic situation, sources of certainty or doubt can be identified with respect to the clarity of the boundary indicated by one's classification. For example, if we work with schizophrenia, how close or distant from the boundary line do we think an individual is? What characteristic would be necessary for that person to cross out of that category into something else, into schizoaffective disorder, into affective disorder, or into nondisorder? These are questions that we carry with us all of the time. As we calibrate ourselves with diagnostic systems such as the DSM-IV, we carry these calibrations with us into each new encounter with a patient. Accordingly, they remain stable or change as we adjust to each new situation.

Principles of the Calculus of Classes and Their Implication for a Local Clinical Science

Cohen and Nagel's (1934) extensive discussion of logic and scientific method included material on the formal relationship between logic and mathematics. This development was relevant to the logical positivist wish to merge logic and empiricism. Ideas included in their discussion are very old and involve the work of Aristotle, Leibniz, Boole, Frege, and numerous others whose abstract contributions now have very concrete and practical application in the operations of computers and the Internet. Throughout this work, particularly that of Boole, there was an effort to develop a new precise language of symbols and operations that, like standard algebra, would render logical analysis precise, unambiguous, and universal. Additionally, the idea of reducing higher-order judgments and principles to their fundamental parts was greatly valued. The assumption was that higher-order reasoning could be understood as built from the basic elements, much like Euclidean geometry can be developed from a set of elementary definitions, axioms, and postulates.

For our purposes, what is interesting about this work is the way it describes some basic assumptions that are involved in categorical and class description. For economy, generality, and precision, symbolic representations are used with letters (e.g., a, b, c) describing terms that define a class, and symbols similar to mathematical symbols (e.g., $+$, $=$) specifying relationships existing between different combinations of descriptive terms. We consider it unlikely that we will convince clinical readers to become deeply involved in symbolically formalizing their thought in the local clinical situation, and it is doubtful that this would be desirable. However, we do wish to show how powerful this form of thought is in raising questions that are indeed relevant to even the most mundane local inquiry.

Table 8.1 presents some basic, presumably elementary principles of the calculus of classes (the term *calculus*, in effect, implying a formal symbolic representation of basic operational assumptions with implications for computation), with verbal interpretations and commentary about the relevance of a principle for the local clinical scientist. In reading the table, note that the symbols look like algebra, and they are related to algebraic formulation, but are not equivalent save for "$=$" signifying equality (in effect, to categories or classes that refer to the same objects). The symbol

"+" indicates logical addition which is equivalent to the set theoretical notion of union (∪) (see Kerlinger, 1986), and the logical operation "or." Thus, a + b can be read "either a or b" [e.g., cats + dogs would be the class (set) "cats or dogs," where both groups of animals are added together to constitute the identified compound class]. The symbol "×" is logical multiplication, which is equivalent to the set theoretical notion of intersection (∩), and the logical operation "and." Thus, a × b (or ab) can be read "both a and b" (e.g., the set of cats with gold markings × cats with black markings would be the class of cats with both gold and black markings, a smaller collection where only members with both designations are selected). Finally, there is the relation of *inclusion*, symbolized by "<" (the "less than" sign in mathematics). The statement a < b reads "a is included in b." Cohen and Nagel noted that the inclusion relation is transitive, meaning that if a < b and b < c, then a < c. It is also nonsymmetrical, meaning that if a < b, it may not be true that b < a with the exception of the situation where a = b.

Table 8.1 shows how the logic of categories considered as classes of objects is important because it addresses fundamental issues in the structure of thinking about collections of objects. Ideas like this can be used to explore the integrity and detail of one's thought about properties presumed to exist in nature. For example, using the laws of thought discussed above (the first three principles in Table 8.1) to assert that alcoholics act a certain way, such as being out of control, implies that (1) alcoholics are different from nonalcoholics with respect to this behavior; (2) an individual cannot be both alcoholic and nonalcoholic and, therefore, presumably cannot both exhibit the behavior and not-exhibit the behavior; and (3) there is nothing in between a clinician's characterization of the alcoholic and the nonalcoholic and, therefore, in his or her understanding of the behavior. Of course, experienced clinicians will immediately acknowledge the need to hedge each of these assertions. Nonetheless, if we accept that merely assigning the category to an individual brings these assumptions to bear, then short of having the facts of the particular usage well worked out, we might be better off avoiding the label. The lack of control may be in the alcohol, or it may reside elsewhere, in which case the overly loose diagnosis is merely a distraction from potentially more productive local inquiry (which is not necessarily equivalent to ignoring the alcoholism, as some might imply).

Table 8.1 provides two basic impressions of the category/class designations we use regularly in our work. First, we often imply clear boundaries when a bit of reflection raises doubt about clarity. Second, the manner in which we organize class designations is related to the ways we are thinking about matters (e.g., the situations in Table 8.1 where order of construct might make a difference). It is important to note that actual everyday categorization may not work exactly this way (e.g., see Rosch & Mervis, 1975). However, the more formal and definitive we, as experts, tend to be with our assertions, the more these historical idealizations raise important questions about the implicit meaning of those assertions. There are many situations, such as diagnosis, where little time is given to hedging an assertion, hence implying clarity of boundary. Even more narrative approaches (Bruner, 1986; Polkinghorne, 1988; Sarbin, 1986)

TABLE 8.1

Principles of the Calculus of Classes with Implications for the Local Clinical Scientist

Principle	Symbolic representation	Interpretation	Usage for the local clinical scientist
Identity	a < a ("a is included in a")	Every class (set) includes itself.	The presumption of identity is built into our use of language to signify objects and events in our world. When objects are assigned similar terminology, then identity with the overall class and its associated meaning is assumed. The class of depressed individuals, for example, is presumed to include itself. Whether we are cognizant of it or not, this property of thought about classes will encourage us to treat class descriptive terms as identical until inconsistencies in such identities become known to us. Often there is confusion about the meaning of conditions that could make presumed identities misleading. Thus, depressed individuals from a college clinic and from a regional medical center may or not be equivalent, although research coming out of both centers may be cast as if identity with the overall class (population) of depressed individuals can be assumed. Homogeneity and heterogeneity of classes is a major concern in psychiatric nosology (Clark, Watson, & Reynolds, 1995). Similarly, clinicians may speak of their work within a setting as if it has implications for a much broader class than they have actually worked with. More precise scrutiny suggests that the class of depressed individuals from a regional hospital, or any other site, contains only itself and not other sites unless additional assumptions are made about population inference and generalizability. We need to understand that the simple assertion of class description does not handle this level of inductive inference for us (see Chapters 4 and 5).
Contradiction	a'a = 0 ("a and not a equals the null set")	The class whose members are both a and not-a is empty.	Our thinking and use of language will tend to make us conform to this principle—to do otherwise would seem self-contradictory. However, the fuzzy nature of classification in clinical science may require us to look more carefully at this. Thus, there may be no one who is both depressed

and not-depressed, but there may be individuals who are mostly depressed but who come alive, or are even happy under some circumstances (e.g., during special visits from a loved one). The principle of contradiction is not violated here because of subtleties in the definition of not-depressed; that is, happy is not necessarily equivalent to not depressed and vice versa. Also note that this idea refers to the structure of the overall class, not a single individual. Local clinical scientists need to pay special attention to the implicit arguments they develop in their own thinking as they classify individuals in various ways, to ensure that complacency with earlier classifications does not restrict their awareness of the changing realities of a case. At the same time they must be wary of contradictions that may be inherent in their usage of their most treasured constructs.

There are few classes in clinical science that conform clearly and simply to this restriction. Yet our tendencies in classifying will be to act as if this is true, especially in our conversation about our work, if not in our actions. Local clinical scientists may benefit from reguarly exploring the "excluded middle" to see how boundaries between their classifications are clear or fuzzy. The issues here are to become aware of fuzziness, to understand why it exists, and to grasp its implications for thought, not to bemoan it because it does not conform neatly to "laws of thought" like those outlined here. Thus, if a patient is disorganized in many areas of life, exploring the excluded middle may lead us to inquire about things we might not otherwise ask about, such as habits with pets or with clothing, revealing pockets of organization that were not included in the initial recognition of disorganization. One could almost define clinicianhood as the endless search for the "middle" that the patient, and usually everyone else, excludes.

| Excluded middle | $a + \prime a = 1$ ("a or not-a equals unity") | The class whose members are either a or not-a is every individual (as long as the categorization is exhaustive). Every individual either is a member of the class or is not, there is nothing in between. |

(continued)

TABLE 8.1 (Continued)

Principle	Symbolic representation	Interpretation	Usage for the local clinical scientist
Commutation	Version 1: ab = ba ("a and b equals b and a") Version 2: a + b = b + a ("a or b equals b or a")	The class whose members are both a and b is the same as that whose members are both b and a. The class whose members are either a or b is the same one whose members are either b or a.	We assume that patients at a clinic who are both depressed and suicidal are the same as those who are both suicidal and depressed. However, sometimes we may be prone to put priority on a characteristic and miss other characteristics that have less priority in our thinking. For example, a set of parents—who themselves have been abused and who are in a parent training program (thereby putting priority on the parenting)—may be treated differently than a set of abused patients who are also parents and in therapy. The parenting may be an important issue for both groups but receive less attention in the latter case. Social cognition research suggests that order can affect our thinking about characteristics (e.g., Wyer & Srull, 1989). Local clinical scientists need to be aware that order in itself may affect judgment but may have no bearing on the actual facts of classes of patients, or other clinical collections, because of the principle of commutation.
Association	Version 1: (ab) c = a (bc) ["(a and b) and c equals both a and (b and c)"; i.e., the result for both is a and b and c] Version 2: (a + b) + c = a + (b + c) ["either (a or b) or c equals either a or (b or c)"; i.e., the result for both is either a or b or c]	The class "both a and b" when combined (and) with c equals a when combined with the set "both b and c." The class "either a or b" in disjunctive (or) relationship with c is equal to the set a in disjunctive relationship with the set "either a or b."	Here again order of properties as they come to us and/or we realize their existence can mislead us in relation to this principle. For example, given an abusive parent (who we can designate as ab), we might be alarmed when alcohol abuse (c) has suddenly come up as an issue. We might treat the discovery of abusiveness (a) in an individual known to be a parent who is alcoholic (bc) somewhat differently. Logically there are no differences between the two when considered in terms of class membership, and there may not be in our dealing with them. But we need to be aware how these different orderings and combinations of phenomena, in sets of individuals and in individuals, may affect our thinking about local clinical situations. Note, for example, that an alcohol treatment center will treat the combination just mentioned differently than will a program for abusive individuals, or one for parenting skills, yet, on the face of it, the same people could be enrolled in any of these programs.

Distribution	Version 1: $(a + b) c = ac + bc$ ["either (a or b) and c equals either (a and c) or (b and c)] Version 2: $ab + c = (a + c)(b + c)$ ["(a and b) or c equals (a or c) and (b or c)"] (note here that this is not at all like standard algebra with numbers)	Version 1: If we combine a set of men and women and dye their hair red, we will have the same result as if we combined the set of men with dyed red hair with women with dyed red hair. Version 2: The set "U.S. citizens who are male (ab) or Canadians (c)" is the same as the set "U.S. citizens or Canadians $(a + c)$ who are also male or Canadians $(b + c)$." The result is always males from the United States and Canadians (note that the Canadians need not be male).	Again the key issues for critical thought have to do with the way we prioritize information we have about a clinical situation. For example, women who have been abused (ab) or their children raise the same issues as women or their children and the abused or their children. Each framing implies a slightly different aspect of the whole, however, and there may be cases where abused women are treated differently from women in general in relation to their children for reasons that are not clearly specified in the classification itself. Critical inquiry is not well served in these situations. The reasons that may exist for giving certain categories priority in the treatment of a patient need to be stated explicitly beyond simply asserting the combination categories used in the classification.
Tautology	Version 1: $aa = a$, ("a and a, equals a") Version 2: $a + a = a$, ("either a or a equals a") (again note the departure from standard algebra in notation)	All elements of a category represent the category.	Here we see the assumption that working with and combining subsets from the category is equivalent to working with the entire category (set). This foundation is essential to the inductive logic that underlies population studies. For example, a control group is only a control to the extent it represents the class of units (persons, objects, events, etc.) for the entire population being studied. Again, intraclass heterogeneity weakens this property of classes.

(continued)

TABLE 8.1 (Continued)

Principle	Symbolic representation	Interpretation	Usage for the local clinical scientist
Absorption	Version 1: $a + ab = a$, ["either a or (a and b) equals a"] Version 2: $a (a + b) = a$, ["a and (either a or b) equals a"]	In the logic of classes, sets of objects may not be perfectly homogeneous in every way, but they still make up a set once a common characteristic is identified.	Consider the characteristics anxiety and obsessionality. All anxious individuals need not be obsessional: If we had information just about anxiety, or if we had information about anxiety and obsessionality, we would still have a set of anxious individuals once that part of the assessment is established and we have collected all of the participants together. Depending on whether or not we attend to similarity or difference, which is a choice we can make consciously in our thinking, the fact of this property of classes can be more or less apparent. Thus, African Americans, Arab Americans, Chinese Americans, and European Americans are all Americans and this is true whether or not any given individual attends to this Constitutional and legal fact. Clearly, the implications of this simple property of classes can be profound under some circumstances. Failure to attend to such facts—perhaps operating under the illusion that some facts can be ignored—such as the case of the internment of Japanese Americans during World War II, can have ramifications that span generations (Nagata, 1993).
Simplification	Version 1: $ab < a$ ("a and b are included in a") Version 2: $a < a + b$ ("a is included in the set (either a or b)"]	This is similar to the principle of absorption in that it emphasizes how sets with common characteristics remain sets even when heterogeneity is present.	The language of classification simplifies the complexity that may actually exist in a situation. Often this can enhance understanding of meaningful similarities. However, if too much heterogeneity is present, then the basis for common classification may be in doubt. This is a continuing problem with psychiatric diagnosis where, in some cases, a simplifying classification may seem strained in relation to other pertinent information about a case (e.g., poverty, social displacement).
Syllogism	$[(a < b)$ and $(b < c)]$ implies $(a < c)$ ("if a is included in b and b is included in c, then a is included in c")	Sets can be nested within sets that are, in turn, nested within larger sets.	This represents the idea of stratification. Higher levels of analysis contain all lower levels, and superordinate classes contain all classes at a lower level. Thus, if insufficient caloric intake is a subclass of dieting, and dieting is a subclass of things that men do, then it is likely that there are men who exhibit insufficient caloric intake. This is only surprising if one believes that men do not have eating disorders. Recent evidence suggests otherwise (e.g., Pope, Katz, & Hudson, 1993). The power of simple ideas like the principle of syllogism is that it encourages us to explore such possibilities in our thinking.

generate extensive categorical designations in the course of narrative development. Enormous confusion can develop when categorical interests, such as those of the legal system, come in contact with the necessary fuzziness of clinical thought. For example, in the case of repressed memory reports (e.g., Loftus, 1993), the absence of needed aggressive attention to the differences between the requests of the courts and the actual strength and relevance of the findings, both from the consulting room and from the scientific laboratory, may have seriously damaged the credibility of our profession. Somehow the repressed memory concept and the times have combined in a situation where professionals often are inattentive to their categorical fuzziness, the important role it plays in the work they do, and its implications for certainty in the context of criminal proceedings (see Trierweiler & Donovan, 1994).

Only heightened awareness of how ideas are being organized locally, quite apart from textbook formulations, will undergird strong, well-grounded clinical analysis. Even in the disjunctive situation, where say a diagnosis might be treated tentatively as an anxiety disorder or an affective disorder, or both, the disjunctive assignment itself narrows the possibilities (e.g., excluding malingering or physical problems from the primary hypothesis) and can be thought of as a categorical assertion in its own right. Again, we are reminded that it is conjunctions and disjunctions of multiple categories that capture the uniqueness we find in the local clinical situation. The principles identified in the calculus of classes compel us to seek out and examine the viability of the implicit assumptions we make about categorical priority and meaning.

Some Examples of Logical Fallacies

It is common for logic and critical thinking texts to present a laundry list of fallacies of thought to watch out for. Here we provide a few of the major ones identified by Cohen and Nagel (1934), and Dauer (1989) that pertain to the evaluation of evidence in clinical contexts. We will include some of those that pertain to talking about cases as well, as outlined by Gambrill (1990) and Meehl (1973). We recommend the reader consult these works to round out the picture of reasoning errors for clinicians. Thinking through the implications of fallacies for particular cases can be a useful way to examine the integrity of one's current thinking and to generate useful alternative hypotheses. It is important to note that there is no implication that fallacious thinking is necessarily wrong, just that it is definitely subject to doubt and a stronger case is needed to achieve the level of certainty one might wish to convey. Note also that many of the fallacies identified below are related to the pervasive tension in categories and classes existing between part–whole distinctions, generality and specificity.

Fallacy of Composition

The fallacy of composition arises when properties of elements are confused with the whole of which they are a part. This is very common in the way clinicians freely generalize from experience (e.g., generalizations are made about suicidal patients based on experience with a few cases). Often such generalizations will be fine and a useful way to concretize one's experience for future reference. However, this thinking opens the door to serious error that must be carefully monitored. For example, because previous suicidal cases have been handled without incident does not justify lowering precautionary standards with the next case. Here, as with many of the other fallacies, much can be accomplished by treating the (fallacious) conclusion as a hypothesis rather than as truth, thereby opening the door to local inquiry.

Fallacy of Division

This is the complement of the fallacy of composition, when properties of a class are considered true of all elements (e.g., a warm and loving family does not ensure that all members are warm and loving, or that all interactions within the family are warm and loving). This fallacy can be seen to operate in statements about diagnostic categories of patients; for example, statements based on a diagnosis such as "these patients have problems with the rigors of occupation and parenting." Again, drawing on general characterizations of groups of patients may be useful in drawing out similarities, and there may even be a level of accuracy in revealing the central tendency within the category, but such thinking can also obscure important variation and comorbidity within the category.

Fallacy of False Disjunction

This is a potential error that arises in assuming that a range of alternatives are necessarily mutually exclusive, usually based on some implicit theory that they will not co-occur (e.g., an impulsive patient in some contexts will not be planful in other contexts, depressed individuals at home will not be enthusiastic at work, meek individuals on the job will not be controlling or aggressive in a relationship, dominant individuals at home will not be pained and innocent in particular problematic situations). This fallacy is particularly notable in situations where a few characteristics are virtually equated with the entire circumstance, meaning that disjunctive assumptions exclude numerous other possibilities. An important psychotherapy example is the situation where the interests of a patient have apparently been thwarted by the actions of a parent, and it is assumed that there are no points of agreement and harmony within that relationship. Patients may often be the primary promulgators of such false disjunctions by ignoring points of agreement with significant others. This can also be an issue in research contexts where choices on a measurement device are stripped of context to achieve generality. For example, to report that a family is extremely argumentative on a numerical scale may force a false disjunction of the given report relative to more specific situations. As a result, the report may not fit the actual experience of individuals in different contexts within the family, even though it may be reliable as a numerical data point (i.e., reliable as an indicator of the family's position relative to other families, but not necessarily as a statement descriptive of various circumstances within the family).

Confusion of Necessary and Sufficient

Communication may be a necessary condition for a happy marriage but it may not be sufficient (happiness implies good communication, but not-happy does not imply not-good communication, or stated positively, good communication does not imply happiness). The message of this example, that there are more things to happiness than good communication (which may be the favored interpretation of the therapist), applies to a great range of phenomena in professional practice.

Genetic Fallacy

This is the tendency to confuse a theoretical or logical order with actual temporal order. For example, in taking a history, the genetic fallacy is involved in an assumption that life domains will always move from the simple to the complex as the child develops, because this is a logical developmental sequence. Some children relate to very complex and difficult situations in their families and may spend substantial portions of adult life interpersonally and familially in much simpler conditions. Intelligent individuals may show great cognitive complexity during their schooling only to become much simpler and intellectually passive if employment and other aspects of life do not draw on their intellectual capacities. Cohen and Nagel (1934) pointed out that the converse of the genetic fallacy, the assumption that temporal order defines theoretical process, is equally problematic in science. For example, a highly intelligent individual who comes of age in an environment that does not call on these gifts, as in the case of many rural poor and working-class Americans and immigrants from poor countries, may change dramatically on entering an environment that nurtures intellectual skills. The same is true for athletic ability or even interpersonal skill that can emerge in the right circumstance, as when an individual meets the right partner. By the same token, marked declines in various areas of functioning can occur when circumstance and tragedy remove favorable conditions. In such cases, temporal order may be less relevant to understanding the case than is the dramatic environmental and cultural shift the individual experiences.

Fallacy of Argument from Ignorance

This is a situation where no evidence is known to refute a proposition; therefore it is assumed to be true. Such thinking can often be found in patients whose view of a situation depends on certain interpretations of the beliefs and intentions of a significant other, say a parent, and it is often taken as factual by clinicians. For example, the gist of a communication in an initial intake session is that a patient is failing in college because his father has taken no interest in him and does not care if he succeeds. Now this might well be an accurate depiction of a lifelong problem, or it could be a tentative interpretation being tried out by the patient for the first time in the therapeutic context. Nonetheless, therapists often bring this type of information to a case conference as a definitive piece of data about the case. If the patient offers no evidence to the contrary—and may or may not actually be able to access it if it existed (e.g., as a contribution to paying for college)—and if the therapist does not explore the meaning and longevity of this interpretation, then its acceptance even as a backdrop for the therapeutic work is grounded in ignorance. Unfortunately, a great deal of clinical data are so grounded, and local clinical scientists need to select information that needs to be explored in depth because of the impact it might have on the course of a treatment.

Fallacy of False Cause

We might call this the correlational fallacy. This is the assumption that because C often occurs with E, therefore, C causes E. Psychologists know that correlation is not equivalent with causation, but we often hear clinicians cite lists of cases where certain observations were perceived to coincide as evidence for interpretations that very much sound causal. For example, marital difficulties are given causal status in the behavior problems of a child, or several cases have been observed where children rebelled against parents who were overly strict about religious matters, so strict religious training is thought to engender rebellion. Unfortunately, the same problem exists in actual correlational studies where, given a correlation less than 1.0, there is no assurance case to case that the asserted coincident properties will actually be observed (Chapter 6 and below). Perhaps such problems are as much related to looseness in our language as to actual causal assumptions, but we could all benefit from greater care about such matters. To admit that one makes causal assumptions, even though they are based on a limited set of contiguous observations, or they are extrapolated from a correlational study, is the first step in setting up one's theory for a stronger test. The causal attribution may actually be correct but have insufficient evidence to support it, and therefore, it is best treated as a hypothesis.

Fallacy of Hasty Conclusion

Hasty conclusions are those drawn on the basis of instances that cannot be assumed to constitute a fair sample. This fallacy is related to the false cause assumption. Ironically, in local realms analysis, one can make a reasonably strong, contextually informed case for a causal relationship (e.g., between the death of a beloved grandparent early in an individual's life and a pervasive sense of apathy and inability to succeed later) that may have no practical generalizability beyond the particular case. This is where conceptualizing the fair sample can be useful in recognizing the limits on one's thinking even if it never leads to an actual study. It may also encourage clinicians to develop their causal hypotheses into forms that are testable. This fallacy also reminds us to pay attention to what might actually be a fair sample (see Chapter 5). On occasion, generalizations about local samples (e.g., a caseload of a clinician in a particular community) may be reasonable and more locally appropriate than would be scientific findings from a national probability sample. On the other hand, this also means that the clinician should not assume that such generalizations pertain to all clinical cases in the larger population.

Heuristics and Biases

Tversky and Kahneman (1974) and Kahneman et al. (1982) described cognitive heuristics that are thought to make information processing more efficient, but which can bias and mislead. Close inspection of this material suggests that, in part, it represents empirical demonstrations of many of the traditional logical fallacies discussed in this section. For example, the *availability heuristic* involves the impact of particularly salient exemplars available in memory on judgment. Turk, Salovey, and Prentice (1988) gave the example of the availability heuristic in the assumed conjunction of violence and psychosis in popular thought, which can be attributed to the prominence of men like Charles Manson or David Berkowitz in thought about psychotic individuals.

The *representativeness heuristic* involves linking judgments or diagnoses to signs thought to be typical or representative in the population without consideration of actual base rates, as in fallacies of composition, division, false disjunction, or hasty conclusion. Thus, spousal abuse is often associated with poverty because of certain assumptions about the nature of lives in poverty, even though it is actually equally represented among the well-to-do.

Anchoring is the undue emphasis placed on information early in an inquiry, again as in the fallacy of false disjunction, that might inhibit ability to respond to new, differing, or contradictory information. Elstein, Shulman, and Sprafka (1978) found crystallization of initial impressions to be a major problem in medical diagnosis. Elstein (1988) proposed that greater use of structured and automated procedures be made to overcome these intuitive weaknesses.

Analytic Incompleteness

Analytic incompleteness refers to the situation that arises when the data of a case are incompletely assessed, often favoring data that fit familiar theory. The representativeness heuristic and confirmatory bias (selecting information that confirms one's beliefs) in judgment tend to lead to emphasis on evidence that fits one's favored theories. Local science demands recognition of incompleteness and effort to develop a broader contextual understanding of cases incompletely handled by standard clinical formulations.

There are numerous other forms of fallacious, even if often convincing, thought and argument, including appeals to emotion (as in many recent contentions about the nature of violence), groupthink (e.g., group emphasis on a popular or interesting perspective quells conversation of a more difficult but incisive perspective), appeal to the irrelevant, failure to consider unreliability of measurement or observation, stereotyping, assuming that incisive thought necessarily contradicts a sympathetic stance, suppression of evidence, *ad hominem* arguments (where a person's view is discredited by discrediting the person), and use of inappropriate analogies. These can readily be observed in virtually any professional conversation dealing with the ambiguities of actual cases. Above all, categories of fallacious thought tell a cautionary tale that merits careful study of professionals because they reveal points in an assertion where additional evidence may be required to strengthen and perhaps modify one's belief.

Fallacies as Tools for Thought, Not Statements about Reality

It is surprising that the traditional training in logic and the concern about fallacious thought have been deemphasized in modern education, particularly doctoral education where logic was an analytical foundation for all we do as practitioners and scientists. Undoubtedly, this reflects a broader loosening and technocratization in our education system that has coincided with the rise of the profession (Barrett, 1978). In any case, the literature on cognitive heuristics has recently raised a number of concerns about clinical judgment that relate to our earlier discussion of quantitative thinking for the local clinical scientist. Therefore, we must digress briefly to point out some questions the local clinical scientist model raises about the applicability of this thinking to professional inquiry. In particular, we wish to underscore that the logical fallacies described herein are tools for examining local inquiry rather than definitive critiques of that inquiry.

The literature on heuristics and biases depends heavily on the assumption that statistical accuracy is the standard against which judgment should be evaluated. The major research paradigm supporting this work involves medical-style diagnosis under extremely limited information circumstances. Although there are situations where this type of judgment approximates reality (e.g., emergencies), there are a great many situations where the facts of a case as presented offer enough to proceed without great concern about specific diagnoses. Indeed, in many of the kinds of judgment situations represented in judgment research, which are tantamount to judgment under "uncertainty" with a capital "U," formal diagnostic judgment is arguably inappropriate to begin with—save where it is justified by other practical concerns such as insurance reimbursement. Most human judges (including professional statisticians) are not good statisticians when it comes to inferences about actual population values of which they have no knowledge. Compounding the problem are all of the difficulties of population definition and measurement discussed in Chapters 5 and 6: Even the best empirical studies rarely are more than preliminary representations of complex phenomena. Thus, even when rates of particular disorders (e.g., substance abuse) are reasonably well established, local base rates and pathways to inquiry into specific cases are virtually never elaborated in empirical studies. (Work dedicated to elaborating these pathways would undoubtedly be useful and could become a guide to more realistic presentation of the limits on the typical scientific research finding for local clinical judgment.)

Certainly, from a policy standpoint, relatively more correct than incorrect decisions are desirable. However, the heuristics research paradigm creates an illusion that ultimate accuracy for diagnostic and other clinical judgment lies in population descriptions and policies, a belief that belies observable complexity in the local clinical situation and that may not be warranted (e.g., few cases of substance abuse, a reasonably clear diagnostic category, are, on closer inspection, simply matters of the impact of substance usage). To the extent reliability studies or population estimates elicit suggestions for blindly uniform response to what is actually an information deficit in the local clinical situation, the patient is poorly served, however well this mode of action may benefit institutional error rates (which are institutional constructions). We must remember that the individual patient with a diagnostic sign for cancer either has the illness or not, quite apart from the population conditional probability associated with that sign (Wright & MacAdam, 1979). (Many clinicians would be dubious about the use of a psychological disorder in the previous sentence, as no doubt would many cancer researchers who question the theory of cancer as a single unitary disorder.) Concerns about such probabilistic properties in populations are of interest to professionals, but they are at best windows to further inquiry, not a definitive foundation for scientifically accurate local judgments.

There often can be surprising consensus among clinicians about the broad contours of clinical cases, but there also can be considerable disagreement. From a local clinical scientific perspective, disagreement is not something to be berated as unscientific, but rather, it may represent the actual state of knowledge, or lack of knowledge, for a case or class of cases. Population frequencies on relevant variables offer one source of information for making judgments, but additional information is virtually always required (Chapters 5 and 6; Lamiell & Trierweiler, 1986). In some complicated cases, certainty in judgment may never be reached, however confident are the expressions of the current clinician in the inevitable long string of clinicians. Therefore, with respect to locally specific judgment, there is reason to doubt that a research paradigm—which is dependent on temporally restricted, structured judgments made in an information vacuum—accurately describes a significant portion of clinician decision making.

We need a stronger science of the relationship between individual judgment and aggregate outcome to resolve these questions. The ultimate standard for the local clinical scientist must be the integrity of the observation base on which decisions are locally grounded, and on the clinician's ability to articulate solid reasoning to informed colleagues and supervisors. If the best that experienced professionals can muster in their individual judgments shows weakness when multiple decisions are aggregated (as in a reliability study, or in a predictive outcome study), then analysis is needed to determine how subclasses of cases (or individual cases) contributed to the observed discrepancy (individual clinicians who are operating in idiosyncratic ways would also be considered here). Our experience suggests that reliability in clinical judgment often hinges on cases that, by their nature, recruit cross-clinician agreement because they fit judgment models quite well (e.g., in the diagnosis of depression) whereas unreliability often originates in fuzzy cases about which agreement within the operative assessment model is difficult or impossible to obtain (such as may be happening in cases of cross-race diagnostic disagreement; e.g., Lawson, 1986; Neighbors & Jackson, 1984). Even researchers strongly committed to the taxonomic integrity of the diagnostic system recognize the important role fuzzy cases play in diagnostic outcome (e.g., Faraone et al., 1996). Research sensitive to the ecological reality of judgment is needed to distinguish judgment errors made between relatively clear and unclear cases and situations (e.g., Rock, Bransford, Maisto, & Morey, 1987). Eliminating this fuzziness by fiat of professional authority, or by structuring judgment instruments such that fuzziness can no longer be registered are unsatisfactory solutions to the scientific problem of understanding the link between individual and aggregate (see Rock, 1994).

Heuristics, biases, and logical fallacies aside, the often uncomfortable relationship that exists between aggregate research findings and the apparent realities of individual cases is one reason we emphasize the didactic goal of using logic to move inquiry forward to new more incisive information, rather than to imply that local judgment is necessarily flawed or that statistical formulations offer certainty about complex and multifaceted clinical situations. We are not alone in this argument. Gigerenzer and colleagues (e.g., Gigerenzer, 1996; Gigerenzer & Murray, 1987) have criticized the extent to which statistical observations and inferences have been equated with correct, or rational, thought in modern decision research, contrary to the beliefs of many influential statistical theorists such as Neyman and Pearson (see also Lamiell, 1995). Undoubtedly, studies of the extremes of judgment under uncertainty are useful for understanding policy behaviors and for revealing situations where logic might assist judgment about aggregates (Kahneman & Tversky, 1996), but a local perspective on information usage and inquiry in real clinical contexts suggests that at best such studies offer an incomplete picture. Overconfidence in statistical thinking and its association with definitive scientific understanding may be one reason· many clinicians are alienated from research practices. We suspect that the conditions that have inhibited science and practice integration will continue to prevail as long as clinicians and scientists are not taught how to think through research problems, both general and local, in other than mechanical ways.

Thus far, we have suggested that the study of logic and critical thought requires that we look deeply at the meaning and applicability of our tools. Next, to elaborate this perspective, we look again at the meaning of the correlation coefficient as viewed in light of some of the material discussed in this chapter.

Logical Doubts about the Interpretive Gist of the Correlation Coefficient

In Chapters 5 and 6 we suggested that problems exist in drawing local inferences from correlational findings insofar as, for any correlation less than one, some cases will show values on the ordered pairs of variables that are in line with the gist of the correlational result and some will not. Our discussion of the tools of logic gives us another way to look at this problem. If we think of the correlation as telling us of the presumably theoretically interesting tendency within a set of ordered pairs of measurements for the z scores on one variable to correspond to the z scores on the other variable, then the following classes of cases will result, assuming a positive correlation in this illustration.

1.   If $r = 1.0$, then comparable to the Euler designation "all Bs are A," all z scores on variable Y are comparable to those found on variable X.

2.   If $0 \leqslant r < 1$, then "some Bs are A," some z scores on Y correspond to those found on X, some do not. This always includes the subsets of ordered pairs where all Bs are A (A ∩ B) and no Bs are A (B ~A and A ~B). Obviously, if the correlation is zero or very small, there is no reason to attribute a relationship between the characteristics identified by the variables. Nonetheless, cases with conjunctions and disjunctions on the various z score magnitudes of the variables exist in any set of observations and, depending on how they come to a particular practitioner, they can create the impression of a correlation (an illusory correlation) in local populations, even when none actually exists there. Note also that correlations may exist in local contexts even when they may not in larger populations.

If a population correlation exists that is greater than zero but less than one, then sometimes this relationship between two variables will provide a correct image of what we will observe in the individual case, and sometimes it will not. We have no prior way of knowing which will be true—although across many cases we will be able to say that, as the correlation gets closer to 1.0, more and more cases congruent with the interpretive gist of a population correlation will be observed. Adding to this interpretive problem is the fact that most practice settings concentrate on only select subpopulations of cases, such as those suffering extremely from a particular condition. For example, we may be concerned about the impact of a high pathology score (e.g., depression) on some other measure. Accurate prediction would involve the identification of accurate conjunctions and disjunctions on levels of characteristics that are described in the population correlation(s).

Consider the situation where we have a high score on a measure of depression and we are predicting the score on interpersonal difficulties. Given a high depression score, a correlation less than one ensures that, as we move across cases, some scores on both measures will be high and some on the interpersonal difficulties will be not as high.

It may help to look again at a diagram of a correlational scatterplot (Figure 8.2). If we roughly identify the midpoints on each variable, the resultant quadrants correspond to the following subclasses of ordered pairs when X designates depression and Y interpersonal difficulties: low X–low Y (no depression–no interpersonal difficulties), high X–high Y (depression and interpersonal difficulties), low X–high Y [no depression–(some) interpersonal difficulties], high X–low Y [(some) depression–no interpersonal difficulties]. Obviously, if we freely apply the idea of relationship often attributed to the correlation, then a problem arises in interpreting individual cases even though there is nothing wrong with the correlation itself (as a measure of an

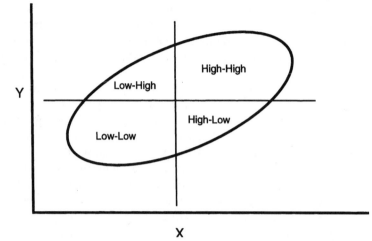

FIGURE 8.2.   Different types of conjunction between values on variables existing in a correlational scatterplot.

aggregate property). The interpretation works for two of the classes of cases (high–high and low–low), but not for the other two (low–high and high–low). This is less a problem as the correlation approaches 1.0 because, as the ellipse gets tighter, the low–high and high–low quadrants become relatively smaller. Also, because the scatterplot is bivariate normal (not visible in the diagram), the problem will generally involve the less extreme examples clustered around the centroid. Still, the problem is not easily dismissed—as clinicians experienced in assessment long have recognized. In effect, the extreme cases we see in professional practices are often extreme as well in their correspondence to the expectations of science.

Even if we are not attempting prediction and can assess the actual levels on two variables of interest in an individual case, there remains an interpretive problem. If we believe that a correlation actually exists based on a compelling theoretical linkage between the sources of variation existing for the variables, as we might in a well-established area where covariation is consistently observed (e.g., the linking between verbal skills and general measures of intelligence), then cases not cooperating with expectations demand explanation. The attribution of random error is not a locally compelling interpretation save in those cases where we have reason to doubt the reliability of our assessments, in which case further inquiry is required. If measurements are trustworthy, our task is to explain the poor fit with theoretical expectation. This can consist of a search for moderator variables and particular context effects. For example, a child may be quite verbal at home but perform poorly at school because of anxiety or subtle discouragement from parents uncomfortable with the achievement of their child. Such particularistic conjunctions of circumstances should be expected for relatively weak aggregate effects; if they did not exist—in effect weakening the observable relationship between variables across cases—then the aggregate effects would be stronger.

Actually, as practitioners know, context always merits careful consideration. To the extent general relationships are not theoretically developed, even cases fitting the correlational "law" need to be assessed locally to develop a stronger qualitative sense of how conjunctions of properties operate. For example, high verbal intelligence may relate to very high school performance in a particular case leading to an acceptance of the implicit aptitude theory, when actually a portion of the impressive school performance might better be accounted for by a weak academic program. This is an instance of the problem that a correlation may reflect the impact of a third, unidentified variable (e.g., Wiggins, 1973). It is good policy always to exercise caution in interpreting local phenomena when a pertinent correlational theory is not well established. This is true in both directions; in deducing particulars from empirical research and in inductively positing general correlations based on series of local observations or on theoretically assumed conjunctions among properties.

At length, the only recommendation we can offer is appropriate caution and humility until the issues associated with extrapolation from correlational findings to particular instances are better worked out. Research to this end is needed in virtually all areas of scientific psychology pertaining to practice.

CONCLUSION

In this chapter we have tried to show that the study of formal logical thought, both as traditionally presented and in recent incarnations, has much to offer a local clinical science. In many ways received view science has dropped the logical ball in the service of aggregated empiricism, particularly in post-World War II U.S. psychology versus earlier in the century. Although this has been productive in many ways, it has played havoc with our basic ability to bring science to the local clinical situation with a modicum of discernment. The cautionary tale told by logic, critical thinking, and scientific skepticism is one of relating to the local clinical situation with openness and care.

We now have covered many tools for observation and analysis. We still need explicit tools for bridging the gap between general clinical and scientific theory and the local clinical situation. This is the topic for the next chapter.

9

Frameworks for Reflective Practice

> The reality exists as a plenum. All its parts are contemporaneous, each is as real as any other, and each as essential for making the whole just what it is and nothing else. But we can neither experience nor think this plenum. What we experience, what comes before us, is a chaos of fragmentary impressions interrupting each other; what we think is an abstract system of hypothetical data and laws.
> —JAMES (1890/1965, pp. 397–398)

> I went to work to learn the shape of the river; and of all the eluding and ungraspable objects that ever I tried to get my mind or hands on, that was the chief.
> —MARK TWAIN, *Life on the Mississippi*, quoted in BARKER (1963)

All professional inquiry can benefit from greater attention to information in the local clinical situation that may not be readily described by traditional assessment practices. General models of reality are needed to guide attention to information in the clinical situation that may be important but unspecified at any given point in time. Standard assessment practices associated with particular theories are special cases of this type of substantive model. For example, behavioral theories emphasize assessment of behavioral realities, cognitive theories emphasize cognitive realities, interpersonal theories emphasize the realities of interpersonal dynamics, and so on. However, none of these theories offer insights into the realms of information in specific situations not addressed directly by their concepts (e.g., assessment of local culture as it pertains to problematic cognitions and behavior). Here we introduce the notion of the heuristic framework as a tool for clarity and specificity in exploring both the known and the unknown, the knowable and the unknowable in the clinical situation.

We will discuss the development of theoretical frameworks for bridging the gap between the generality of scientific theories and the specificity of the local clinical situation. We have suggested throughout that all scientific methodology, when properly considered, raises possibilities for achieving the science–practice bridge. Methodology, however, is a creative and evaluative tool; we still must have ways of bringing the substance of theory to bear on the substance of local observation.

Schön (1983) called the process of linking theory and action in the professions,

259

reflective practice. In this chapter we will consider some of Schön's arguments, which, consistent with the local clinical scientist model, suggest that inquiry in the practice context is something more than applied science. We will then expand on ideas about theoretical frameworks that can be found in the literature on qualitative research methods (e.g., Miles & Huberman, 1994; Chapter 7), paying particular attention to their value as heuristic devices for guiding inquiry. Finally we will offer two examples of frameworks. The first provides a useful perspective on the major focus of this book, namely, the very personal and local elements of professional inquiry. The second is a framework for understanding memory narratives in psychotherapy that is consistent with scientific perspective on perception and memory without oversimplifying local complexities. At the end of the chapter, we argue for the development of local practice communities in which framework generation is an ongoing part of professional development, and in which explicit frameworks guide practice in particular problem domains and link local practices to more general theory and scientific research.

THE REFLECTIVE PRACTITIONER

Schön (1983) unpacked some of the implications of cognitivist and social constructionist thinking for the problem of professional practice. He called the dominant epistemology of practice *technical rationality.* This is the view that the practitioner is a technician of science. Science creates knowledge that addresses problems found in professional practice and, therefore, the practitioner's job is to assess these problems and implement the solution(s) suggested by science. As we suggested in Chapter 1, this view has had a prominent place in the scientist-practitioner model and led to the overwhelming emphasis on practice evaluation, as opposed to substantively oriented inquiry, as the overarching scientific goal for clinical science.

Technical rationality claims a knowledge base that is specialized, clearly bounded, scientific, and standardized (Schön, 1983, p. 23).[1] Scientifically grounded professional action derives from higher-level scientific formulations. Applied science consists of a hierarchy of principles in which general scientific formulations are the highest and concrete applications are the lowest. (See Chapters 4, 5, and 6 for some of the background logic for this viewpoint.) In this view, (1) effectiveness is considered a technical pursuit of preestablished ends, (2) scientific rigor in practice is thought to be derived from the rigor and control established in research-based theory and experimentation rather than in terms of the practice itself, and (3) knowing and doing are separate such that action has no independent status other than as an implementation or test of a preestablished technical formulation (Schön, 1983). Such hierarchical thinking is evidenced in recent versions of the diagnostic system (e.g., the DSM-IV; American Psychiatric Association, 1994) and in manualized approaches to psycho-

---

[1]Schön is referring to any professional who claims to draw on a scientific knowledge base.

therapy intervention and training (Luborsky, 1993). Emphasis on crisp, standardized boundaries in the categories used in applied scientific work (see Chapter 8) has become extreme. For example, discussions of the DSM-IV present reliability as a major standard for both scientific legitimacy and clinical utility with little regard for validity (e.g., Williams, Gibbon, First, & Spitzer, 1992). Crisp categories are claimed even in the face of limited empirical evidence and multiple reasons to question their validity (Clark et al., 1995; Good, 1992; Kirk & Kutchins, 1992; Wakefield, 1992).

Experienced practitioners know that there are serious problems with this viewpoint, particularly as it preempts more complete representation of the actual complexities of practice (Trierweiler & Stricker, 1992). Schön (1983) suggested that the heavy emphasis on problem solving in applied science leads to an underemphasis on the problem setting, that often vague and uncertain context within which decisions are actually made about problems to be solved and goals to be achieved. He used case material from a variety of professions, including psychotherapy and engineering design, to show that practice is actually "reflection-in-action" (Schön, 1983, p. 44). Contrary to the image of clear and standardized science, knowing and doing are not separable in the ways traditionally framed. In actual practice, problems do not present themselves as givens, awaiting the enlightened examination of the practitioner (see also Stricker & Trierweiler, 1995; Trierweiler & Stricker, 1992). Rather, problems and their solutions are constructed in the local clinical situation (Hoshmand, 1994; D. R. Peterson & R. L. Peterson, in press; Stricker & Trierweiler, 1995; Trierweiler & Stricker, in press).

Useful categorical and interventional tools, which may be rooted in scientific research, are rarely applicable in textbook form. Instead, professionals often must work in a world of uncertainty, openness, and local variety not identified in the general formulation. Practitioners manage the conflict between images of rigor and relevance in professional science by various hedges, by "cutting the practice situation to fit professional knowledge" (Schön, 1983, p. 44). Aspects of the plenum—which is the local clinical situation—that do not fit professional categories are ignored, "junk categories" (Schön, 1983, p. 44) are used to explain away a failure of professional knowledge (e.g., the patient was uncooperative), or the professional makes the situation manageable by simplifying (or in some cases complicating) matters into familiar forms (Schön, 1983).

We concur with the general thrust of this perspective. Our profession might hope to provide interventions solidly grounded in science, but our knowledge base is rarely up to the task. The ideal of practice as a strictly applied science (McFall, 1991) has not been realized in our profession and probably never will be. For one thing, many of the activities of the professional that clients value are not clearly delineated in science, and may be incompatible with scientific generalities insofar as they are locally specific. Several other professions have confronted similar barriers to completely scientifically specified practice (Beutler, Williams, Wakefield, & Entwhistle, 1995). Moreover, as we have noted, scientific generalizations often decay, are imprecisely coordinated with actual observations in the local clinical situation, and are often incomplete descriptions of the human complexities professionals confront (Stricker & Trierweiler, 1995).

A realistic aspiration to scientific practice requires that we move beyond simplistic notions about the direct linear application of scientific findings to a homogeneous universe of applicability, which is a professional image that D. R. Peterson (1991) considered to be a preprofessional stage of development for psychology. Rather, local clinical scientists, as reflective practitioners, need to confront the actual complexities of the local clinical situation directly. Often, scientifically based theory will be useful; however, which theory is most relevant will not always be predictable without careful local assessment. As Cronbach (1975a) suggested, all application of theory involves a test of a local hypothesis (see Chapter 6). When a given theory is not useful, then skills in local inquiry and problem recognition and solving will be needed. Schön's image of the reflective practitioner is fitting in this regard.

Still, although we agree with Schön that existing professional practices involve tacit knowledge and local decision processes, and that these are an essential feature of professional skill, we also believe that current practices can be improved by further development of scientific forms of thought in the exploration of local circumstances. Reflective action can be as wrongheaded as naive scientism if the practitioner fails to connect with the realities of the local clinical situation. Next we discuss framework development as a tool for monitoring reflective action that can both aid the implementation of the kind of methodological thinking we are advocating in this book and as a means of bridging substantive research and theory into the realities of local circumstances.

FRAMEWORKS FOR REFLECTIVE PRACTICES

Most psychological theories are nonspecific and there may be considerable variety in the ways proponents of the same theory actually operate. Correspondingly, proponents of allegedly different theories may actually work quite similarly. The imprecision and variety of concepts associated with practice suggest that, rather than operating from strong theories, which would involve precise predictions about the nature of phenomena and relationships among phenomena (Meehl, 1978; Chapter 6), we actually operate more from conceptual frameworks. As discussed in Chapter 7, a framework is a set or system of ideas that draws attention to certain phenomena and to particular aspects of phenomena in the local clinical situation. Thus, the ideas of resistance, of transference and countertransference, or of conditioned response are miniframeworks for organizing and interpreting certain observations in the local clinical situation. Such frameworks are often thought to have both descriptive and explanatory properties. However, in this context we wish to emphasize the ways frameworks serve to gather attention to particular phenomena.

The major criterion for a good framework, as we use the term here, is that it have heuristic value. *Heuristic value* means that a framework moves inquiry forward into meaningful new territory by drawing attention to particular phenomena, by encouraging empirical elaboration, and by raising as many new questions as it answers. Most importantly, a good framework will keep the professional ever aware both of what is known and not known in the clinical situation.

There are no precise rules for framework development. Therefore, we shall illustrate the concept of framework with two examples.

Example 1: Professional Inquiry as a Personal Process

This book has concentrated on the problem of localizing scientific inquiry. Accordingly, our first framework example explores inquiry as a process of personal judgment and action in confronting the local clinical situation (Figure 9.1). Such a framework is applicable both to analyzing how a professional comes to know the local clinical situation and as an aid in focusing discussion and debate with other practitioners about professional issues. It pulls together many of the basic ideas we have outlined in this book.

The framework describes a transaction between the professional and the information reality presented by the clinical situation. Time and experience flow from top to bottom in Figure 9.1. The professional enters into the situation, is affected by it, and affects it as time progresses. This transaction is represented as a two-level cyclical process where (1) interpretation is developed out of experience and knowledge in a process of mutual influence and (2) actions are taken based on interpretations that are, themselves, influenced by their justification and impact on a chosen audience for the inquiry and the intervention. In turn, the whole cycle of interpretation and action is affected by the realities of circumstances—including both local properties of the professional and of the situation—as experience advances in time.

This model of the inquiry process is consistent with basic presentations of scientific inquiry and with research models of cognition and action (e.g., Ericsson & Simon, 1993; Miller et al., 1960; Neisser, 1976). The two overarching components are the *apprehension process*, which refers to the observational and interpretive portion of inquiry, and the *argument process*, which refers to the assertion and action portion of the inquiry and related intervention. The apprehension process refers to periods of opening up, observing, and considering (cf. Cronbach, 1982); the argument process refers to a closing down based on what has been determined to be true in one's inquiry, and acting based on ongoing observation and analysis. These are described in greater detail below. The operations of these two processes may vary in length of time depending on context and, indeed, they will often take place simultaneously. Nonetheless, it is useful to keep the two separate in that the subjective and action sides of inquiry differ in important ways, e.g., in their being public or private (see below).

The Apprehension Process

The apprehension process describes a way of looking at all aspects of experiencing, noticing, attending, recognizing, and interpreting that might take place in professional inquiry. It involves an attitude of opening the inquiry and of considering

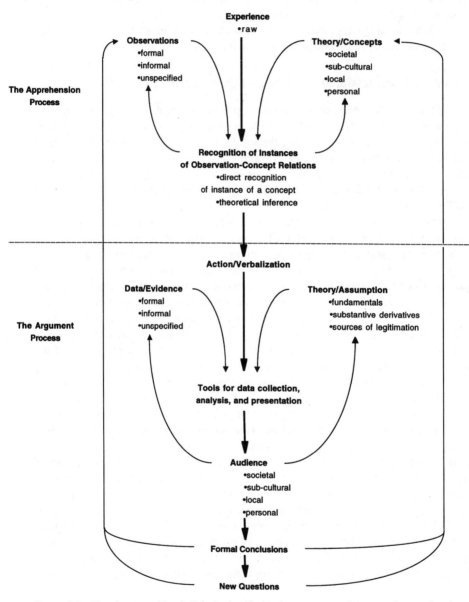

FIGURE 9.1. The elements of local clinical scientific inquiry as a personal process: the apprehension–argument model.

possibilities based on what is observed. Apprehension begins at the moment of onset of a clinical encounter (e.g., the clinician receives a telephone inquiry from the patient, notes that an appointment has been set, or receives a letter of referral).

Raw Experience. Following theoretical models that have been developed that address experience (e.g., Heider, 1958; Schutz, 1962; Weick, 1969), the top of Figure 9.1 begins with experience in raw form. It is unlikely that much of our experience is actually raw in the sense of uninterpreted (see Chapter 3)—for most of life we are surrounded by very recognizable objects and events and we tend to avoid situations where too much is uninterpretable given what we already know. However, the idea of raw experience captures the implication that human interaction always contains phenomena that are neither directly known nor even knowable to the participants (e.g., Nisbett & Wilson, 1977). Most importantly, it captures the notion that there are phenomena that are in principle interpretable in experience even though in practice they may not be accessible (e.g., the actual experience of other people in the interaction in all of its nuance and complexity). Clinicians often learn to interpret patients' nonverbal behavior, countenance, and emotional reactions to various situations as an indirect window to some of this material not given directly in the patient's presentation of self.

Observations. On entering the situation, the professional immediately begins making observations, here referring to sensorially noticed events. Some of these are formal and preinterpreted (as in related to formal professional inquiry), such as those following from a more or less standard sequence of questions the clinician may ask a new patient. Some are informal, as in observations related to commonsense practices and common courtesy. An example might be observations that follow from any event not intrinsic to the treatment setting, such as the patient's reaction to another individual she happened to see in the waiting room. Finally, some are not specified, meaning they are not particularly notable observations at all and may have no meaning until circumstances call them to attention [e.g., a child enters wearing jeans, not a particularly noteworthy (unspecified) event until sometime later when it emerges that his informal manner of dress is a significant bone of contention between the child and his very formal father]. Sometimes whole patterns and sequences of observations—even those previously treated as unrelated—might be conjoined and reinterpreted when significant reason for doing so emerges.

Theory. Application of formal and informal theory to the events observed in the local clinical situation is fundamental to professional inquiry, as we argued in the preceding chapter. Theories entail linguistic concepts and the associations that exist among them. The model suggests that this linking of concepts to local realities involves the several levels of local information setting identified in Chapter 3. Some concepts are general to the entire professional interaction (e.g., formal diagnostic categories or symptom recognition). We have labeled such concepts, which will often be found in the broader discourse of science and the organized professional community, the societal level. These are concepts developed and disseminated within the general science setting of local information we described in Chapter 3.

The other settings—local cultures, unique information, and the space-time local—are variously specified in the remaining categories in Figure 9.1 (subcultural information, local information, and personal information). For example, an individual's way of expressing his understanding and values concerning relationships may be based in community-specific social trends, interpretations, and knowledge (e.g., within the culture of young professionals in a particular community). This would be a subcultural theory of relationships and a local cultural issue to be assessed by the practitioner. Such local interpretations may or may not be represented in the larger society (e.g., semiurban communities may reflect more traditional views of relationships than large urban or multinational communities even as they share many interests and qualities of appearance). There will also be concepts that are even more locally represented. For example, going to a certain restaurant in a rural community may have local implication not immediately apparent to an outsider; a reference to a particular location in a town, such as a swimming area on a local river, may carry meaning and interpretive implication that extends beyond the outward event described—as when the swimming area is a place where teens spend time coming of age. Understanding these local theories and the concepts they engender, many of which may take the form of encapsulated narratives (Bruner, 1986; Polkinghorne, 1988), can have major impact on the direction taken in a professional inquiry.

Finally, personal theories are also a part of inquiry, some originating in the experience of the professional and some in that of the client. These encompass both the idiographic and space-time local settings of information described in Chapters 2 and 3, depending on the specificity of the point of the inquiry. The major feature of this level is that personal theories involve the impact of the particulars of unique experience on the process of the inquiry. A professional who understands the unique viewpoint and theories of the client can use this understanding to better grasp the broader information provided in an inquiry. Similarly, the professional would do well to grasp his or her own personal theories and their implications for inquiry. For example, a professional who believes she has not done well in her own relationships may inappropriately put limits on what she believes her patients can achieve or she may unconsciously draw attention away from such matters.

Experience of Instances of Observation–Concept Relationships.   Recognition of linkages between theoretical concepts and the observations available in a situation is the major outcome of the apprehension process. It is the point of recognition where the clinician experiences the understanding of something that had previously been unclear. For example, a patient's cryptic conversation about communication problems suddenly suggests hidden sexual difficulties, or a series of classroom problems is belatedly recognized as linked to labor difficulties for teachers rather than to student behavior. This understanding can be very direct, as in the recognition of particular instances of a concept, or it can follow a more indirect, inferential reasoning process. As we suggested in the last chapter, this is one point where logic may be useful in establishing and evaluating alternative possibilities for important recognitions and inferences in an inquiry. To the extent the practitioner orients from the empirical, observation–concept linkages are extrapolations from observations. To the extent the inquiry is theory driven, observation–concept linkages are extrapolations from theoretical formulations.

As shown in Figure 9.1, recognition feeds back to affect future observation and the theory used in interpreting the situation. Thus, if a clinician comes to recognize a young woman presenting about her depression as a case of marital conflict, then that recognition will affect future attention to observational events and to the theories recruited to understand observations. Alternatively, if the same situation is interpreted as related to lifelong issues of character development, then both theory and observation will proceed accordingly.

The Argument Process

The argument process is inherent in all professional action, as well as in verbal discourse about professional issues. As used here, the term *argument* refers to the act of arguing, which according to one *Webster's Dictionary* definition is "to maintain; contend" or to "persuade by giving reasons." In this model, all professional behavior is an expression of, and therefore an argument for, some relevant view of reality. Arguments may be explicit, as in clearly formed verbal arguments framing a particular view of a case; or implicit, as in the case where one's actions presume a particular viewpoint but the details of the reasoning are not explicated. The emphasis here is on how the practitioner is aware of and justifies a construction rather than on its substance. Regardless, professional expressions and actions, along with those of the client, contribute to the mutual construction of the clinical situation. For example, even before directly contacting a patient, the clinician enacts (argues for) the role of expert who will listen and evaluate the situation the patient presents. Such arguments can be found in the cultural trappings of professional life (e.g., offices with comfortable furniture, phonebook listings, professional licenses), and in professional manner and comportment (greetings, discussions of payment, levels of disclosure). A gentle supportive manner, dignified distance, and incisive intellectual probing are all parts of the argument process that may be enacted by a professional. Within this context of basic stylistic communication, the professional also enacts the current status of her theory of the situation at its current level of development.

An argument is a micro unit of the local social construction of the reality of the clinical situation. The argument process always implies the expression of theoretical assumptions (e.g., one can express classical psychoanalytic assumptions by suggesting that a patient lie down on a couch) that are presented and verified by particular types of inquiry and evidence; in effect, a paradigm is enacted where one's assumptions imply the data to be sought and vice versa. Professional actions and verbalizations take place in relation to an audience that affects how arguments are expressed and legitimized. In turn, depending on audience reaction, these actions lead to conclusions that may lead to new inquiry, repetitions of successful actions, and new actions (see below).

Data/Evidence.   In the argument context, data refer to the transformation of actual observations into evidence that might support a particular interpretation of the case. Here is the point where the clinician actually isolates and identifies the significance of particular facts and observations in support of a developing understanding of the clinical situation. The clinician might report this material as evidence in support of a case formulation. Mirroring the above discussion of observations, data/evidence can be formally elaborated, as when a set of symptoms and their observational basis are formally identified and recorded as evidence in support of a diagnosis. Also, evidence can be informal, such as noting a guarded sarcasm in the tone of voice of one member of a troubled couple as informal support for doubts about the couple's viability. Finally, like observations themselves, evidence can be unspecified until reason emerges for doing so. For example, a patient who is severely conflicted about sexual identity may offer veiled evidence to this effect in describing relationships that are not yet revealed to be unsatisfactory. The clinician may actually note these observations but not identify their significance until the interpersonal rapport has sufficiently developed and further evidence is revealed.

Theory/Assumptions.   The argument process is the place where theories are realized in actual expressions or actions that describe the meaning of the theory in the particular clinical context. These expressions may involve fundamentals and substantive derivatives, such as explication and enactments corresponding to the basic interpersonal problems associated with an interpersonal analysis of a particular problem such as self-mutilation (e.g., Benjamin, 1996) or depression (Safran & Segal, 1990). Another example might be the extension of a basic interpretation of a conflict developing in early childhood, which may be fundamental to a particular psychodynamic theory, to a current troubling relationship for the patient. The expression of one's theories and assumptions also involves the mustering of particular sources of legitimation in support of one's argument. Thus, depending on orientation, some therapists will draw more on empirical observations to support propositions whereas others will cite the writings of a recognized authority of the particular approach or the viewpoint of a valued supervisor.

Tools for Data Collection, Analysis, Interpretation, and Presentation.   Theoretical enactments and their supporting evidence come together in tools for data collection, analysis, interpretation, and presentation. Often these tools, such as the face-to-face interview, are taken-for-granted parts of the clinical process. Such tools imply particular data forms, analytical trajectories, and possibilities for formal and informal presentation of one's findings. For example, an interview will emphasize verbal data, self-disclosure, interpretation on the part of the patient, interpretive analysis within the context of the clinical intervention, and narrative presentation—as is common in case presentations.

In earlier chapters, we have suggested that the tools of scientific methodology offer guidelines for useful inquiry in the local clinical situation. If one thinks in terms of experimental control, even if not practically possible (see Chapter 4), then the relationship between theory and data may be modified and advanced in particular instances. Statistical thinking, qualitative methods, and logical analysis are other tools that might have operational significance in linking theory to data in particular situations. In Chapter 4 we gave an example of the relevance of statistical regression for considering the local meaning of extreme observations. If it is believed that unreliability of measurement (or observation) in a particular instance leads to a sense of the measurement's extremity, then assessing urgency or severity of the problem by other means may be necessary. For example, consider a situation where a panicked father presents the problems of a teen in extremely urgent terms. If the child echoes the parent's presentation or offers no detailed commentary, then friends of the child, other family members, or teachers might offer helpful perspectives on the situation. Similarly, direct assessment of the child's true feelings about the situation may clarify matters such that not only is the extreme measurement understood, but new information of great importance to understanding the case can emerge. For example, in one of our cases an otherwise closed and distant teen opened and became an active participant in her treatment when it became clear that the therapist was not necessarily interpreting the situation with the same dire severity as the parents and other interested adults.

Audience. Unlike the private world of thought and the apprehension process, the realm of argument is public in its outcome. Professional actions can and will be contemplated by interested parties. The scientific and authoritative tools we have developed in our profession are designed to satisfy the various audiences interested in our profession. As shown in Figure 9.1, an audience can be considered to function at various levels of society, as did the theory/concept node in the apprehension process. In so doing, an audience sets limits on the freedom of the professional's actions/ verbalizations in particular contexts and determines the nature of the professional's interactions with the local clinical situation. More specifically, the audience limits the types of evidence that can convincingly be brought to bear in support of a theory and, in turn, the types of theory that can be credibly expressed in any given professional activity. As professionals we are surrounded by multiple audiences that quite literally set limits on our behavior and ways of viewing the world.

As a practitioner enacts a theory of the situation, such enactment is designed to connect with a particular audience at a particular time. Thus, at a national conference, a professional audience may be interested in general issues of theory and research that would not be of interest to an audience with a more local focus, such as a patient population—of course, there also may be overlap in the interests of these constituencies. Presentations to the professional audience must be made along particular communication channels, such as publication of books and articles, convention presentations, talks, case presentations, and the like. More local audiences focus on specific information of local relevance, such as case formulations conducted within a particular context of group supervision, or within a particular ward of a hospital. As with any theory, audiences, and the interests they engender, can be very personal in nature. Some of the perspectives a clinician holds may never be presented to anyone outside the very private confines of therapy itself. Within the limits of confidentiality, aspects of the patient's life and beliefs can reasonably be presented in a case presentation, but other aspects, such as the actual events of particular interactions, are the stuff of dialogue between patient and therapist that may never be seen or heard by anyone else. For example, it is common for individuals to assume they have free will at some level—though society increasingly attempts to shed doubt on this prospect. A professional may accept and even encourage this viewpoint in many contexts. However, as an academic topic, this idea of free will is highly controversial and often will be avoided in academic conversations. A case presentation may likewise avoid the topic and concentrate on an endless array of other matters, even though this belief may be of great importance to both patient and therapist.

Each audience determines the nature and scope of the data that may be discussed and translated through theory (Miles & Huberman, 1994). One outcome of the stratification of audience is that some important events may never be well described by general theories (e.g., a deeply moving spiritual moment in an otherwise mundane circumstance) and, conversely, important aspects of theory may never be realizable in the local clinical situation because the relevant data never emerge (e.g., a patient never shows her angry side because, for unknown reasons, the right moment never occurs in her therapy). Moreover, there may exist impediments to translating important data into more general scientific theories because the linkages between local realities and theories are not well worked out or because the necessary theory does not exist at a particular time (i.e., appropriate audience is lacking, e.g., the impact of cultural issues on therapy was largely unrecognized in professional circles until quite recently).

Formal Conclusions and New Questions. The output of the argument process is conclusions and new questions for further inquiry and action. Figure 9.1 suggests that these outcomes feed back into the theory and observational content of the apprehension process. In effect, the practitioner's current inquiry and actions affect future understanding of the case as it develops in time.

Usage of the Apprehension–Argument Model

Why do we need abstractions such as this? There are three activities that can follow from such a model. First, we need some tool, or goad, to assist reflection on what we are doing. It is one thing to reflect in terms of a substantive model of a situation, such as reflecting on a diagnosis in terms of the DSM-IV or considering a dream in light of one's grasp of Jungian theory, it is another thing actually to step back and reflect on one's whole process, including the theories and conditions that one brings to a clinical situation and the observations that have influenced the current interpretation. Psychologists have long suggested the need for metareflection on the professional's own perspective and values (e.g., Rappaport, 1977), but how one should accomplish and benefit from such reflection has not been elaborated.

The theoretical tools implicit in methodological practices offer a means for metareflection when they are elaborated in guiding theoretical frameworks. The philosophical model described in Chapter 3 is one such framework that describes a broader vision of clinical phenomena than might otherwise be investigated. The apprehension–argument model is another heuristic tool that might be considered based on our entire discussion of methodological thought for a local clinical science. Each of these models could be used in clinical inquiry, for example, as tools for clinical supervision.

Second, having opened oneself to reflection, more specific categories to guide reflective inquiry are needed. The elements of the apprehension–argument model can assist inquiry without implicitly endorsing or negating a particular substantive theory. For example, evidence may suggest that a patient's current difficulties originate in long-term conflicts between self-idealization and fear of abandonment. Obviously, such a formulation, by its nature, already reflects certain theoretical commitments. In reflecting on this theory, the apprehension–argument model invites consideration of how the theory came to be linked to certain observations and how this process might have affected the actions of both the therapist and the patient over the course of their interaction. Reflection might lead to recognition of the external reality of some abandonment fears, but not others. For example, a patient from a working-class background may be perceived by kindred as self-aggrandizing if she expresses upward mobility in certain fashion—such as speaking a certain way or buying particular types of clothing. On the other hand, her inhibition about accepting the fact of her authority as a corporate executive may be less grounded in external local reality and more in the internal subjective reality of her experience of her life and work. Gender issues may also be involved in such a scenario.

In moving down the model to reflect on the existing argument process, the clinician may come to recognize that his manner and questions have not allowed for the possibility that the patient's material has some basis in external reality. That is, in focusing only on the patient's subjectivity (and for some therapists the unconscious), the time-extended ecological reality for the patient may be poorly understood. Put differently, if the audience for the therapist's actions—either implicit or explicit—has primarily been like-minded colleagues or supervisors as well as the patient, then other cultural, local, and personal realities may have gone unheeded. For example, the patient may be uncomfortable with the therapy itself as an expression of upper-class values, a side of her not recognized thus far in the therapy.

We consider any situation where reflection leads to an expanded sense of the possibilities for understanding clinical data as a positive outcome even though nothing else in the work may change. At length, successful reflection can lead the therapist to choice points wherein new questions are framed, leading to modification of approach or to continuation along the existing path, but with eyes open to alternative interpretations of the case.

Finally, in the spirit of the Boulder Conference, the third function of the apprehension–argument model is to encourage the development of new substantive theory and observation. Application of a framework like this to specific cases might deepen and extend the clinician's understanding of a particular substantive problem, not only in light of what the literature says about that problem, but also in light of the professional's actual experience of the problem in the local clinical situations that comprise his practice. Well-formulated reflective questions can lead to fruitful exploration of the psychological literature for relevant theory and research, to grasping research perspectives that might not be clearly linked to clinical perspectives, and to the development of theory that not only helps one grasp local situations but also actually suggests new avenues for research.

The exploration of new approaches might begin locally in a debate between clinicians operating from different viewpoints. Reflection on the debate may suggest that the arguments proposed by each side address different audiences (e.g., relevance to treatment of a working-class as opposed to an upper-middle-class population), or different assumptions about basic evidence (e.g., behavior versus experienced affect). Rather than simply fueling additional debate—which many clinicians find unproductive—such analyses would ideally lead to additional investigation of the differences in the information and phenomena addressed in the argument and set a foundation for productive integration of perspectives (Gold & Stricker, 1993; Stricker, 1997; Stricker & Gold, 1993).

The apprehension–argument model is a general guide for inquiry into what has been recognized in the clinical situation and for evaluating this information in light of what might be observed therein. More specific theoretical formulations will accomplish similar goals for more specific substantive questions. Next we look at a formal model for interpersonal memory that links to theory of basic perceptions and cognitive process and the research literature on memory.

Example 2: The Ecological Foundations of Interpersonal Memory

The research literature on memory emphasizes its fallibility (Loftus, 1993). The clinical literature, on one hand, emphasizes the lack of historical truth in memory (e.g., Bonanno, 1990) and, on the other hand, the truth of repressed memories and their powerful emotional impact on current functioning (Loftus, 1993). There is a vociferous debate about how to conceptualize the veracity of memories and about the implications that might be drawn from memory reports (e.g., whether perpetrators of abuse, as reflected in once-repressed memories, should be prosecuted solely based on memory claims) (e.g., Loftus, 1993; Ofshe & Waters, 1994; Terr, 1994).

The problem with the literature on a topic such as this is that the theoretical models and issues being discussed may not correspond well to the realistic needs of professionals in most everyday circumstances. To the extent models of clinical processes are not represented in the literature in forms that are useful to professionals, professionals must take on the task of translating the available material into the local clinical situation. Framework development is a means to this end.

Trierweiler and Donovan (1994) recently presented a framework dealing with the problem of interpersonal memory narratives. Interpersonal memories were defined as memory narratives describing personal episodes from an individual's life that involve other people. Consistent with recent research literature, the model accepts that memory narratives can be fallible in a variety of ways, including distorting actual events in the person's life, but it also accepts that some narratives are more accurate and thoroughly descriptive than others. Thus, the problem for the clinician becomes one of interpreting the meaning and implications of some temporally distal event based solely on a current narrative offering.

This framework assumes that understanding the past at some level is important. Many clinicians describe being solely interested in the current presentation and having no interest in what actually transpired. Although we can accept that a here-and-now focus has a place in practice, we find the notion of having no commitment whatsoever to the truth value of historical material implausible. Clinicians regularly justify case formulations and treatment plans with narrative information drawn from the patient's memory. Therefore, the memory problem cannot be avoided. One can be concerned about the veracity of certain aspects of a presentation without preempting particular interpretations of the events described.

The ecological foundations model represents two areas of concern for clinicians: (1) the information needed in principle for a memory narrative to be a complete account of an event and (2) the management of the technical problems various theoretical and empirical concerns raise for clinical inquiry. The model bridges the gap between extreme views of memory that insist on vague notions of an objective reality, the description of which is usually not achievable or would require means not available to the clinician, and views that treat recollections as constructions not necessarily attached to an underlying reality. It is one of a class of heuristic models that might be developed based on the current knowledge in this area.

In the following discussion we simplify Trierweiler and Donovan's presentation to illustrate the conceptualization and application of a substantive framework.

Figure 9.2 presents a simple model of memory found in traditional research, which we can use to represent aspects of Trierweiler and Donovan's (1994) model. The research participant is exposed to a stimulus (such as a word, a nonsense syllable, or a sequence of numbers) for some period of time and within some context, a period of time elapses, and a memory test is conducted to assess the extent to which the presented material can be reproduced. This simple paradigm, which treats memory as a kind of bin in which important information is retained, has generated an enormous

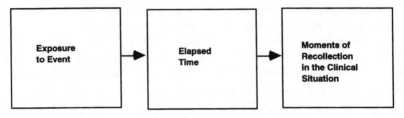

FIGURE 9.2.   A simple research-based model of the ecological foundations of interpersonal recollection in psychotherapy.

amount of research over several decades. Yet it is surprising how seldom its basic implications are considered in the clinical context.

The model involves three basic elements: exposure, a time interval, and a recollection. How are these aspects of memory relevant to the clinical setting? Clinicians are often dubious about memory research because it focuses on simple stimuli in the service of experimental control. However, the lack of direct representation of clinical situations does not mean that the model itself is irrelevant. Indeed, a great deal can be learned about interpersonal memory by the attempt to extrapolate such a simple model to the real world of memories of psychotherapy patients (e.g., Bower 1981). Such a model can be used to describe theoretical components of apprehension and argument, as described earlier, that need to be assessed and acted on in the local clinical situation. It suggests phenomena, which exist in principle even though they may be difficult to access, that might be fruitfully integrated into a larger understanding of local circumstances (e.g., a particular momentary observation in the treatment interaction).

Exposure.   Trierweiler and Donovan (1994) discussed the need to understand the actual perception of an interpersonal event as it happened in real time. Obviously this is a difficult proposition and frankly impossible for an event that occurred some time in the past. Nonetheless, consideration of exposure reveals some constraints that must be placed on a memory narrative were it actually to represent an interpersonal event in the past. In particular, there are limits on what can actually be experienced at a particular point in time that may constrain what can be said about the event later.

Trierweiler and Donovan drew on Gibson's theory of perception (1966, 1986; see also Baron & Misovich, 1993) as a model because it focuses on perception as a continuous dynamic process where properties of a perceiver interact with structure in the physical world. They suggested, for example, that if one were to track an event in detail through time, the perceiver's eyes would be seeing some things available in proximity to the event and not others. For example, a child looking into the eyes of a parent may be experiencing a somewhat different circumstance than one who cannot see the parent's eyes but can only hear a voice or feel physical contact. As long as events referenced in a narrative actually transpired in space and time, then the perceiver's eyes necessarily saw some things and not others. Although this fact would be relatively trivial for perceiving simple objects, which can be reperceived over and over even years after the event (which is why physical evidence is accorded such importance in criminal investigations), it can have major implications for understanding interpersonal event perception as represented in a narrative. For example, it raises questions about what might have been perceived but was not, or about what was perceived but is not currently represented in the existing narrative.

Unfortunately, things may be even more complex than this. If we add perceptions of subjectivity to the perceptual field, including both that of the patient and his interpretation of the subjectivity of the other person in the interaction, then the original experience becomes all the more relevant to understanding the meaning of the experience in memory. For example, a teenager who tells of being disgusted with the appearance and actions of his father at the dinner table may be referencing a moment when the father was actually trying unsuccessfully to manage an argument with his wife. Add to this a real moment during that same day at school when the teen was feeling unlikable and second-rate compared with some more popular (in his perception) acquaintances, then the event described takes on a clinically interesting complexity. If we were able to replay this entire scene and ask the parents to describe what happened, and we were to find that the father was actually experiencing a sense of inferiority in relation to his wife, whom he always perceived as being from a higher class than himself, then family themes, particularly those in the father–son relationship, may be very fruitful to explore. Emotional overlaps such as this are not uncommon in family therapy but they may exist unnoticed if the clinical inquiry does not open them up.

Elapsed Time. Considering the interval between an event and its recollection also raises clinically interesting issues. Typically in memory experiments the interval between exposure and memory test is controlled, with distractions or instructions of various kinds to enhance or inhibit rehearsal that might affect recall. This is no less true in the reality of interpersonal memory, it is just not often considered. As suggested in memory studies, if something has been schematized, it is recognized and memorable (e.g., Wyer & Srull, 1989). If not, it may be forgotten rather quickly. However, the important thing here is that interpretations and consideration of events do not stop with the physical space-time boundaries of the event, even though we tend to talk about events as if this is true (Miller & Johnson-Laird, 1976). Rather, people can forget events until some reason brings them back to attention, they can think about and try to understand the interpersonal events of their lives, or they can even talk to others about them. Indeed, talk about events from memory can lead to new interpersonal events that can have considerable psychological significance in their own right. The assumption that conversations about important matters in life have a major interpersonal impact in their own right is paramount to psychotherapy considered as a "talking cure." It is particularly relevant to the notion that interpersonal events in the therapy relate to the significant events of everyday life, thus allowing for enhanced understanding or corrective experience (Gold & Stricker, 1993).

Consideration of the actual circumstances that existed for an individual in recollecting an event at times prior to the current exploration may reveal "rehearsal" or interpretation effects of great importance to a treatment. For example, the literature argues that if individuals are experiencing false memories of abuse and other traumatic circumstances, then these may be false because they were created, not in the past, but in some other moment of looking at the past in a particular fashion, such as after reading a book (e.g., Loftus, 1993). If so, the reading of the book must either have led to generation of memories that never existed or to modification of the interpretation of some actual memory (e.g., imagined episodic content is added to a memory of an actual circumstance). Reinterpretation of the past may be as important to the treatment as are the events described.

The very words used to describe a situation may be a function of intervening learning or actual recollections of the event. For example, much of what teens will say about their parents may speak as much to how their peer group evaluates adult behavior, or how media evaluate adult actions, as it does about the teen's own views. Trierweiler and Donovan (1994) suggested that, despite overwhelming problems that exist in exploring these interpolative memories and interpretations, doing so can be of great benefit under some circumstances. For example, a teen describing an interaction with his father may use terminology reflecting his peer culture that, in turn, leaves out important information for a clinical understanding of the actual events. The father's patting the young man on the head endearingly (from the father's perspective) as he proceeded to act in other ways that are described as embarrassing for the youth, which is the substance of the original narrative, may not be brought up at all as part of the event if only those things discussed, or discussible, with peers are considered. Yet, this simple, momentary act can wholly change the clinician's understanding of an event by suggesting something about the parent's motives in acting in particular ways.

Many salient events of life are like this. For example, as children grow they learn that Santa Claus is a myth and they must, therefore, reinterpret all salient Santa memories. As they grow older still, they may come to realize that Santa is not a body but perhaps a cultural spirit and, as such, may be inclined, once again, to reinterpret the past. Any such reinterpretations—events of realization, doubt, and pain in their own right, which are presumed to have actually happened in space and time—are of great interest in the attempt to grasp the current story's relationship with an actual past. As long as the practitioner maintains an open-inquiring stance, similar to that described above in discussing the apprehension–argument model, then the likelihood of premature and ultimately unsupported interpretations of events in the past and present will be reduced.

Moments of Recollection in the Clinical Situation.   Clinicians are perhaps most aware of the significance of the impact of conditions existing in the therapy on the information revealed. The conditions of the treatment, which also involve significant events, are the memory test. Depending on local context, such as the patient's recent experience, or the particular direction the clinician pursues in an inquiry, the information revealed can be influenced to more or less clarity or detail. Trierweiler and Donovan (1994) pointed out that the interpersonal circumstances are particularly important in the retrieval of salient interpersonal memories. In the example above, the teen may reveal different information depending on whether he sees the therapist as an agent of the parents or as a personal helper. Moreover, he may only provide information to the extent that it seems relevant to his view of what is expected, which is quite different from the completely free association the therapist might wish for. If the therapist's memory test (implicit or explicit) does not seek specific details, patients will not necessarily provide them. Unlike the laboratory memory test, where a major objective is to provide a uniform cue across participants for the retrieval of the target information, clinical situations are complex in ways that can make retrieval variable even when directed toward the same event at different times. As the relationship between therapist and patient develops, and issues arise around their interpersonal interactions, new perspectives and even new information can be brought in about events already discussed. Trierweiler and Donovan suggested that this is one reason to encourage practitioners to seek more detail, as we have been describing, so that the implications of recollected events for the current therapy, and vice versa, might be better understood.

For example, a patient's recollecting feeling out of place with her family during holiday visits may provide additional evidence for a therapist's observation that she is beginning to deal with the implications of settling into the therapy and of her nascent recognition of the person she becomes in this new open context. The particulars of single events of "feeling out of place" can be extremely informative for inferences about the actual subjective experience of this phenomenon and how it relates to a personal and interpersonal sense of self.

Our examples reflect an interpersonal stance toward the analysis of memory in psychotherapy, which we believe is also a scientific stance inasmuch as all memory retrieval and narrative generation involve an interpersonal communication process. However, the basic analysis of the memory retrieval design applies to any theoretical perspective. Inquiry into behavioral memory can also be affected by the kinds of questions asked, the patient's perspective toward the inquiry, and his or her sense of what is relevant to the treatment and what is not. As anthropologists have long recognized, inquiry depends on the development of a workable relationship between the informant and the researcher. In this country we depend on the acceptance of professionalism and expert status, but as difficult patients often demonstrate, this position cannot always be assumed in our work and we must adjust accordingly.

Framework Development

Practitioners will always be instruments of science to some degree (Singer et al., 1992). It is widely accepted in our training lore that becoming a professional psychologist requires more than a good mind and ambition, but also openness, the development of personal style and personality in the context of being a therapist, and the use of self and one's personal background in executing one's role (e.g., Raimy, 1950; see Chapter 1). The texture of one's life and personal background become intertwined with the experience of professional work such that it does not intrude on the psychological needs of the client. At once, there is need to recognize and cross diverse boundaries while retaining enough aspects of the self that the personal genuineness—which is so important to the psychotherapist—is not lost. This is a scientific achievement insofar as it involves coming to grips with the realities of self, other, the ambiguities of history and personal narrative, and the power and limitations of our professional traditions. The development of personal frameworks can assist this professional development.

Framework development can also help professionals communicate with the public about their work and address insufficiencies in their favored theories. Clinicians need to be local scientists but they will also need to find ways to bring their local science into the public sphere, as do all traditional scientists. Local clinical scientists must assist researchers in investigating the general implications of clinical interventions and, in turn, in bringing general science back down into local realms.

It is left to the readers to determine how to select or create frameworks that compellingly describe their own work. Framework development is a process of creative scholarship, observation, and dialogue with professional colleagues. There are many useful examples in the scientific and clinical literature, which are often presented as definitive theories for particular phenomena. For our purposes, the ultimate certainty of a particular framework is less important than its heuristic value in leading to good questions and useful observations.

Any complete system of ideas has potential to be a useful framework, the development of which is the creative, generative aspect of local clinical science. For example, in the scientific literature Triandis (1972) presented an exceptional framework for cross-cultural studies that could readily be applicable (extrapolated) to cultural analyses in local contexts. Weick (1969) discussed a penetrating theory of organizing that can guide thought about dyads or organizations. Cronbach (1982) presented a UTOS (Units, Treatments, Observations, and Settings) model that is quite compatible with the objectives of a local clinical science. His model is a framework for considering issues of design and execution of an evaluation in any context. Although aspects of it are quite abstract, the UTOS model could be useful in both formal and informal assessments in the local clinical situation. For example, if we (1) treat memory narratives as units for evaluation, (2) explore the conditions for generating the narrative (contexts, questions, language usage, and so on) as naturally occurring treatments, (3) make careful reflective assessments of narrative events as observations, and (4) interpret this entire endeavor in terms of overarching properties of the therapy setting as time passes, we will be implementing the spirit of Cronbach's exceptional model. The reader is encouraged to examine Cronbach (1982) for additional detail.

A virtually endless array of other meritorious frameworks exist in our diverse and intellectually exciting literature. The limits that exist seem only those of time, our ability to grasp the significance of a well-developed perspective, and our prejudices about what should be the driving force in the field. Affective issues can also be elaborated in frameworks (e.g., Yalom, 1989). These have tended to be less clearly elaborated, but greater elaboration of issues that have been associated with transference and countertransference and so on would undoubtedly be productive for affective observation and inquiry.

Framework development, like the development of a nomological net (Chapter 6), involves identification of important constructs or descriptive elements and the relationships that exist between them. As in qualitative research strategies (Chapter 7), visual displays will greatly facilitate this work. The elements of a framework can be found in the empirical and theoretical literature, but also in simplest descriptions of local phenomena that a clinician recognizes as important to his work. Often these very important, locally meaningful constructs will not be recognized formally in the literature (e.g., the myth and common experience associated with a nearby mountain that is prominent on the horizon in a community, or elements of the local experience of a declining economy).

Frameworks as Tools for Community Discourse

Kuhn (1970, 1974) made his concept of paradigm more precise by reframing it as a disciplinary matrix, a constellation of group commitments. This revision emphasized the reality of the people involved in scientific progress, their actions and interactions. Consistent with social constructionist thinking, the disciplinary matrix also includes theory, means of communication, training modes and expectations, and ways of conceptualizing and solving problems (Kuhn, 1974). If we accept that professional psychology is multiply paradigmatic—which is essentially Kuhn's description of a preparadigmatic science—then different groups of people, operating at various levels in the profession, collect around different perspectives.

A discourse community is any group, actual or potential, that takes responsibility for articulating and developing important ideas in the field. Any group of psychologists with interests in particular ideas can be thought to exist as a discourse community. They may be identifiable as represented on membership rosters of groups espousing particular perspectives, engaging in various forms of debate, or managing particular problems (e.g., licensing boards). Or, they may be implicit, as in the large group implied by the widespread acceptance of certain ideas manifested through organized activities (e.g., acceptance of the importance of ethical principles for the profession) or, conversely, by a general lack of support for particular initiatives or political agenda advanced by more active members. These groups may be represented formally in the literature, in research studies, in formal theoretical expositions, or in divisions of national organizations. They may or may not be formally identified by a name. They may exist via shared training approaches, training programs, or clinical facilities. More importantly for the present discussion, they exist as local, formal and informal affiliations of like-minded professionals who view themselves as operating from common interests and perspectives.

Advancing Local Science through Explicating the Views of Local Discourse Communities

We encourage these various communities, and the individual clinicians within, to pay greater attention to explicating their operative clinical frameworks with special attention to how they actually use these frameworks in their work. These frameworks should have a local focus, including other information that may accompany a theoretically oriented intervention but which may not be represented clearly in the formal literature (e.g., information about the particular populations of patients in a treatment facility or particular practice). Framework articulation might be accomplished as part of a professional development exercise and become the basis for a continuing process of self- and community scrutiny of one's work. It could also become a vehicle for incorporating material from the research literature into one's thinking.

Each practitioner is a contributor to the local realization of a theory. Some theories will create greater sharedness in behavior and interpretation among practitioners than others. Science may or may not be determinative depending on its relationship to the local information setting, which includes characteristics of the practitioner. It is our thesis that in addition to enhancing scientific practice, we will understand this relationship better when we have a broader understanding of how professionals actually operate. To this end, professionals and researchers can use their framework development efforts to compare and contrast their work, to come together in local discourse communities where they can consider alternative conceptualizations, where they can press one another for more and more clarity and less personally biased viewpoints, where mutual respect for different positions can be articulated, and where the continuing development of members can be documented and affirmed within the culture of professional psychology. If formalized, such communities could function as mediating structures between the university and professional communities.

We must continue to seek a generally applicable science. However, this may not be equivalent simply to endorsing current scientific practices. Status quo academic science has not solved the science–practice gap in the past and it may not be the best for advancing the quality of local science. For one thing, general science tends to create competition when sharing of ideas may be more functional. What if we were to dispense with the need to proclaim the truth value of our favored perspective, and the eternal need to argue for our work and differentiate ourselves from others? We believe that expanding the idea that intellectual and scientific ferment is to the good of the profession, and practicing this on a local level, perhaps as part of professional development activities, could greatly enhance the actual scientific practices of our profession. In this way, the diversity, which is our strength, might be realized in forms that benefit both general scientists and practitioners.

CONCLUSION

Scientist–philosopher Polanyi (1958) pointed out that science involves a personal side. There are aspects of objects and events that are assumed to be true, though never observed directly. He termed this nondirectly given component, *tacit knowledge*. Local clinical scientists depend heavily on the accuracy and viability of our tacit assumptions about meaning in the local clinical situation. Tacit assumptions abound in the attempt to grasp the subjective experience of clients. It may be that psychological interventions are so unique in clients' experience that accuracy in observation, judgment, and formulation is not all that important. Alternatively, we may be accurate enough in our understanding that intervention is valued despite all of the scientific problems we face in assessing subjectivity. Whatever the case, it does seem that the experience of being understood and accepted by a therapist is enormously powerful for clients. This power can be enhanced as we achieve increasingly accurate understanding of the events of our clients' lives.

Similarly, we need to explore ourselves and our profession more deeply and realistically. In this chapter we have suggested that practitioners articulate their operative frameworks in as clear and explicit a language as possible and that they continue to develop these personal theories throughout their careers. We have also proposed that this work take place with colleagues in self-identified discourse communities. In this way the currently hidden, personal component of our local clinical science can be explored, both by ourselves and by our colleagues. In turn, framework development, although not a panacea, can be one mechanism for bringing general science into local contexts, and the converse, for bringing local complexity to the body of questions, methods, and possible answers being explored by science.

10

Conclusion

In a recent presentation to the American Psychological Association, Stricker (1997) drew on concepts from Kuhn's (1970; see Chapter 3) theory of scientific revolutions to discuss how science and practice in psychology might be compatible paradigms.

> If [the term] *paradigm* is taken to mean shared theory and rules of inquiry, then science and practice are two separate and connected activities. Science is an epistemological undertaking and practice is a praxis that seeks to apply the body of knowledge developed in scientific explorations. Thus, science and practice are not competing paradigms, under this definition, in that they do not seek to explain the same aspect of reality. Rather, they are, or should be, complementary and synergistic approaches to that reality. In this view, science and practice are not candidates for commensurability, but rather are, or can be, extensions of one another. They are both components within larger paradigms. Why, then is there so much difficulty with the scientist-practitioner model, and why is it that practitioners frequently eschew reliance on science? (p. 444)

As we have seen, the study of research methodology illuminates the problems in science–practice integration, while, at the same time, it offers renewed hope. On the one hand, science is an epistemological endeavor, historically rooted in the quest for certainty. It drives ideas and observations to their extremes in the hope of uncovering basic principles and structural limits in nature (e.g., Manicas & Secord, 1983). Scientists can be aggressive, contentious, exceedingly skeptical, and uncompromising in this work. On the other hand, as a contribution to history and culture, science has given us a complex and elegant set of conceptual tools for analyzing any situation, tools that become especially powerful when implemented with an open mind and questioning attitude, when pretensions to certainty are put aside in the search for hidden messages in the local clinical situation.

In this book we have suggested four settings of local information to be assessed [the local instantiation of general scientific concepts, the local culture(s), the locally unique, and the space-time local]. In Chapter 3 we suggested that these be examined using three trajectories for information gathering and analysis (information in the empirical realm, information that we understand and interpret via theory and a practice paradigm, and information that describes and interprets a sociocultural context for the inquiry that must be treated realistically). Other organizing frameworks, linked to differing methodological interests and strategies, were discussed throughout the book. Taken together, these frameworks represent a powerful set of conceptual tools for discerning and creative inquiry into all types of clinical situations. But beyond the tools themselves, methodology concerns attitude and thought. We close the book with a recapitulation of some of the attitudinal implications of research thinking for the local clinical scientist.

AN OPEN ATTITUDE TOWARD INQUIRY

Our professional theories need to be framed in terms of the local situation (Chapter 9). For example, many psychotherapeutic viewpoints exist, each having particular strengths in particular local circumstances (e.g., a behavioral intervention may be better for targeting and modifying specific behaviors, whereas a family perspective may be needed to enhance an entire approach to childrearing). We are now in a period where trainees are less often indoctrinated into a single perspective; there is interest in theoretical integration (e.g., Stricker & Gold, 1993). Once the professional accepts that a reality surrounds the local clinical situation that may not be completely specified by any single perspective, then the task becomes one of establishing the best possible approximation of an accurate inquiry. All tools of research help this process of selecting relevant and compelling theory.

Many wonder why scientific data are not more strongly heeded in various areas of practice (e.g., Hollon, 1996; Strupp, 1986). History suggests that data have not always carried the same persuasive power as a well-structured argument in our profession—nor, for that matter, in our science. Given psychotherapy's long history of mavens and gurus, we must encourage psychologists at the highest levels of training to consider carefully what the authorities were actually saying, and to keep reconsidering it throughout their careers, even as their respect and awe for the creativity and incisiveness of a theorist may increase. All science benefits from the mutual efforts of the theorist and the researcher. The local clinical scientist's task is to remain aware and, at the same time, evaluative of both sources of conceptual tools.

Scientists sometimes act as though current fashions have definitively replaced other viewpoints when rarely is this the case. Change in fashion is not equivalent to scientific progress, and scientists must be wary of tendencies to limit viewpoints based more on fashion than on evidence. (For example, economic considerations in the health care system may lead to greater interest in short-term interventions, but this does not necessarily supplant the relevance of long-term interventions. However, change provoked by economic conditions may well lead to new understanding of how some goals can be accomplished in a shorter time frame than previously thought.) More to the point, the basic question is, how does a particular perspective, new or old, inform an inquiry into a particular clinical situation?

The art and science of practice combine in each instance of professional observation. There is art in the skill needed to gain proximity to phenomena of interest; there is science in the care, method, doubt, and disciplined attention used to investigate what must be true in this case, in the world in which science suggests we live. We must be able to ask questions that are consistent with what is known in science, and that draw on professionally acceptable theory concerning matters yet to be fully understood by science. Even more, whenever science does not offer an exhaustive understanding of the clinical situation, then we must fill in the blanks of our understanding using some model of reality. Having explicit frameworks on hand for such situations can greatly facilitate reflective inquiry (Chapter 9).

When our source of general knowledge involves aggregated data, we must translate this knowledge to the individual level. Conversely, when knowledge comes from other individual cases, we must ever be alert to limits on its generalizability and applicability to the current situation. Sometimes our perspective will span several cases—as in making disposition decisions in an emergency room—and policies that offer the best overall outcome across the many cases will be desirable. However, as we have argued throughout the book, this will never be enough for, even in the context of a good scientifically grounded policy, the other local information settings that exist in any clinical inquiry will require attention.

IMPLICATIONS FOR PROFESSIONAL IDENTITY

Professionals need to move beyond platitudes about our work being too unique and too complex for science, but at the same time, we must not underestimate the complexity that does in fact surround every psychological intervention. The only methods that science can produce to attune to these levels, short of those that actually deal with physical systems (e.g., blood tests for DNA), will be methods that guide thought and decisions in single cases based on careful use of knowledge, observation, and logic. It will be exactly the kind of science outlined by Peirce, and Doyle over a century ago in the Sherlock Holmes mysteries, where all observation, recognition (judgment), and inference were carefully wrought to illuminate a deeper meaning in unique circumstances (see Truzzi, 1983).

Local clinical science is like the naturalistic science of the nineteenth century, like the particularistic analysis of Darwin, and more a reflective practice than the consensus building process that characterizes general science or simply applied science (Howard, 1986; Kanfer, 1990; D. R. Peterson, 1991, 1995; D. R. Peterson & R. L. Peterson, in press; Stricker & Trierweiler, 1995). Consensus is possible in local science, but it typically will be achieved after a formulation has been developed and has proven its worth, not during each step in an inquiry, as is often alleged to be true in the more time-extended and conservative pathways of general science. As a naturalist, the local clinical scientist inevitably stands between two not always compatible or complementary forces. One is the nature of phenomena in the world, their complexity, clarity, openness to analysis, and apprehensibility; the other is the ease with which consensus can be established given the local conditions, and their correspondence with the ideal conditions described by our theories and research-based models.

In many cases, local scientific inquiry will be very much like existing practice traditions that have an underlying scientific ethic. Nonetheless, this similarity is not grounds for resting on the status quo: All practice traditions can benefit from intensifying the observational and logical linkages that are drawn regularly between major theoretical tenets and the commonsense reality of the local clinical situation. The local clinical scientist conducts an inquiry such that similarly informed observers might arrive at a similar understanding of the evidence and draw similar conclusions. In practice, this often will have as much to do with the way information is organized and presented as with the information itself. As in qualitative research strategies (Chapter 7), where pathways to data collection, analysis, and presentation are often crafted to the problem at hand, a local clinical scientist places special emphasis on the relationship between properties of the data and the conclusions drawn.

Too often, existing beliefs are simply taken for granted, thereby inhibiting careful reflective inquiry. Established beliefs will serve us well much of the time; it is important to apply our beliefs as systematically and thoroughly as possible. Still, we must remain ever alert to changing conditions and open to the possibility that circumstances are not well captured by existing beliefs. On occasion, this diligence will require active suspension of beliefs so as to allow other explanations to emerge and to allow oneself to be influenced by evidence.

More often than not, the practitioner will need to avoid precipitous conclusions (Chapter 8), enacting a tentative stance until sufficient evidence emerges to support still tentative conclusions. Of course, tentativeness must be applied within the limits of acceptable professional practice, where appropriate action often must be taken in timely fashion despite some uncertainty. Nonetheless, the goal must be to act as needed while avoiding strong conclusions until the requisite evidence emerges. In clinical conferences, for example, an ethic of not jumping to conclusions would allow us to be speculative while understanding we are withholding judgment until more evidence is in, even as we gather potentially testable hypotheses from our colleagues.

BACK TO THE FUTURE

More attention is needed to the problems outlined in this book. We need more explicit training for practitioners in the attitudinal and methodological forms of thought and analysis that science afford us. Some of this will necessarily involve looking back beyond existing rhetoric to our historical roots—as we have begun to do in this book—to uncover the actual reasoning that supports current practices. We believe that history provides a necessary tonic for contemporary overstatement in the health professions. Additionally, research must be undertaken on how professional thought can be improved separate from the dogmatic, authority-based, schools-of-thought form of training that presently exists. We need to deal directly with the problem of our students, once trained, wishing to go off into their own corners never to be bothered again by new ways of looking at clinical issues.

The logic of science and the logic of professional inquiry are quite compatible.

Indeed, one can imagine a whole subdiscipline being built around unpacking and articulating this compatibility. Professional psychologists are human, and we must cope with the realities of markets and shifting political winds. However, as clinical scientists we must endeavor to move beyond the apathy, despair, conceptual indolence, and political preoccupation attendant on hollow claims of certainty, be they based in scientific research, clinical experience, or political rhetoric.

Scientist-practitioner status is an achievement that requires a lifetime of professional development. It is the aspiration to become a wise scholar, observer, theoretician, and healer. It requires the careful and mindful crafting of a professional identity that fosters openness while using all available conceptual tools and pragmatic concerns as a basis for action. Such an identity is something to be nurtured and sustained from within, as well as expressed via the external trappings and privileges of professional life. In particular, scientist-practitioner status is not equivalent to one's job, nor to any credential. Academic researchers who also do clinical work are not the only models for this achievement. The laboratory researcher who generates models of clinical realities and elaborates their clinical implications, perhaps never engaging in direct service delivery, can craft an identity as a scientist-practitioner. Similarly, the professional in individual or group practice, working to make her interventions as decisive and effective as they might be, developing her personal theories of how local cases can be best conceptualized, although never conducting formal scientific research, can also claim allegiance to the scientist-practitioner model.

The scientist-practitioner identity is a matter of thought, of using the tools of science to ask questions to take one closer to relevant qualities of reality—qualities that extend beyond oneself. Such qualities need not be permanent, they may be moving and changing with time, and they may be difficult to access directly, as in the actual subjectivity of a patient at a particular moment in time. Nonetheless, we need to use the tools of science to track down such phenomena, perhaps never being sure that we have attained full understanding. Following the tradition of our forebears in realistic fashion, we must demonstrate how academic pursuits can help to bring ourselves and our clients closer to the realities of our shared humanity. In this way, the hopes of Boulder may be realized in their unending pursuit by all professional psychologists.

References

Allen, M. J., & Yen, W. M. (1979). *Introduction to measurement theory.* Monterey, CA: Brooks/Cole.

Allport, G. W. (1961). *Pattern and growth in personality.* New York: Holt, Rinehart & Winston.

Allport, G. W. (1967). *The person in psychology.* Boston: Beacon Press.

American Psychiatric Association. (1994). *Diagnostic and statistical manual of mental disorders* (4th ed.). Washington, DC: Author.

American Psychological Association, Committee on the Scientific and Professional Aims of Psychology. (1965). Preliminary report. *American Psychologist, 20,* 95–100.

American Psychological Association, Committee on Training in Clinical Psychology. (1947). Recommended graduate training program in clinical psychology. *American Psychologist, 2,* 539–558.

Andreasen, N. C., Arndt, S., Alliger, R., Miller, D., & Flaum, M. (1995). Symptoms of schizophrenia: Methods, meanings, and mechanisms. *Archives of General Psychiatry, 52,* 341–351.

Argyris, C., Putnam, R., & Smith, D. M. (1985). *Action science: Concepts, methods and skills for research and intervention.* San Francisco: Jossey–Bass.

Auden, W. H. (1991). Shorts II. In E. Mendelson (Ed.), *W. H. Auden: Collected poems* (pp. 853–859). New York: Vintage Books.

Ayer, A. J. (1952). *Language, truth, and logic.* New York: Dover.

Baars, B. J. (1986). *The cognitive revolution in psychology.* New York: Guilford Press.

Bakan, D. (1956). Clinical psychology and logic. *American Psychologist, 11,* 655–662.

Bakan, D. (1966). The test of significance in psychological research. *Psychological Bulletin, 66,* 423–437.

Barker, R. G. (Ed.). (1963). *The stream of behavior: Exploration of its structure and content.* New York: Appleton–Century–Crofts.

Barkow, J. H., Cosmides, L., & Tooby, J. (1992). *The adapted mind: Evolutionary psychology and the generation of culture.* London: Oxford University Press.

Barlow, D. H. (1981). On the relation of clinical research to clinical practice: Current issues, new directions. *Journal of Consulting and Clinical Psychology, 49,* 147–155.

Barlow, D. H. (1996). Health care policy, psychotherapy research, and the future of psychotherapy. *American Psychologist, 51,* 1050–1058.

Barlow, D. H., Hayes, S. C., & Nelson, R. O. (1984). *The scientist practitioner: Research and accountability in clinical and educational settings.* New York: Pergamon Press.

Baron, J. (1994). *Thinking and deciding* (2nd ed.). London: Cambridge University Press.

Baron, J. B., & Sternberg, R. G. (Eds.). (1987). *Teaching thinking skills: Theory and practice.* San Francisco: Freeman.

Baron, R. M., & Misovich, S. J. (1993). Dispositional knowing from an ecological perspective. *Personality and Social Psychology Bulletin, 19,* 541–552.

Barrett, W. (1978). *The illusion of technique.* Garden City, NY: Anchor Books.

Bateson, G. (1972). *Steps to an ecology of mind.* New York: Ballantine Books.

Bateson, G. (1979). *Mind and nature: A necessary unity.* New York: Dutton.

Belar, C. D., & Perry, N. W. (1992). National conference on scientist-practitioner education and training for professional practice of psychology. *American Psychologist, 47,* 71–75.

Belenky, M. F., Clinchy, B. M., Goldberger, N. R., & Tarule, J. M. (1986). *Women's ways of knowing: The development of self, voice, and mind.* New York: Basic Books.

Bem, D. J., & Allen, A. (1974). On predicting some of the people some of the time: The search for cross-situational consistencies in behavior. *Psychological Review, 81,* 506–520.

Benjamin, L. S. (1996). *Interpersonal diagnosis and treatment of personality disorders* (2nd ed.). New York: Guilford Press.

Berger, P. L., & Luckman, T. (1966). *The social construction of reality: A treatise on the sociology of knowledge.* New York: Doubleday.

Berkowitz, L., & Donnerstein, E. (1982). External validity is more than skin deep: Some answers to criticisms of laboratory experiments. *American Psychologist, 37,* 245–257.

Beutler, L. E., Williams, R. E., Wakefield, P. J., & Entwhistle, S. R. (1995). Bridging scientist and practitioner perspectives in clinical psychology. *American Psychologist, 50,* 984–994.

Bhaskar, R. (1978). *A realist theory of science* (2nd ed.). Brighton, England: Harvester Press.

Bhaskar, R. (1979). *The possibility of naturalism: A philosophical critique of the contemporary human sciences.* Atlantic Highlands, NJ: Humanities Press.

Bishop, J. E. (1993, February 4). Study confirms most ulcers are caused by a bacterium, curable by antibiotics. *The Wall Street Journal,* pp. B4, B6.

Bonanno, G. A. (1990). Remembering and psychotherapy. *Psychotherapy, 27,* 175–186.

Boneau, C. A. (1992). Observations on psychology's past and future. *American Psychologist, 47,* 1586–1596.

Borger, G. (1995, August 14). What do women want? *U.S. News and World Report, 118,* 23.

Boring, E. G. (1929). *A history of experimental psychology.* New York: Appleton–Century.

Bourg, E. F., Bent, R. J., McHolland, J., & Stricker, G. (Eds.). (1989). Standards and evaluation in the education and training of professional psychologists: The National Council of Schools of Professional Psychology Mission Bay Conference. *American Psychologist, 44,* 66–72.

Bower, G. H. (1981). Mood and memory. *American Psychologist, 31,* 129–148.

Brown, D. R., Ahmed, F., Gary, L. E., & Milburn, N. G. (1995). Major depression in a community sample of African Americans. *American Journal of Psychiatry, 152,* 373–378.

Bruner, J. (1973). *Beyond the information given: Studies in the psychology of knowing* (J. M. Anglin, Ed.). New York: Norton.

Bruner, J. (1986). *Actual minds, possible worlds.* Cambridge, MA: Harvard University Press.

Bruner, J. (1990). *Acts of meaning.* Cambridge, MA: Harvard University Press.

Burke, E., & Foxley, E. (1996). *Logic and its applications.* Englewood Cliffs, NJ: Prentice–Hall.

Buss, D. M. (1992). Mate preference mechanisms: Consequences for partner choice and intrasexual competition. In J. H. Barkow, L. Cosmides, & J. Tooby, *The adapted mind: Evolutionary psychology and the generation of culture* (pp. 249–266). London: Oxford University Press.

Bynum, W. F., Browne, E. J., & Porter, R. (Eds.). (1981). *Dictionary of the history of science.* Princeton, NJ: Princeton University Press.

Campbell, D. T. (1957). Factors relevant to the validity of experiments in social settings. *Psychological Bulletin, 54,* 297–312.

Campbell, D. T., & Fiske, D. W. (1959). Convergent and discriminant validation by the multitrait–multimethod matrix. *Psychological Bulletin, 56,* 81–105.

Campbell, D. T., & Stanley, J. C. (1963). *Experimental and quasi-experimental designs for research.* Chicago: Rand McNally.

Cattell, R. B. (1944). Psychological measurement: Normative, ipsative, interactive. *Psychological Review, 51,* 292–303.

Chaplin, J. P. (1985). *Dictionary of psychology* (2nd rev. ed.). New York: Dell.

Chapman, L. J., & Chapman, J. P. (1969). Illusory correlation as an obstacle to the use of valid psychodiagnostic signs. *Journal of Abnormal Psychology, 74,* 271–280.

Clark, L. A., Watson, D., & Reynolds, S. (1995). Diagnosis and classification of psychopathology: Challenges to the current system and future directions. *Annual Review of Psychology, 46,* 121–153.

Cohen, J. (1994). The earth is round (p<.05). *American Psychologist, 49,* 997–1003.

Cohen, L. H., Sargent, M. M., & Sechrest, L. B. (1986). Use of psychotherapy research by professional psychologists. *American Psychologist, 41,* 198–206.

Cohen, M. R., & Nagel, E. (1934). *An introduction to logic and scientific method*. New York: Harcourt, Brace.

Comte, A. (1880). *A general view of positivism* (J. H. Bridges, trans.). London: Reeves & Turner.

Cook, T. D., & Campbell, D. T. (1979). *Quasi-experimentation: Design and analysis issues for field settings*. Boston: Houghton Mifflin.

Cooley, C. H. (1930). *Sociological theory and social research, being selected papers of Charles Horton Cooley*. New York: Holt.

Coombs, C. H. (1964). *A theory of data*. New York: Wiley.

Coyne, J. C., & Gotlib, I. H. (1983). The role of cognition in depression: A critical appraisal. *Psychological Bulletin, 94*, 472–505.

Creighton, J. E., & Smart, H. R. (1932). *An introductory logic* (5th ed.). New York: Macmillan Co.

Cronbach, L. J. (1957). The two disciplines of scientific psychology. *American Psychologist, 12*, 671–684.

Cronbach, L. J. (1975a). Beyond the two disciplines of scientific psychology. *American Psychologist, 30*, 116–127.

Cronbach, L. J. (1975b). Five decades of public controversy over mental testing. *American Psychologist, 30*, 1–13.

Cronbach, L. J. (1982). *Designing evaluations of educational and social programs*. San Francisco: Jossey–Bass.

Cronbach, L. J. (1984). *Essentials of psychological testing* (4th ed.). New York: Harper & Row.

Cronbach, L. J., & Gleser, G. (1953). Assessing similarity between profiles. *Psychological Bulletin, 50*, 456–473.

Cronbach, L. J., Gleser, G. C., Nanda, H., & Rajaratnam, N. (1972). *The dependability of behavioral measurements: Theory of generalizability for scores and profiles*. New York: Wiley.

Cronbach, L. J., & Meehl, P. E. (1955). Construct validity in psychological tests. *Psychological Bulletin, 52*, 281–302.

Cushman, P. (1990). Why the self is empty: Toward a historically situated psychology. *American Psychologist, 45*, 599–611.

Darwin, C. (1968). *The origin of species* (J. W. Burrow, Ed.). London: Penguin Books. (Original work published 1859)

Dauer, F. W. (1989). *Critical thinking*. London: Oxford University Press.

Dawis, R. V. (1987). Scale construction. *Journal of Counseling Psychology, 34*, 481–489.

Denzin, N. K., & Lincoln, Y. S. (Eds.). (1994). *Handbook of qualitative research*. Beverly Hills, CA: Sage.

Donner, F. (1982). *Shabono*. New York: Dell.

Doyle, A. C. (1891–1892). The adventures of Sherlock Holmes. In *The original illustrated Sherlock Holmes*. Secaucus, NJ: Castle. (Reprinted from issues of *The Strand*)

Ehrlich, E., Flexner, S. B., Carruth, G., & Hawkins, J. H. (1979). *Oxford American dictionary*. New York: Avon Books.

Eliot, T. S. (1943). *Four quartets*. New York: Harcourt Brace Jovanovich.

Elstein, A. S. (1988). Cognitive processes in clinical inference and decision making. In D. C. Turk & P. Salovey (Eds.), *Reasoning, inference, and judgment in clinical psychology* (pp. 17–50). New York: Free Press.

Elstein, A. S., Shulman, L. S., & Sprafka, S. A. (1978). *Medical problem solving: An analysis of clinical reasoning*. Cambridge, MA: Harvard University Press.

Ennis, R. H. (1987). A taxonomy of critical thinking dispositions and abilities. In J. B. Baron & R. G. Sternberg (Eds.), *Teaching thinking skills: Theory and practice* (pp. 9–26). San Francisco, Freeman.

Epstein, S. (1983). Aggregation and beyond: Some basic issues in the prediction of behavior. *Journal of Personality, 51*, 360–392.

Ericsson, K. A., & Charness, N. (1994). Expert performance: Its structure and acquisition. *American Psychologist, 49*, 725–747.

Ericsson, K. A., & Simon, H. A. (1993). *Protocol analysis: Verbal reports as data* (rev. ed.). Cambridge, MA: MIT Press.

Eysenck, H. J. (1952). The effects of psychotherapy: An evaluation. *Journal of Consulting Psychology, 16*, 319–324.

Faraone, S. V., Blehar, M., Pepple, J., Moldin, S. O., Norton, J., Nurnberger, J. I., Malaspina, D., Kaufman, C. A., Reich, T., Cloninger, C. R., DePaulo, J. R., Berg, K., Gershon, E. S., Kirch, D. G., & Tsuang, M. T. (1996). Diagnostic accuracy and confusability analyses: An application to the diagnostic interview for genetic studies. *Psychological Medicine, 26*, 401–410.

Finkelhor, D. (1979). *Sexually victimized children*. New York: Free Press.

Flexner, A. (1925). *Medical education: A comparative study*. New York: Macmillan Co.

Frank, J. B. (1991). *Persuasion and healing: A comparative study of psychotherapy* (3rd ed.). Baltimore: Johns Hopkins University Press.

Freud, S. (1959). The question of lay analysis. In J. Strachey (Ed., Trans.), *The standard edition of the complete psychological works of Sigmund Freud* (Vol. 20, pp. 176–258). London: Hogarth Press.

Galton, F. (1965). On the inheritance of intelligence. In R. J. Herrnstein & E. G. Boring (Eds.), *A source book in the history of psychology* (pp. 414–420). Cambridge, MA: Harvard University Press. (Original work published 1869, *Hereditary genius: An inquiry into its laws and consequences*, Chapter 3)

Gambrill, E. (1990). *Critical thinking in clinical practice: Improving the accuracy of judgments and decisions about clients*. San Francisco: Jossey–Bass.

Garner, W. R., Hake, H. W., & Eriksen, C. W. (1956). Operationism and the concept of perception. *Psychological Review, 63*, 149–159.

Gay, P. (Ed.). (1989). *The Freud reader*. New York: Norton.

Geertz, C. (1973). *Interpretation of cultures*. New York: Basic Books.

Geertz, C. (1983). *Local knowledge: Further essays in interpretive anthropology*. New York: Basic Books.

Geiger, G. (1992). Philosophy and social change. *Antioch Review, 50*, 15–27. (Original work published 1941, *Antioch Review, 1*)

Geiselman, R. E., Fisher, R. P., MacKinnon, D. P., & Holland, H. L. (1985). Eyewitness memory enhancement in the police interview: Cognitive retrieval mnemonics versus hypnosis. *Journal of Applied Psychology, 70*, 401–412.

Gergen, K. J. (1973). Social psychology as history. *Journal of Personality and Social Psychology, 26*, 309–320.

Gergen, K. J. (1985). The social constructionist movement in modern psychology. *American Psychologist, 40*, 266–275.

Gergen, K. J. (1991). *The saturated self: Dilemmas of identity in contemporary life*. New York: Basic Books.

Gergen, K. J. (1992). Toward a postmodern psychology. In S. Kvale (Ed.), *Psychology and postmodernism* (pp. 17–30). Beverly Hills, CA: Sage.

Gibson, J. J. (1966). *The senses considered as perceptual systems*. Boston: Houghton Mifflin.

Gibson, J. J. (1986). *The ecological approach to visual perception*. Hillsdale, NJ: Erlbaum.

Gigerenzer, G. (1996). On narrow norms and vague heuristics: A reply to Kahneman and Tversky (1996). *Psychological Bulletin, 103*, 592–596.

Gigerenzer, G., & Murray, D. J. (1987). *Cognition as intuitive statistics*. Hillsdale, NJ: Erlbaum.

Glaser, B. G., & Strauss, A. L. (1967). *The discovery of grounded theory: Strategies for qualitative research*. Chicago: Aldine.

Goffman, E. (1974). *Frame analysis: An essay on the organization of experience*. New York: Harper & Row.

Gold, J. R., & Stricker, G. (1993). Psychotherapy integration with personality disorders. In G. Stricker & J. R. Gold (Eds.), *Comprehensive handbook of psychotherapy integration* (pp. 323–336). New York: Plenum Press.

Goldfried, M. R. (1984). Training the clinician as scientist-practitioner. *Professional Psychology: Research and Practice, 15*, 477–481.

Goldfried, M. R. (1991). Research issues in psychotherapy integration. *Journal of Psychotherapy Integration, 1*, 5–25.

Goldfried, M. R., & Wolfe, B. E. (1996). Psychotherapy practice and research: Repairing a strained alliance. *American Psychologist, 51*, 1007–1016.

Good, B. J. (1992). Culture, diagnosis and comorbidity. *Culture, Medicine & Psychiatry, 16*, 427–446.

Gove, P. B., et al. (Eds.). (1971). *Webster's seventh new collegiate dictionary*. Springfield, MA: Merriam.

Graham, J. R. (1977). *The MMPI: A practical guide*. London: Oxford University Press.

Grünbaum, A. (1992). Freud's theory: The perspectives of a philosopher of science. In R. B. Miller (Ed.), *The restoration of the dialogue: Readings in the philosophy of clinical psychology* (pp. 366–387). Washington, DC: American Psychological Association. (Original work published 1983, *American Philosophical Association Proceedings, 57,* 5–31)

Guba, E. G., & Lincoln, Y. S. (1994). Competing paradigms in qualitative research. In N. K. Denzin & Y. S. Lincoln (Eds.), *Handbook of qualitative research* (pp. 105–117). Beverly Hills, CA: Sage.

Guralnik, D. B., et al. (Eds.). (1973). *Webster's new world dictionary of the American language.* New York: Popular Library.

Hare-Mustin, R. T., & Maracek, J. (1986). Autonomy and gender: Some questions for therapists. Special issue: Gender issues in psychotherapy. *Psychotherapy, 23,* 205–212.

Harré, R. (1986). *Varieties of realism: A rationale for the natural sciences.* Oxford: Blackwell.

Harré, R., & Secord, P. F. (1973). *The explanation of social behavior.* Totowa, NJ: Littlefield, Adams.

Hayes, W. L. (1981). *Statistics* (3rd ed.). New York: Holt, Rinehart & Winston.

Headland, T. N., Pike, K. L., & Harris, M. (1990). *Emics and etics: The insider/outsider debate.* Beverly Hills, CA: Sage.

Heider, F. (1958). *The psychology of interpersonal relations.* New York: Wiley.

Heider, F., & Simmel, M. (1944). An experimental study of apparent behavior. *American Journal of Psychology, 57,* 243–259.

Hoch, E. L., Ross, A. O., & Winder, C. L. (Eds.). (1966). *Professional preparation of clinical psychologists.* Washington, DC: American Psychological Association.

Hollon, S. D. (1996). The efficacy and effectiveness of psychotherapy relative to medications. *American Psychologist, 51,* 1025–1030.

Hoshmand, L. T. (1994). *Orientation to inquiry in a reflective professional psychology.* Albany: State University of New York Press.

Hoshmand, L. T., & Polkinghorne, D. E. (1992). Redefining the science–practice relationship and professional training. *American Psychologist, 47,* 55–66.

Howard, G. S. (1986). The scientist-practitioner in counseling psychology: Toward a deeper integration of theory, research, and practice. *The Counseling Psychologist, 14,* 61–105.

Hoyningen-Huene, P. (1993). *Reconstructing scientific revolutions: Thomas S. Kuhn's philosophy of science* (A. T. Levine, Trans.). Chicago: University of Chicago Press.

Hughes, D., Seidman, E., & Williams, N. (1993). Cultural phenomena and the research enterprise: Toward a culturally anchored methodology. Special issue: Culturally anchored methodology. *American Journal of Community Psychology, 21,* 687–703.

Hull, C. L. (1951). *Essentials of behavior.* New Haven, CT: Yale University Press.

Hume, D. (1955). *An inquiry concerning human understanding* (C. Hendel, Ed.). Indianapolis, IN: Bobbs-Merrill. (Original work published 1748)

Jacobson, N. S., & Truax, P. (1991). Clinical significance: A statistical approach to defining meaningful change in psychotherapy research. *Journal of Consulting and Clinical Psychology, 59,* 12–19.

Jacoby, R. (1986). *The repression of psychoanalysis: Otto Fenichel and the political Freudians.* Chicago: University of Chicago Press.

James, W. (1950). *The principles of psychology* (Vol. II). New York: Dover. (Original work published 1890)

James, W. (1965). On the limitations of associationism. In R. J. Herrnstein & E. G. Boring (Eds.), *A source book in the history of psychology* (pp. 388–399). Cambridge, MA: Harvard University Press. (Original work published 1890, *The principles of psychology* (Vol. II, Chapter 28). New York: Holt)

Kahneman, D., Slovic, P., & Tversky, A. (1982). *Judgment under uncertainty: Heuristics and biases.* London: Cambridge University Press.

Kahneman, D., & Tversky, A. (1996). On the reality of cognitive illusions. *Psychological Bulletin, 103,* 582–591.

Kanfer, F. H. (1970). *Learning foundations of behavior therapy.* New York: Wiley.

Kanfer, F. H. (1990). The scientist-practitioner connection: A bridge in need of constant attention. *Professional Psychology: Research and Practice, 21,* 264–270.

Kaplan, A. (1964). *The conduct of inquiry.* New York: Chandler.

Kelly, G. A. (1963). *A theory of personality: The psychology of personal constructs*. New York: Norton.

Kerlinger, F. N. (1986). *Foundations of behavioral research* (3rd ed.). New York: Holt, Rinehart & Winston.

Kiesler, D. J. (1966). Some myths of psychotherapy research and the search for a paradigm. *Psychological Bulletin, 65*, 110–136.

Kiesler, D. J. (1982). Confronting the client–therapist relationship in psychotherapy. In J. C. Anchin & D. J. Kiesler (Eds.), *Handbook of interpersonal psychotherapy* (pp. 274–295). New York: Pergamon Press.

Kirk, S. A., & Kutchins, H. (1992). *The selling of DSM: The rhetoric of science in psychiatry*. New York: Aldine De Gruyter.

Koch, S. (1959). *Psychology: A study of a science* (Vol. 3). New York: McGraw–Hill.

Kuhn, T. S. (1970). *The structure of scientific revolutions* (2nd ed.). Chicago: University of Chicago Press.

Kuhn, T. S. (1974). Second thoughts on paradigms. In F. Suppe (Ed.), *The structure of scientific theories* (pp. 459–482). Urbana: University of Illinois Press.

Kuhn, T. S. (1977). The essential tension: Tradition and innovation in scientific research. In T. S. Kuhn (Ed.), *The essential tension: Selected studies in scientific tension and change* (pp. 225–239). Chicago: University of Chicago Press.

Lakoff, G., & Johnson, M. (1980). *Metaphors we live by*. Chicago: University of Chicago Press.

Lamiell, J. T. (1981). Toward an idiothetic psychology of personality. *American Psychologist, 36*, 276–289.

Lamiell, J. T. (1987). *The psychology of personality: An epistemological inquiry*. New York: Columbia University Press.

Lamiell, J. T. (1995). Rethinking the role of quantitative methods in psychology. In J. A. Smith, R. Harre, & L. Van Langenhove (Eds.), *Rethinking methods in psychology* (pp. 143–161). Beverly Hills, CA: Sage.

Lamiell, J. T., & Trierweiler, S. J. (1986). Personality measurement and intuitive personality judgments from an idiothetic point of view. *Clinical Psychology Review, 6*, 471–492.

Lao Tzu. (1963). *Tao te ching: The classic book of integrity and the way*. D. C. Lau (Trans.). Middlesex, England: Penquin Books.

Lawson, W. B. (1986). Racial and ethnic factors in psychiatric research. *Hospital and Community Psychiatry, 37*, 50–54.

Lazarus, R. S. (1984). On the primacy of cognition. *American Psychologist, 39*, 124–129.

Levi, D. S. (1991). *Critical thinking and logic*. Salem, WI: Sheffield.

Levine, F. M., Sandeen, E., & Murphy, C. M. (1992). The therapist's dilemma: Using nomothetic information to answer idiographic questions. *Psychotherapy, 29*, 410–415.

Levinson, D. J., Darrow, C. N., Klein, E. B., Levinson, M. E., & McKee, B. (1978). *The seasons of a man's life*. New York: Knopf.

Lewin, K. (1975). *Field theory in social science: Selected theoretical papers*. Westport, CT: Greenwood Press.

Lincoln, Y. S., & Guba, E. G. (1985). *Naturalistic inquiry*. Beverly Hills, CA: Sage.

Loftus, E. F. (1993). The reality of repressed memories. *American Psychologist, 48*, 518–537.

Luborsky, L. (1993). Recommendations for training therapists based on manuals for psychotherapy research. *Psychotherapy, 30*, 578–580.

Luria, A. R. (1981). *Language and cognition* (J. V. Wertsch Ed.). Washington, DC: Winston.

Lykken, D. T. (1968). Statistical significance in psychological research. *Psychological Bulletin, 70*, 151–159.

MacCorquodale, K., & Meehl, P. E. (1948). On the distinction between hypothetical constructs and intervening variables. *Psychological Review, 55*, 95–107.

Mahoney, M. J. (1991). *Human change processes: The scientific foundations of psychotherapy*. New York: Basic Books.

Manicas, P. T., & Secord, P. F. (1983). Implications for psychology of the new philosophy of science. *American Psychologist, 38*, 399–413.

Mannheim, K. (1936). *Ideology and utopia*. New York: Harcourt, Brace & World.

Markus, H. (1983). Self-knowledge: An expanded view. *Journal of Personality, 51*, 543–565.

Markus, H., & Nurius, P. (1986). Possible selves. *American Psychologist, 41*, 954–969.

McFall, R. M. (1991). Manifesto for a science of clinical psychology. *The Clinical Psychologist, 44*, 75–88.

McHolland, J. D. (1992). National council of schools of professional psychology core curriculum conference resolutions. In R. L. Peterson, J. D. McHolland, R. J. Bent, E. Davis-Russell, G. E. Edwall, E. Magidson, K. Polite, D. L. Singer, & G. Stricker (Eds.), *The core curriculum in professional psychology* (pp. 155–166). Washington, DC: American Psychological Association.

McNemar, Q. (1969). *Psychological statistics* (4th ed.). New York: Wiley.

Mead, H. (1934). *Mind, self, & society from the standpoint of a social behaviorist* (C. W. Morris, Ed.). Chicago: University of Chicago Press.

Meehl, P. E. (1954). *Clinical versus statistical prediction: A theoretical analysis and review of the evidence.* Minneapolis: University of Minnesota Press.

Meehl, P. E. (1960). The cognitive activity of the clinician. *American Psychologist, 15,* 19–27.

Meehl, P. E. (1970). Nuisance variables and the *ex post facto* design. In M. Radner & S. Winokur (Eds), *Minnesota studies in the philosophy of science,* IV (pp. 373–402). Minneapolis: University of Minnesota Press.

Meehl, P. E. (1973). Why I do not attend case conferences. In P. E. Meehl (Ed.), *Psychodiagnosis: Selected papers* (pp. 225–302). Minneapolis: University of Minnesota Press.

Meehl, P. E. (1978). Theoretical risks and tabular asterisks: Sir Karl, Sir Ronald, and the slow progress of soft psychology. *Journal of Consulting and Clinical Psychology, 46,* 806–834.

Meehl, P. E. (1994). Subjectivity in psychoanalytic inference: The nagging persistence of Wilhelm Fliess' Achensee question. *Psychoanalysis and Contemporary Thought, 17,* 3–82.

Meehl, P. E. (1995). Bootstraps taxometrics: Solving the classification problem in psychopathology. *American Psychologist, 50,* 266–275.

Meehl, P. E., & Golden, R. R. (1982). Taxometric methods. In P. C. Kendall & J. N. Butcher (Eds.), *Handbook of research methods in clinical psychology* (pp. 127–181). New York: Wiley.

Meehl, P. E., & Rosen, A. (1955). Antecedent probability and the efficiency of psychometric signs, patterns or cutting scores. *Psychological Bulletin, 52,* 194–216.

Messick, S. (1980). Test validity and the ethics of assessment. *American Psychologist, 35,* 1012–1027.

Michotte, A. (1946). *La perception de la causalité.* Paris: J. Vrin.

Miles, M. B., & Huberman, A. M. (1994). *Qualitative data analysis: A sourcebook of new methods* (2nd ed.). Beverly Hills, CA: Sage.

Miller, G. A., Galanter, E., & Pribram, K. H. (1960). *Plans and the structure of behavior.* New York: Holt, Rinehart & Winston.

Miller, G. A., & Johnson-Laird, P. N. (1976). *Language and perception.* Cambridge, MA: Harvard University Press.

Miller, R. B. (1992a). Introduction to the philosophy of clinical psychology. In R. B. Miller (Ed.), *The restoration of the dialogue: Readings in the philosophy of clinical psychology* (pp. 1–28). Washington, DC: American Psychological Association.

Miller, R. B. (Ed.). (1992b). *The restoration of the dialogue: Readings in the philosophy of clinical psychology.* Washington, DC: American Psychological Association.

Mills, C. W. (1959). *The sociological imagination.* London: Oxford University Press.

Mischel, W. (1969). On continuity and change in personality. *American Psychologist, 24,* 1112–1118.

Mishler, E. G. (1986). *Research interviewing: Context and narrative.* Cambridge, MA: Harvard University Press.

Morse, J. M. (1994). Designing funded qualitative research. In N. K. Denzin & Y. S. Lincoln (Eds.), *Handbook of qualitative research* (pp. 202–235). Beverly Hills, CA: Sage.

Nagata, D. K. (1991). The transgenerational impact of the Japanese-American internment: Clinical issues in working with children of former internees. *Psychotherapy, 28,* 121–128.

Nagata, D. K. (1993). *Legacy of injustice: Exploring the cross-generational impact of the Japanese American internment.* New York: Plenum Press.

Neighbors, H. W., & Jackson, J. S. (1984). The use of informal and formal help: Four patterns of illness behavior in the black community. *American Journal of Community Psychology, 12,* 629–644.

Neisser, U. (1976). *Cognition and reality: Principles and implications of cognitive psychology.* San Francisco: Freeman.

Nietzsche, F. (1954). *Thus spoke Zarathustra: A book for all and none.* In W. Kaufman (Trans.), *The portable Nietzsche* (pp. 103–442). New York: Viking Press.

Nisbett, R. E., & Wilson, T. D. (1977). Telling more than we can know: Verbal reports on mental processes. *Psychological Review, 84,* 231–259.

Nunnally, J. C. (1967). *Psychometric theory.* New York: McGraw–Hill.

Ofshe, R., & Waters, E. (1994). *Making monsters: False memories, psychotherapy, and sexual hysteria.* New York: Scribner's.

O'Leary, K. D., & O'Leary, S. (Eds.). (1972). *Classroom management: The successful use of behavior modification.* New York: Pergamon Press.

Orne, M. T. (1962). On the social psychology of the psychological experiment: With particular reference to demand characteristics and their implications. *American Psychologist, 17,* 776–783.

O'Sullivan, J. J., & Quevillon, R. P. (1992). 40 years later: Is the Boulder model still alive? *American Psychologist, 47,* 67–70.

Patton, M. Q. (1990). *Qualitative evaluation and research methods* (2nd ed.). Beverly Hills, CA: Sage.

Paul, G. L. (1967). Strategy of outcome research in psychotherapy. *Journal of Consulting Psychology, 31,* 109–118.

Paul, I. H. (1978). *The form and technique of psychotherapy.* Chicago: University of Chicago Press.

Paulos, J. A. (1995). *A mathematician reads the newspaper.* New York: Basic Books.

Peirce, C. S. (1955). The fixation of belief. In J. Buchler (Ed.), *Philosophical writings of Peirce* (pp. 5–22). New York: Dover. (Original work published 1877, *Popular Science Monthly, 5,* 358–387)

Peirce, C. S. (1955). How to make our ideas clear. In J. Buchler (Ed.), *Philosophical writings of Peirce* (pp. 23–41). New York: Dover. (Original work published 1878, *Popular Science Monthly*)

Peirce, C. S. (1955). Critical common-sensism. In J. Buchler (Ed.), *Philosophical writings of Peirce* (pp. 290–301). New York: Dover. (Original work published 1905, *The Monist, 5,* 438–446, 453, 457)

Peirce, C. S. (1955a). The scientific attitude and fallibilism. In J. Buchler (Ed.), *Philosophical writings of Peirce* (pp. 42–59). New York: Dover. (Excerpted from notes circa 1896–1899)

Peirce, C. S. (1955b). Abduction and induction. In J. Buchler (Ed.), *Philosophical writings of Peirce* (pp. 150–156). New York: Dover. (Excerpted from notes circa 1901 and Lectures on Pragmatism at Harvard, 1903)

Peirce, C. S. (1955c). *Philosophical writings of Peirce* (J. Buchler, Ed.). New York: Dover.

Penrose, R. (1989). *The emperor's new mind: Concerning computers, minds, and the laws of physics.* New York: Penguin Books.

Pervin, L. A. (1980). *Personality: Theory, assessment, and research* (3rd ed.). New York: Wiley.

Peterson, D. R. (1968). *The clinical study of social behavior.* New York: Appleton–Century–Crofts.

Peterson, D. R. (1985). Twenty years of practitioner training in psychology. *American Psychologist, 40,* 441–451.

Peterson, D. R. (1991). Connection and disconnection of research and practice in the education of professional psychologists. *American Psychologist, 46,* 422–429.

Peterson, D. R. (1995). The reflective educator. *American Psychologist, 50,* 975–983.

Peterson, D. R., & Peterson, R. L. (in press). Ways of knowing in a profession: Toward an epistemology for the education of professional psychologists. In R. L. Peterson, D. R. Peterson, & J. C. Abrams (Eds.), *Standards for education in professional psychology.* Washington, DC: American Psychological Association.

Peterson, R. L. (1992). The social construction of the core curriculum in professional psychology. In R. L. Peterson, J. D. McHolland, R. J. Bent, E. Davis-Russell, G. E. Edwall, E. Magidson, K. Polite, D. L. Singer, & G. Stricker (Eds.), *The core curriculum in professional psychology* (pp. 23–36). Washington, DC: American Psychological Association.

Peterson, R. L., McHolland, J. D., Bent, R. J., Davis-Russell, E., Edwall, G. E., Magidson, E., Polite, K., Singer, D. L., & Stricker, G. (Eds.). (1992). *The core curriculum in professional psychology.* Washington, DC: American Psychological Association.

Phillipson, M. (1972). Phenomenological philosophy and sociology. In P. Filmer, M. Phillipson, D. Silverman, & D. Walsh, *New directions in sociological theory* (pp. 119–163). London: Collier–Macmillan.

). *Thought and language*. Cambridge, MA: MIT Press.

On theory, practice, and the nature of integration. In R. B. Miller (Ed.), *The* dialogue: Readings in the philosophy of clinical psychology (pp. 418–433). American Psychological Association. (Original work published 1984, H. Arkowitz s.), *Psychodynamic therapy and behavior therapy: Is integration possible?*)

). The concept of mental disorder: On the boundary between biological facts and *merican Psychologist*, *47*, 373–388.

n, J. H., & Jackson, D. D. (1967). *Pragmatics of human communication: A study in tterns, pathologies, and paradoxes*. New York: Norton.

kland, J. H., & Fisch, R. (1974). *Change: Principles of problem formulation and tion*. New York: Norton.

Systematic observational methods. In G. Lindzey & E. Aronson (Eds.), *The handbook ology* (2nd ed., pp. 357–451). Reading, MA: Addison–Wesley.

The social psychology of organizing. Reading, MA: Addison–Wesley.

oward a competency-based core curriculum in professional psychology: A critical . Peterson, J. D. McHolland, R. J. Bent, E. Davis-Russell, G. E. Edwall, E. Magidson, Singer, & G. Stricker (Eds.), *The core curriculum in professional psychology* (pp. 13– n, DC: American Psychological Association.

). *Learning from strangers: The art and method of qualitative interview studies*. New ess.

6). *Language, thought, and reality: Selected writings of Benjamin Lee Whorf* (J. B. Cambridge, MA: MIT Press.

1). *Street corner society: The social structure of an Italian slum (3rd rev. ed.)*. Chicago: Chicago Press.

73). *Personality and prediction: Principles of personality assessment*. Reading, MA: esley.

d.). (1996). *The five-factor model of personality: Theoretical perspectives*. New York: ess.

ll, M., & Vang, E. (1992). *SYSTAT: Statistics* (Version 5.2 ed.). Evanston, IL: SYSTAT. & Collins, C. (1995). US socioeconomic and racial differences in health: Patterns and s. *Annual Review of Sociology*, *21*, 349–386.

Gibbon, M., First, M. B., & Spitzer, R. L. (1992). The Structured Clinical Interview for (SCID): II. Multisite test–retest reliability. *Archives of General Psychiatry*, *49*, 630–636.

(1904). *History and natural science*. Strasbourg: J. H. Ed. Heitz (Heitz & Mündel). (J. T. npublished translation, October 1991.)

ann, S. A., Leff, J. P., & Nixon, J. M. (1978). The concept of a "case" in psychiatric surveys. *Psychological Medicine*, *8*, 203–217.

5). On the inadequacy of mental tests. In R. J. Herrnstein & E. G. Boring (Eds.), *A source e history of psychology* (pp. 442–445). Cambridge, MA: Harvard University Press. (Origi- ublished 1901, *The Psychological Review Monograph Supplements*, *3*, 4, 27, 29, 34–36.)

. (1958). *The blue and brown books*. New York: Harper & Row.

& MacAdam, D. B. (1979). *Clinical training and practice: Diagnosis and decision in patient* ford: Churchill Livingstone.

& Srull, T. K. (1989). *Memory and cognition in its social context*. Hillsdale, NJ: Erlbaum.

(1989). *Love's executioner and other tales of psychotherapy*. New York: Basic Books.

airchild, H. H., Weizmann, F., Wyatt, G. E. (1993). Addressing psychology's problems with *merican Psychologist*, *48*, 1132–1140.

(1984). On the primacy of affect. *American Psychologist*, *39*, 117–123.

H. J. (1996). *Fuzzy set theory and its applications* (3rd ed.). Boston: Kluwer.

Pike, K. L. (1967). *Language in relation to a unified theory of the structure of human behavior* (2nd rev. ed.). The Hague: Mouton.

Poincaré, H. (1952). Science and method. New York: Dover.

Polanyi, M. (1958). *Personal knowledge: Towards a post-critical philosophy*. Chicago: University of Chicago Press.

Polanyi, M. (1992). Logic and psychology. In R. B. Miller (Ed.), *The restoration of the dialogue: Readings in the philosophy of clinical psychology* (pp. 50–69). Washington, DC: American Psychological Association. (Original work published 1967, *American Psychologist*, *33*, 27–43)

Polkinghorne, D. (1983). *Methodology for the human sciences: Systems of inquiry*. Albany: State University of New York Press.

Polkinghorne, D. E. (1988). *Narrative knowing and the human sciences*. Albany: State University of New York Press.

Pope, H. G., Katz, D. L., & Hudson, J. I. (1993). Anorexia nervosa and "reverse anorexia" among 108 male bodybuilders. *Comprehensive Psychiatry*, *34*, 406–409.

Popper, K. R. (Trans.). (1959). *The logic of scientific discovery*. New York: Harper & Row.

Raimy, V. C. (Ed.). (1950). *Training in clinical psychology*. Englewood Cliffs, NJ: Prentice–Hall.

Rappaport, J. (1977). *Community psychology: Values, research, and action*. New York: Holt, Rinehart & Winston.

Rappaport, J. (1992, August). Science, practice, and the implications of question asking. In G. Stricker (Chair), *Education miniconvention—Research training for the clinical psychologist*. Symposium conducted at the meeting of the American Psychological Association, Washington, DC.

Reber, A. S. (1989). Implicit learning and tacit knowledge. *Journal of Experimental Psychology: General*, *118*, 219–235.

Rock, D. L. (1994). Clinical judgment survey of mental-health professionals: I. An assessment of opinions, ratings, and knowledge. *Journal of Clinical Psychology*, *50*, 941–950.

Rock, D. L., Bransford, J. D., Maisto, S. A., & Morey, L. (1987). The study of clinical judgment: An ecological approach. *Clinical Psychology Review*, *7*, 645–661.

Rodnick, E. H. (1966). Comments on the "Boulder" model. In E. L. Hoch, A. O. Ross, & C. L. Winder (Eds.), *Professional preparation of clinical psychologists* (pp. 21–23). Washington, DC: American Psychological Association.

Rogers, C. R. (1955). Persons or science? A philosophical question. *American Psychologist*, *10*, 267–278.

Rorty, R. (1979). *Philosophy and the mirror of nature*. Princeton, NJ: Princeton University Press.

Rorty, R. (1982). *Consequences of pragmatism*. Minneapolis: University of Minnesota Press.

Rosch, E., & Mervis, C. (1975). Family resemblances: Studies in the internal structure of categories. *Cognitive Psychology*, *7*, 573–605.

Rosenthal, R. (1976). *Experimenter effects in behavioral research* (2nd ed.). New York: Irvington.

Rosenwald, G. C., & Ochberg, R. L. (Eds.) (1992). *Storied lives: The cultural politics of self-understanding*. New Haven, CT: Yale University Press.

Runkel, P. J., & McGrath, J. E. (1972). *Research on human behavior: A systematic guide to method*. New York: Holt, Rinehart & Winston.

Runyan, W. M. (1982). *Life histories and psychobiography: Explorations in theory and method*. London: Oxford University Press.

Rychlak, J. F. (1981). *A philosophy of science for personality theory*. Huntington, NY: Robert E. Krieger.

Safran, J. D., & Segal, Z. V. (1990). *Interpersonal process in cognitive therapy*. New York: Basic Books.

Sampson, E. E. (1985). The decentralization of identity: Toward a revised concept of personal and social order. *American Psychologist*, *40*, 1203–1211.

Sarason, S. B. (1971). *The culture of the school and the problem of change*. Boston: Allyn & Bacon.

Sarbin, T. R. (Ed.). (1986). *Narrative psychology: The storied nature of human conduct*. New York: Praeger.

Schact, T. E. (1985). DSM-III and the politics of truth. *American Psychologist*, *40*, 513–521.

Schacter, S., & Singer, J. (1962). Cognitive, social and physiological determinants of emotional state. *Psychological Review*, *69*, 379–399.

Schmidt, F. L. (1992). What do data really mean? Research findings, meta-analysis, and cumulative knowledge in psychology. *American Psychologist, 47*, 1173–1181.

Schön, D. A. (1983). *The reflective practitioner: How professionals think in action.* New York: Basic Books.

Schutz, A. (1962). Common-sense and scientific interpretation of human action. In M. Natanson (Ed.), *Collected papers I: The problem of social reality by Alfred Schutz* (pp. 3–47). The Hague: Nijhoff.

Schutz, A. (1963). Concept and theory formation in the social sciences. In M. Natanson (Ed.), *Philosophy of social sciences: A reader* (pp. 231–249). New York: Random House.

Schutz, A. (1967). *The phenomenology of the social world.* Evanston, IL: Northwestern University Press.

Schutz, A. (1970). *Reflections on the problem of relevance* (R. M. Zaner, Ed.). Westport, CT: Greenwood Press.

Shakow, D. (1948). Clinical training facilities: 1948. *American Psychologist, 3*, 317–318.

Shakow, D. (1976). What is clinical psychology? *American Psychologist, 31*, 553–560.

Singer, D. L., Peterson, R. L., & Magidson, E. (1992). The self, the student, and the core curriculum: Learning from the inside out. In R. L. Peterson, J. McHolland, R. J. Bent, E. Davis-Russell, G. E. Edwall, E. Magidson, K. Polite, D. L. Singer, & G. Stricker (Eds.), *The core curriculum in professional psychology* (pp. 133–139). Washington, DC: American Psychological Association.

Singer, J. L. (1980). The scientific basis of psychotherapeutic practice: A questions of values and ethics. *Psychotherapy: Theory, Research, and Practice, 17*, 372–383.

Skeat, W. W. (Ed.). (1989). *An etymological dictionary of the English language.* London: Oxford University Press.

Skinner, B. F. (1971). *Beyond freedom and dignity.* New York: Knopf.

Skinner, B. F. (1974). *About behaviorism.* New York: Knopf.

Skinner, B. F. (1987). Whatever happened to psychology as the science of human behavior? *American Psychologist, 42*, 780–786.

Smith, M. L., Glass, G. V., & Miller, T. I. (1980). *The benefits of psychotherapy.* Baltimore: Johns Hopkins University Press.

Sperber, D., & Wilson, D. (1986). *Relevance: Communication and cognition.* Cambridge, MA: Harvard University Press.

Stern, D. N. (1985). *The interpersonal world of the infant: A view from psychoanalysis and developmental psychology.* New York: Basic Books.

Stevens, S. S. (1976). Psychology and the science of science. In M. H. Marx & F. E. Goodson (Eds.), *Theories in contemporary psychology* (2nd. ed., pp. 2–31). New York: Macmillan Co. (Original work published 1939, *Psychological Bulletin, 36*, 221–263.

Stevens, S. S. (1951). Mathematics, measurement, and psychophysics. In S. S. Stevens (Ed.), *Handbook of experimental psychology* (pp. 1–49). New York: Wiley.

Stigler, S. M. (1986). *The history of statistics: The measurement of uncertainty before 1900.* Cambridge, MA: Harvard University Press.

Stiles, W. B. (1993). Quality control in qualitative research. *Clinical Psychology Review, 13*, 593–618.

Strauss, A., & Corbin, J. (1994). Grounded theory methodology. In N. K. Denzin & Y. S. Lincoln (Eds.), *Handbook of qualitative research* (pp. 273–285). Beverly Hills, CA: Sage.

Stricker, G. (1970). Mathematics and statistics in psychology. *Professional Psychology, 1*, 275–277.

Stricker, G. (1992). The relationship of research to clinical practice. *American Psychologist, 47*, 543–549.

Stricker, G., & Cummings, N. A. (1992). The professional school movement. In D. K. Freedheim (Ed.), *History of psychotherapy: A century of change* (pp. 801–828). Washington, DC: American Psychological Association.

Stricker, G. (1997). Are science and practice commensurable? *American Psychologist, 52*, 442–448.

Stricker, G., & Gold, J. R. (Eds.). (1993). *The comprehensive handbook of psychotherapy integration.* New York: Plenum Press.

Stricker, G., & Gold, J. R. (1996). Psychotherapy integration: An assimilative, psychodynamic approach. *Clinical Psychology: Science and Practice, 3*, 47–58.

Stricker, G., & Keisner, R. H. (1985a). The relationship between research and practice. In G. Stricker & R. H. Keisner (Eds.), *From research to clinical practice* (pp. 3–14). New York: Plenum Press.

Stricker, G., & Keisner, R. H. (Eds.). (1985b). *F...*

Stricker, G., & Trierweiler, S. T. (1995). The loc... *American Psychologist, 50*, 995–1002.

Strupp, H. H. (1981). Clinical research, clinical p... *and Clinical Psychology, 49*, 216–219.

Strupp, H. H. (1986). Psychotherapy: Research, ... *American Psychologist, 41*, 120–130.

Sue, S., & Zane, N. (1987). The role of culture a... reformulation. *American Psychologist, 42*, 3...

Sullivan, H. S. (1954). *The psychiatric interview.*...

Suppe, F. (1974). The search for philosophic unde... *structure of scientific theories* (pp. 3–232). U...

Suzuki, D. T. (1960). *Manual of Zen Buddhism.* N...

Taylor, S., Koch, W. J., Woody, S., & McLean, P. (19... related? *Journal of Abnormal Psychology, 105*...

Terr, L. (1994). *Unchained memories: True stories of t...* Books.

Torgerson, W. S. (1958). *Theory and methods of sca...*

Triandis, H. C. (1972). *The analysis of subjective cu...*

Triandis, H. C. (1977). *Interpersonal behavior.* Mont...

Trierweiler, S. J. (1987). Practitioner training: A model... 410–411.

Trierweiler, S. J., & Donovan, C. M. (1994). Exploring... therapy: Interpersonal affordance, perception, and... *Review, 14*, 301–326.

Trierweiler, S. J., Nagata, D. N., & Banks, J. V. (1995). Co... *video reconnaissance methodology.* University of M...

Trierweiler, S. J., & Stricker, G. (1992). The research and ev... scientist. In R. L. Peterson, J. McHolland, R. J. Bent, E... Polite, D. L. Singer, & G. Stricker (Eds.), *The core cu...* 113). Washington, DC: American Psychological Asso...

Trierweiler, S. J., & Stricker, G. (in press). Designing standa... Implications of the local clinical scientist model. In R... (Eds.), *Standards for education in professional psycho...* cal Association.

Truzzi, M. (1983). Sherlock Holmes: Applied social psycho... *sign of three: Dupin, Holmes, Peirce* (pp. 55–80). Bloc...

Tyron, W. W. (1979). The test-trait fallacy. *American Psycho...*

Tufte, E. R. (1983). *The visual display of quantitative inform...*

Tufte, E. R. (1990). *Envisioning information.* Cheshire, CT: C...

Turk, D. C., & Salovey, P. (Eds.), (1988). *Reasoning, inference,...* York: Free Press.

Turk, D. C., Salovey, P., & Prentice, D. A. (1988). Psychotherapy... In D. C. Turk & P. Salovey (Eds.). *Reasoning, inference, a...* 1–14). New York: Free Press.

Tversky, A., & Kahneman, D. (1971). Belief in the law of small num...

Tversky, A., & Kahneman, D. (1974). Judgment under uncertain... 1124–1131.

Ullmann, L. P., & Krasner, L. (1975). *A psychological approc...* Englewood Cliffs, NJ: Prentice–Hall.

Underwood, B. J. (1949). *Experimental psychology.* New York: A...

Underwood, B. J. (1957). *Psychological research.* New York: App...

Vygotsky, L. S. (1962...

Wachtel, P. L. (1992... *restoration of t...* Washington, DC... & S. Messer (E...

Wakefield, J. C. (199... social values. A...

Watzlawick, P., Beav... *interactional p...*

Watzlawick, P., We... *problem resolu...*

Weick, K. E. (1968)... *of social psyc...*

Weick, K. E. (1969...

Weiss, B. (1992)... history. In R... K. Polite, D. ... 21). Washingt...

Weiss, R. S. (1994... York: Free P...

Whorf, B. L. (19... Carroll, Ed.)...

Whyte, W. F. (198... University o...

Wiggins, J. S. (1... Addison–W...

Wiggins, J. S. (E... Guilford Pr...

Wilkinson, L., ...

Williams, D. R.... explanation...

Williams, J. B.,... DSM-III-R...

Windelband, W... Lamiell, u...

Wing, J. K., M... population...

Wissler, C. (19... book in th... nal work...

Wittgenstein,...

Wright, H. J.,... care. O...

Wyer, R. S.,... Yalom, I. D...

Yee, A. H., ... race. A...

Zajonc, R. ...

Zimmerman...

Index

When page numbers are followed by *f* or *t*, readers can find the subject cited in the figure or table, respectively, on that page.